GYNAECOLOGY ILLUSTRATED

GYNAECOLOGY
ILLUSTRATED

MATTHEW M. GARREY

MB DPH FRCOG

Royal Samaritan Hospital for Women, Glasgow

A. D. T. GOVAN

MD PhD FRCP(G) FRCP(Ed) FRCOG FRCPath

Royal Samaritan Hospital for Women, Glasgow

C. H. HODGE

MB FRCS(Ed) FRCOG

Larkfield Hospital, Greenock

ROBIN CALLANDER

FFPh MMAA AIMBI

Medical Illustration Unit, University of Glasgow

CHURCHILL LIVINGSTONE

EDINBURGH AND LONDON

1972

ISBN 0 443 00914 7

Printed in the British Commonwealth

PREFACE

'Gynaecology Illustrated' is offered to the student with the same intention as 'Obstetrics Illustrated': to provide him with an informative and easily assimilated textbook combining general principles with some technical detail, and using illustration wherever possible. The gynaecologist should be a surgeon whose skill is based on a solid knowledge of the anatomy, physiology and pathology of the reproductive system, and diseases and abnormalities are considered in the light of this belief. Gynaecological operations are described in as much detail as will help the student to understand them although not perform them, and to appreciate something of what the patient is being asked to endure; and we have tried throughout to inculcate an informed and enlightened attitude towards a group of patients whose complaints are peculiarly likely to have an emotional background.

We are indebted to many of our colleagues for information and advice, and we should like to acknowledge with gratitude the assistance of Professor G. R. Bishop of Glasgow University who read and made many corrections to the section on the physical basis of radiotherapy; and the assistance of Dr T. B. Brewin of the Department of Radiotherapy, and Dr Ivan Draper of the Department of Neurology for a similar service in respect of their own specialties. We should also like to thank Mrs Elizabeth Callander for her work on the index; and Miss Sheila Anderson who has been a most efficient and enthusiastic secretary.

Glasgow, 1972

Matthew M. Garrey
A. D. T. Govan
C. H. Hodge
Robin Callander

CONTENTS

1. EMBRYOLOGY OF THE REPRO-
    DUCTIVE TRACT   1
    Development of the ovary   ...   3–5
    Development of uterus and
        fallopian tubes 6, 7
    Development of external geni-
        talia 8, 9
    Development of testis...   10, 11
    Development of male external
        genitalia 12, 13

2. ANATOMY OF THE REPRO-
    DUCTIVE TRACT   15
    Perineum   16
    Vulva 17, 18
    Bartholin's gland   19
    Muscles of the perineum   ...   20
    Urogenital diaphragm   21
    Anatomy of the pelvis...   ...   22
    Muscles of the pelvis   23
    Pelvic diaphragm   24
    Pelvic fascia   25
    Vagina   26–28
    Uterus   29–35
    Fallopian tube   36
    Broad ligament   37
    Ovary   38–40
    Changes in the genital tract
        with age   41
    Blood supply of the pelvis   42–44
    Lymphatic drainage of the
        genital tract   45
    Nerves of the pelvis   46
    Autonomic nerve supply of the
        pelvis   47

3. PHYSIOLOGY OF THE REPRO-
    DUCTIVE TRACT   49
    Ovulation   51–53

Endometrial cycle   54
Cyclic changes in vagina and
    tube   55
Cyclic ovarian hormonal
    changes   56
Control of ovulation   ...   57–59
Action of ovarian hormones ...   60
Ovarian hormones and vaginal
    smear   61
The menopause   ...   62, 63

4. EXAMINATION OF THE
    PATIENT   65
    Taking the history   66
    Normal menstrual history   ...   67
    Abnormal menstrual history ...   68
    Complaints of pain   69
    Examination of the breasts   ...   70
    Abdominal examination   71–73
    Examination of the vulva   ...   74
    Bimanual pelvic examination ...   75
    Speculum examination   76, 77
    Laparoscopy   78–80
    Lymphography and gynaeco-
        graphy   81

5. ABNORMALITIES OF MENSTRU-
    ATION   83
    Dysfunctional uterine bleeding 84–87
    Total hysterectomy   ...   88, 89
    Subtotal hysterectomy   ...   90
    Abnormal vaginal bleeding   ...   91
    Amenorrhoea   92–95
    Primary pituitary hypofunction   96
    Secondary pituitary hypo-
        function   97
    Adreno-genital syndrome   98–100
    Lactation-amenorrhoea syn-
        drome   101

Polycystic ovary disease   102–104
Genetic causes of amenor-
   rhoea 105–107
Laboratory detection of genetic
   defects 108
Turner's syndrome 109
Sex chromosome additions ... 110
Testicular feminisation ... 111
Cryptomenorrhoea 112
Virilism 113
Hirsutism 114, 115
Dysmenorrhoea 116
Primary spasmodic dysmenor-
   rhoea 117
Secondary congestive dys-
   menorrhoea 118
Treatment of dysmenorrhoea 119
Presacral neurectomy 120
Pre-menstrual tension 121

6. CONGENITAL ABNORMALITIES 123
Abnormalities of ovary and tube 125
Abnormalities of the tube and
   uterus 126
Abnormalities of uterus ... 127
Abnormalities of the vagina ... 128
Abnormalities of the vulva ... 129

7. DISEASES OF VULVA AND
   PERINEUM 131
Vulval dystrophy—Kraurosis 132, 133
Leukoplakia 134, 135
Lichen planus 136
Localised scleroderma and
   Lichen simplex 137
Cyst of Bartholin's gland 138, 139
Simple tumours of the vulva 140–142
Carcinoma of the vulva 143–149
Simple vulvectomy 150
Diseases of the urethra 151–153
Operations on the perineum ... 154
Repair of deficient perineum ... 155
Repair of complete tear ... 156

Operation for enlarging the
   vaginal outlet 157

8. DISEASES OF VAGINA 159
Vaginal discharge ... 160–165
Cysts of the vagina 166
Carcinoma of vagina ... 167, 168
Plastic surgery of the vagina 169, 170

9. DISEASES OF CERVIX 171
Cervical erosion 173
Ectropion of cervix and trachel-
   orrhaphy 174
Conisation of cervix 175
Cervical polyps and chronic
   cervicitis 176
Specific infections 177
Squamous metaplasia 178
Dysplasia 179
Carcinoma in situ ... 180, 181
Prognosis in dysplasia and
   carcinoma in situ 182
The positive smear in pregnancy 183
Carcinoma of the uterine cervix 184
Histology 185, 186
Aetiology 187
Spread 188
Symptoms 189
Differential diagnosis 190
Clinical staging 191, 192
Treatment 193
Results of treatment 194
Indications for surgery ... 195
Combined radiotherapy and
   surgery 196
Scheme of treatment of cervical
   carcinoma 197
Carcinoma of the cervical stump 197
X-rays 198, 199
Linear accelerator 200
Betatron 201
Gamma rays 202, 203
Effects of irradiation 204

Radiotherapy of cervical carcinoma 205
Radiation dosage 206
External radiation ... 207, 208
Radioactive isotopes 209
Intracavitary irradiation ... 210
Techniques of intracavitary application 211
The Stockholm method ... 212
The Manchester method ... 213
Protection of normal tissue ... 214
Dosage to bladder and rectum 215
Afterloading technique ... 216
Preparation for radiotherapy ... 217
Early complications 218
Late complications 219
Radiosensitivity and radio-resistance 220
Operations for cervical carcinoma 221
Radical hysterectomy ... 222, 223
Radical vaginal hysterectomy 224, 225
Pelvic exenteration ... 226, 227
Combined abdomino-vaginal operation 228
Preparation for radical surgery 228
Complications of radical surgery 229
Pain in advanced cancer 230, 231
Colposcopy 232

10. DISEASES OF UTERUS 233
Uterine polyps 235
Fibroids 236–239
Adenomyosis 240
Carcinoma of the endometrium 241
Histology 242
Spread 243
Staging 244
Clinical features 245
Treatment 246, 247
Recurrence 248
Sarcoma of the uterus ... 249, 250

11. DISPLACEMENTS OF UTERUS 251
Backward displacements of the uterus 253, 254
Symptoms of displacement ... 255
Treatment of displacement 256, 257
Sling operations on uterus ... 258
Chronic inversion of the uterus 259–261
Uterovaginal prolapse ... 262, 263
Cervicovaginal prolapse ... 264
Prolapse of the posterior wall 265
Cervical prolapse 266
Changes following prolapse ... 267
Clinical features of prolapse ... 268
Differential diagnosis of prolapse 269
Pessary treatment ... 270, 271
Anterior colporrhaphy (and repair of cystocele) ... 272, 273
Repair of uterine prolapse 274, 275
Posterior colpoperineorrhaphy 276
Repair of enterocele ... 277, 278
Repair by vaginal hysterectomy 279, 280
Le Fort's operation for prolapse 281
Selection of patients for operation 282
Post-operative complications ... 283
Late complications 284

12. STRESS INCONTINENCE ... 285
Physiology of micturition 286–288
Causes of stress incontinence ... 289
Disturbed bladder function ... 290
Frequency 291
Investigation of incontinence 292–294
Surgical treatment 295
Physiotherapy 296
Vaginal urethroplasty 297
Aldridge's operation ... 298, 299
Moir's operation 300

Millin's operation 301
Marshall - Marchetti - Kranz operation 302
Other urethropexy techniques 303
Interposition operations ... 304
Electrical control of stress incontinence 305, 306

13. THE URETER 307
Anatomy 308, 309
Blood supply 310
Injury to the ureter ... 311, 312
Prevention of injury ... 313, 314
Ureter in vaginal operations ... 315
Repair of damaged ureter 316–318
Treatment of damaged ureter 319
Urinary diversion operations 320, 321
Complications of diversion procedure 321
The ileal conduit 322

14. FISTULA 323
Urinary fistula 324
Causes 325
Pathology 326
Symptoms 327
Examination 328
Treatment 329
Operative treatment ... 330, 331
The flap-splitting technique ... 332
Vaginal vault fistula 333
Urethral fistula 334
Interposition operations ... 335
Interposition of the gracilis muscle 336, 337
Interposition of the rectus muscle 338
Interposition of omental fat (Method of Bastiaanse) ... 339
Transvesical repair 340

15. DISEASES OF BROAD LIGAMENT AND FALLOPIAN TUBE 341
Broad ligament cysts ... 342, 343
Carcinoma of fallopian tubes ... 344
Sterilisation 345, 346
Restoring tubal patency 347, 348
Ectopic pregnancy 349
Sites of implantation 350
Rupture of the tube 351
Diagnosis of tubal pregnancy 352, 353
Treatment 354

16. DISEASES OF THE OVARY ... 355
Clinical features of ovarian tumours 356
Physical signs 357, 358
Differential diagnosis ... 359–362
Torsion of the pedicle ... 363, 364
Rupture of ovarian cyst 365, 366
Extraperitoneal development of ovarian tumours 367
Surgical treatment of ovarian tumours 368, 369
Dealing with the tumour pedicle 370
Mucinous cystadenoma ... 371
Serous cystadenoma 372
Ovarian tumours 373
Germ cell tumours ... 374, 375
Carcinoma of the ovary ... 376
Krukenberg tumour 377
Clinical staging of malignant tumours 378
Cytotoxic drugs 379
Hormone-producing tumours 380
Androgen-producing tumours 381, 382
Other hormone-producing tumours 383

17. SEXUAL PROBLEMS 385
Infertility 386
Investigation of the wife 387, 388

Tests for ovulation ... 389–391
Hsterosalpingography ... 392, 393
Induction of ovulation with clomiphene 394
Induction of ovulation with gonadotrophins ... 395, 396
Causes of infertility in the male 397
Dyspareunia 398
Apareunia 399
Oral contraceptives ... 400–403
Intra-uterine contraceptive devices (IUCD) ... 404, 405
The vaginal diaphragm ... 406
Rhythm method 407
Medico-legal problems 408, 409

18. ABORTION 411
Abortion 412, 413
Classification 414
Dilatation and curettage ('D and C') 415
Complications of dilatation ... 416
Incomplete abortion 417
Abdominal hysterotomy ... 418
Therapeutic abortion ... 419–423
Habitual abortion ... 424, 425
Septic abortion 426
Septic shock 427
Possible mechanism of septic shock 428
Treatment of circulatory failure 429–431
Hydatidiform mole 432

Hormonal effects of mole ... 433
Clinical features of mole 434, 435
Invasive mole 436
Choriocarcinoma ... 437–439
Treatment of choriocarcinoma 440, 441

19. ENDOMETRIOSIS AND PELVIC INFLAMMATION 443
Endometriosis 445–447
Pelvic inflammation ... 448, 449
Salpingo-oophoritis 450
Pelvic cellulitis 451, 452
Abscess formation in pelvic cellulitis 453
Gonorrhoea 454, 455
Syphilis 456, 457
Chancroid 458
Lymphogranuloma inguinale ... 458
Granuloma inguinale 459
Diagnosis of syphilis 460
Genital tuberculosis ... 461–463
Venous thrombosis 464
Sites of formation 465
Clinical features ... 466, 467
Diagnosis 468, 469
Treatment 470
Complications of anticoagulants 471
Surgical treatment of venous thrombosis 472, 473
Pulmonary embolism 474
Management of pulmonary embolism 475

CHAPTER 1
EMBRYOLOGY OF THE REPRODUCTIVE TRACT

DEVELOPMENT OF THE OVARY

The germ cells which will eventually inhabit the gonads originate from the primitive hind gut. They appear around the 25th day.

By 30 days the gut complete with mesentery is formed. The germ cells now migrate from the gut to the root of the mesentery.

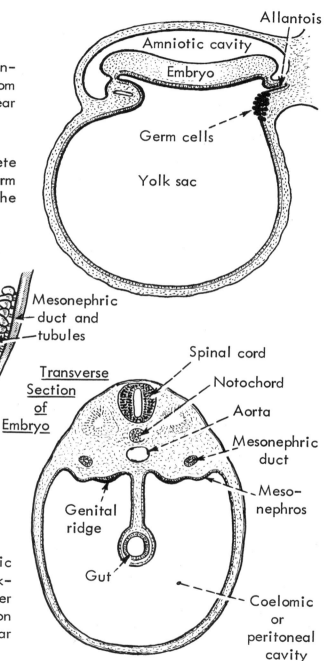

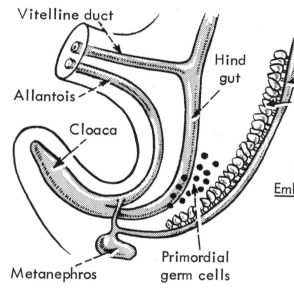

At the same time the coelomic epithelium proliferates and forms thickenings, the genital ridges, together with the underlying mesenchyme on either side of the mesenteric root near the developing kidney.

3

DEVELOPMENT OF THE OVARY

At this stage the primitive gonad (genital ridge) consists of mesoderm (coelomic epithelium plus mesenchyme) covered by coelomic epithelium. The germ cells now migrate from the root of the mesentery to the genital ridge.

The coelomic epithelium growing into the genital ridge forms so-called sex cords which enclose each germ cell.

Up to this time, around the 7th week, the gonad is of indifferent type, male being indistinguishable from female.

The germ cells and most of the sex cord cells remain in the superficial part, the future cortex of the ovary. The cords lose contact with the surface epithelium and form small groups of cells each with its germ cell, a primitive follicle. Some of the sex cord cells grow into the medulla. These tend to regress and form rudimentary tubules, the rete.

As the ovary grows it projects increasingly into the peritoneal (coelomic) cavity, thus forming a mesentery.

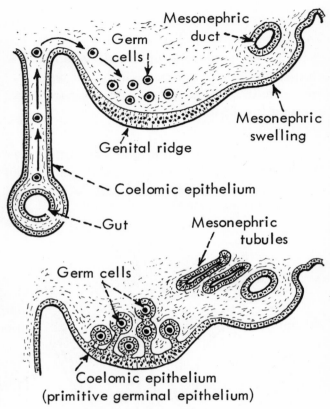

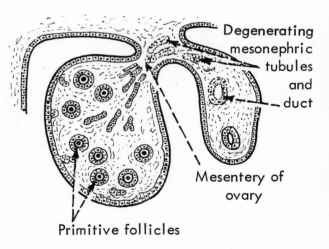

DEVELOPMENT OF THE OVARY

At the same time the ovary descends extraperitoneally in the abdominal cavity. Two ligaments develop and these may help to control its descent, guiding it to its final position and preventing its complete descent through the inguinal ring in contrast to the testes. The first structure is the suspensory ligament attached to the anterior (cephalic) pole of the ovary and connecting it with its site of origin, the genital ridge.

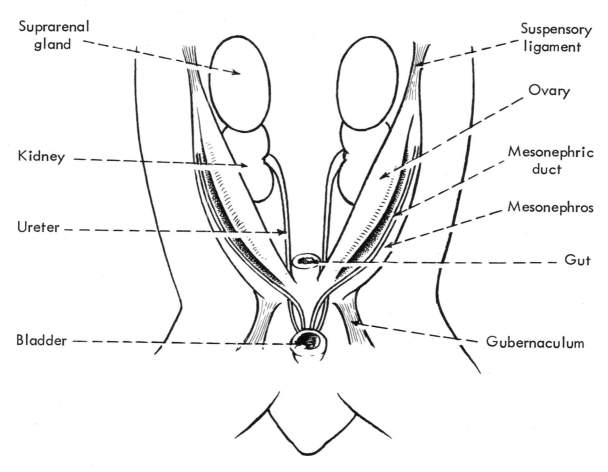

Another ligament or gubernaculum develops at the posterior or caudal end of the ovary. At first attached to the genital ridge it later becomes attached to the developing uterus and follows the latter.

DEVELOPMENT OF UTERUS AND FALLOPIAN TUBES

When the embryo reaches a size of 10mm at 35–36 days a longitudinal groove appears on the dorsal aspect of the coelomic cavity lateral to the Wolffian (mesonephric) ridge.

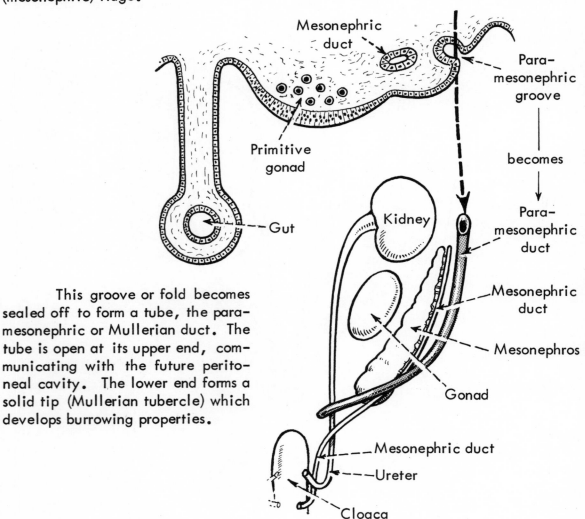

This groove or fold becomes sealed off to form a tube, the para-mesonephric or Mullerian duct. The tube is open at its upper end, communicating with the future peritoneal cavity. The lower end forms a solid tip (Mullerian tubercle) which develops burrowing properties.

DEVELOPMENT OF UTERUS AND FALLOPIAN TUBES

The Mullerian ducts from either side grow in a caudal direction, extra-peritoneally. They also bend medially and anteriorly and ultimately fuse in front of the hind gut. The mesonephric duct becomes involved in the walls of the para-mesonephric ducts.

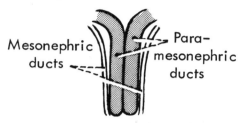

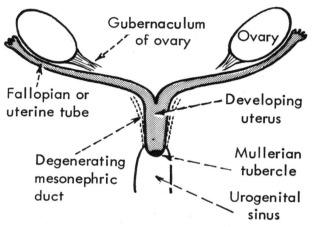

At first there is a septum separating the lumina of the two ducts. Later the septum disappears and a single cavity is formed, the uterus. The upper parts of both ducts retain their identity and form the fallopian tubes.

While this is happening the ovary is also affected. Its gubernaculum is ultimately attached to the Mullerian duct at the cornu of the developing uterus. Its effect is to pull the ovary medially so that its long axis becomes horizontal.

The lower end of the fused Mullerian ducts beyond the uterine lumen remains solid, proliferates and forms a solid cord. This cord will canalise to form the vagina which opens into the urogenital sinus.

At the point of entry into the urogenital sinus part of the Mullerian tubercle persists and forms the hymen.

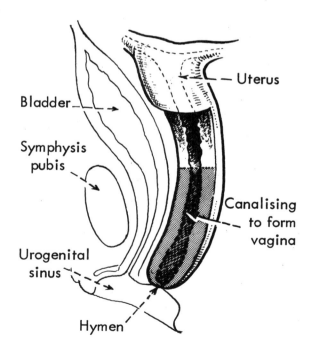

DEVELOPMENT OF EXTERNAL GENITALIA

At an early stage the hind gut and the various urogenital ducts open into a common cloaca.

A septum (uro-rectal) grows down between the allantois and the hind gut during the 5th week.

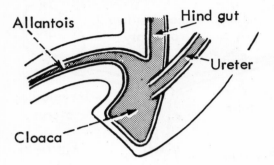

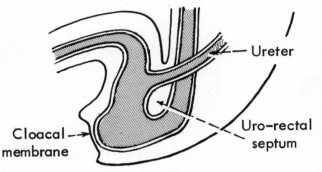

Eventually this septum fuses with the cloacal membrane dividing the cloaca into two compartments – the rectum dorsally and the urogenital sinus ventrally. At the same time the developing uterus grows down and makes contact with the urogenital sinus.

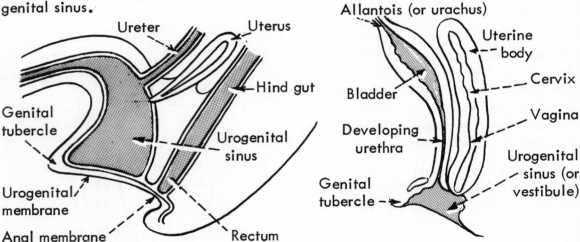

At the end of the 7th week the urogenital membrane breaks down so that the urogenital sinus opens on to the surface.

The developing uterus and vagina push downwards and cause an elongation and narrowing of the upper part of the urogenital sinus. This will form the urethra.

DEVELOPMENT OF EXTERNAL GENITALIA

Meanwhile on the surface of the embryo around the urogenital sinus five swellings appear. At the cephalic end a mid-line swelling grows, the genital tubercle, which will become the clitoris. Posterior to the genital tubercle and on either side of the urogenital membrane a fold is formed – urethral folds. Lateral to each of these a further swelling appears – the genital or labial swelling. These swellings approach each other at their posterior ends, fuse and form the posterior commissure. The remaining swellings become the labia minora.

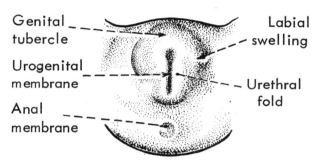

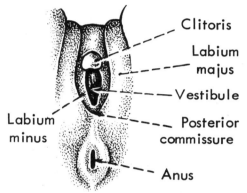

Certain small but clinically important glands are formed in and around the urogenital sinus.

In the embryo epithelial buds arise from the urethra and also from the epithelium of the urogenital sinus. In the male these two sets of buds grow together and give rise to the glands of the prostate. They remain separate in the female the urethral buds forming the urethral glands and the urogenital buds giving rise to the para-urethral glands of Skene. The ducts of the latter open into the vestibule on either side of the urethra.

Two other small glands arise by budding from the epithelium of the posterior part of the vestibule, one on either side of the vaginal opening. These are the greater vestibular or Bartholin's glands. Similar smaller glands also arise in the anterior portion of the vestibule.

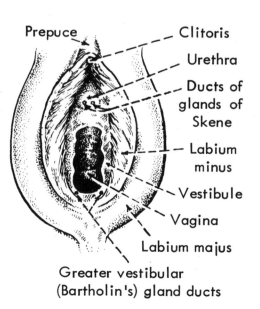

DEVELOPMENT OF TESTIS

Some consideration must be given to the development of the male genital organs in view of the anomalies which may arise either due to organisational defects, endocrine influences or genetic abnormalities.

TESTIS   The early development of the organs of reproduction is the same in both male and female up to the 6th-7th week.   Around this time the male gonad develops radial fibrous tissue bundles which divide the specialised tissue into cords. These cords of mesoderm enclose the germ cells, extend into the medulla and join to form the rete tubules.

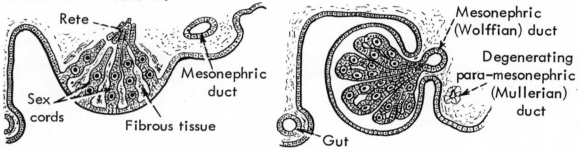

The rete tubules make contact with the mesonephric ductules and thus join with the mesonephric (Wolffian) duct which becomes the main sex duct of the male. In the meantime a paramesonephric (Mullerian) duct forms as in the female, but this subsequently degenerates and plays no functional role in the male.   The mesonephric body also degenerates.

The mesonephric duct which becomes the main sex duct or ductus deferens, opens into the urogenital sinus.
The proximal part of this mesonephric duct becomes greatly elongated and convoluted to become the epididymis.   At the distal end near its junction with the urogenital sinus the duct becomes dilated to form an ampulla from which the seminal vesicle arises.   The ultimate portion of the duct forms the ejaculatory duct.

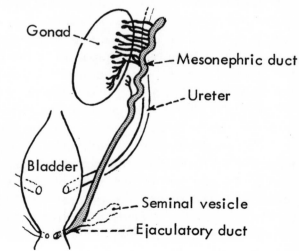

DEVELOPMENT OF TESTIS

DESCENT OF TESTIS

The posterior end of the testis is continuous with a band which runs round the abdominal wall to reach the inguinal region. At this point the band becomes attached to a mass of mesenchyme which will form the inguinal canal and which is continuous with the genital swelling. This structure thus formed becomes the gubernaculum testis. Although the body elongates the gubernaculum does not and thus the testis descends in a relative sense and comes close to the inguinal region. At the sixth month a diverticulum of the coelomic lining (peritoneum) is formed – the processus vaginalis. This grows into the gubernaculum, helping to form the inguinal canal, extending downwards, distending the genital swelling to form the scrotum. The testis follows along this line pushing the processus vaginalis before it. The processus vaginalis eventually becomes the tunica vaginalis.

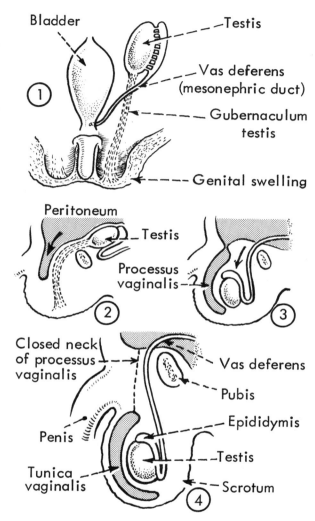

PROSTATE

The development of the prostate has already been indicated (page 9). Small epithelial buds arise from the urethra and from the urogenital sinus. Coming together they surround the urethra as it issues from the bladder. The ejaculatory ducts also pass through these buds to join the urethra. A small saccule, the prostatic utricle, develops from the region of the Mullerian tubercle which is on the dorsal wall of the urethra. This is thought by some to be the masculine equivalent of the uterus.

DEVELOPMENT OF MALE EXTERNAL GENITALIA

The earlier stages of development of the external genitalia are the same in both sexes. The same five swellings appear in the male around the cloaca (page 9).

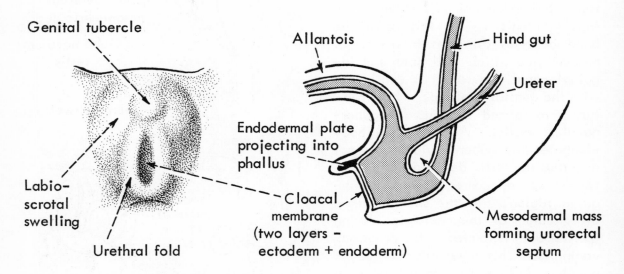

Genital tubercle

Allantois

Hind gut

Ureter

Endodermal plate projecting into phallus

Labio-scrotal swelling

Cloacal membrane (two layers – ectoderm + endoderm)

Urethral fold

Mesodermal mass forming urorectal septum

The genital tubercle elongates to form a phallus. Meanwhile a projection arises from the endoderm lining the interior of the cloaca and pushes into the mesenchyme of the phallus.

A groove appears on the under surface of the phallus – the primitive urethral groove.

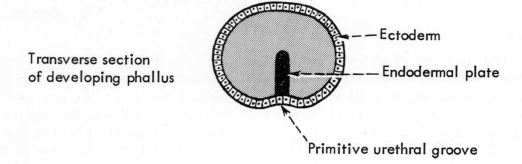

Transverse section of developing phallus

Ectoderm

Endodermal plate

Primitive urethral groove

DEVELOPMENT OF MALE EXTERNAL GENITALIA

As in the female a mesodermal mass, the urorectal septum, grows downwards and separates the urogenital sinus from the rectum and anus. The urogenital portion of the cloacal membrane disintegrates so that an open gutter is formed through which the urine drains. This gutter is continuous anteriorly with the primitive urethral groove on the phallus.

The ectoderm on the under surface of the phallus disappears, exposing the underlying endodermal plate.

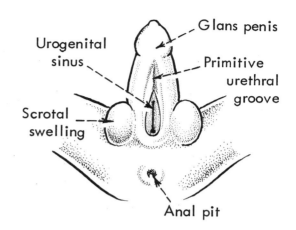

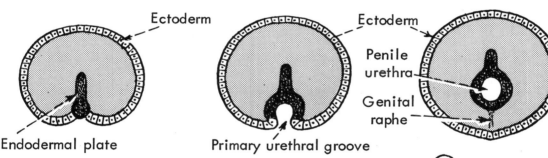

The endodermal plate becomes hollowed to form the primary urethral groove.

The hollow endodermal plate is drawn back into the body of the phallus and in the process it forms a tube. The ectodermal surface is restored.

At the same time the urethral folds are approximated and ultimately fuse.

The testes descend into the labio-scrotal swellings which become distended and move medially to form the scrotum.

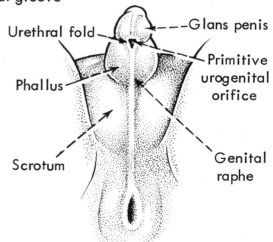

13

CHAPTER 2
ANATOMY OF THE REPRODUCTIVE TRACT

THE PERINEUM

THE PERINEUM (Gk. 'around the natal area')

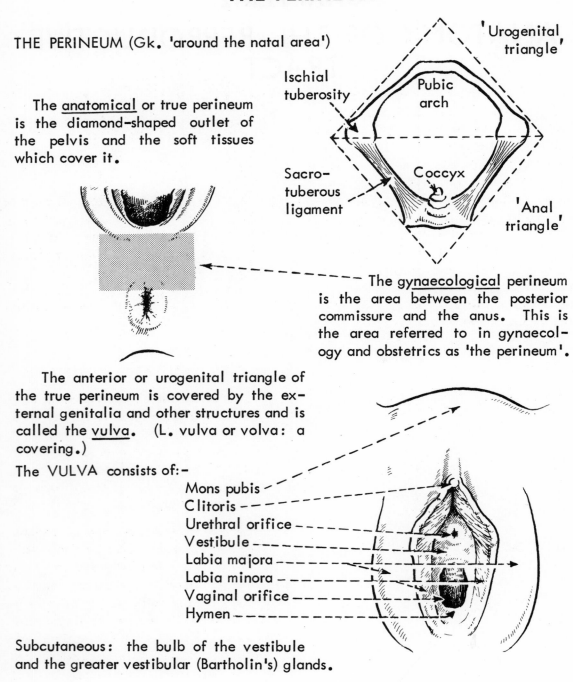

The <u>anatomical</u> or true perineum is the diamond-shaped outlet of the pelvis and the soft tissues which cover it.

'Urogenital triangle'

Ischial tuberosity

Pubic arch

Sacro-tuberous ligament

Coccyx

'Anal triangle'

The <u>gynaecological</u> perineum is the area between the posterior commissure and the anus. This is the area referred to in gynaecology and obstetrics as 'the perineum'.

The anterior or urogenital triangle of the true perineum is covered by the external genitalia and other structures and is called the <u>vulva</u>. (L. vulva or volva: a covering.)

The VULVA consists of:—

Mons pubis
Clitoris
Urethral orifice
Vestibule
Labia majora
Labia minora
Vaginal orifice
Hymen

Subcutaneous: the bulb of the vestibule and the greater vestibular (Bartholin's) glands.

THE VULVA

MONS PUBIS AND LABIA MAJORA

The mons pubis is a pad of fatty tissue overlying the symphysis pubis and covered by skin and pubic hair. The labia are folds of skin and fat which pass from the mons back to the perineum. The lateral labial surfaces are pigmented and hairy, the inner smooth and containing many sebaceous, sweat and apocrine glands which give off the smell peculiar to the vulva.

The substance of the labia consists of vascular fatty tissue with many lymphatics, and also vestigial remnants of the dartos muscle. (The labium is the homologue of the scrotum.)

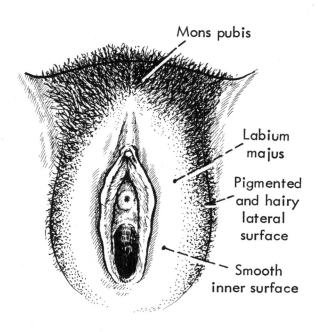

CLITORIS AND LABIA MINORA

The clitoris is the vestigial homologue of the penis and is formed the same way from two corpora cavernosa and a glans of spongy erectile tissue which has a copious blood supply from the clitoral artery. The clitoris is highly innervated.

The labia minora are two cutaneous folds enclosing the urethral and vaginal orifices. Anteriorly each divides to form a hood or prepuce, and a frenulum for the clitoris. Posteriorly they unite in a frenulum or fourchette which is obliterated by the delivery of a baby. The labia minora contain no fat but many sebaceous glands.

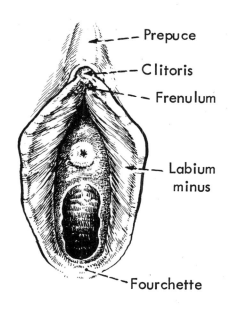

17

THE VULVA

The VESTIBULE is the area between the labia minora. It is perforated by the urethral and vaginal orifices and the ducts of Bartholin's glands. The fossa navicularis between the vagina and the fourchette is, like the fourchette, obliterated by childbirth. The lesser vestibular glands are mucosal glands discharging on to the surface of the vestibule.

The EXTERNAL URETHRAL ORIFICE is in the healthy state a small protuberance with a vertical cleft. The tiny orifices of the paraurethral

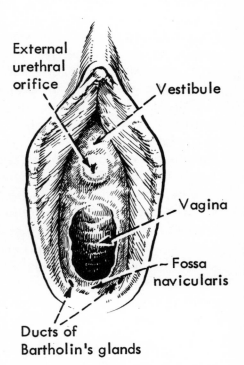

External urethral orifice
Vestibule
Vagina
Fossa navicularis
Ducts of Bartholin's glands

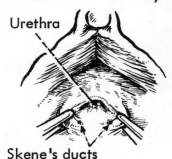

Urethra
Skene's ducts

(Skene's) ducts lie just inside or outside the meatus. The paraurethral glands are homologues of the prostate and form a system of tubular glands surrounding most of the urethra.

The VAGINAL ORIFICE is a midline aperture incompletely closed by the HYMEN. The hymen is a thin fold of tissue lined by squamous epithelium with a small hole (sometimes several) for the passage of menstrual blood. It is ruptured by coitus and more or less obliterated by childbirth. A few tags of skin are left called carunculae myrtiformes. The appearances of the hymen are unreliable as medicolegal evidence, whether of virginity or childbirth.

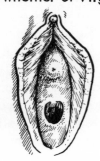

Normal virgin hymen

Hymen after coitus (or after using tampons)

Carunculae myrtiformes

BARTHOLIN'S GLAND

The BULB of the VESTIBULE consists of two masses of erectile tissue on either side of the vagina, lying beneath the skin and bulbospongiosus muscle but superficial to the perineal membrane. They are connected anteriorly by a narrow transverse strip and are the homologue of the bulb of the penis.

BARTHOLIN'S (GREATER VESTIBULAR) glands are the homologues of the bulbourethral (Cowper's) glands in the male but lie superficial instead of deep to the perineal membrane. Each gland is partly covered by the erectile tissue of the bulb and drains by a duct about 2cm long which opens into the vaginal orifice lateral to the hymen. Bartholin's gland is not palpable in the healthy state.

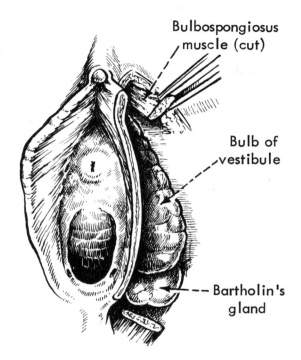

The erectile tissue of the bulb becomes tumescent during sexual excitement and the glands secrete a mucoid discharge which acts as a lubricant.

Histology of Bartholin's Gland

The gland is formed of racemose glands lined with columnar or cuboid epithelium. The duct demonstrates the very intimate embryological connection between genital and urinary tracts by being lined with transitional epithelium.

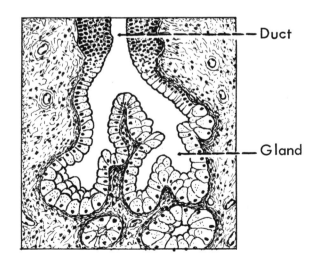

MUSCLES OF THE PERINEUM

Ischiocavernosus

This muscle compresses the root of the clitoris during sexual excitement, to produce erection by venous congestion.

Bulbospongiosus

This muscle conceals the vestibular bulb and Bartholin's glands. Its function is to diminish the vaginal orifice during coitus.

Trasversus Perinei Superficialis

A feeble muscle which helps to fix the perineal body.

Sphincter Ani Externus

Normally in a state of contraction to keep the anus closed. It also helps to fix the perineal body.

The <u>Perineal Body</u> is a fibromuscular node between anus and vagina with attachments to 8 muscles.

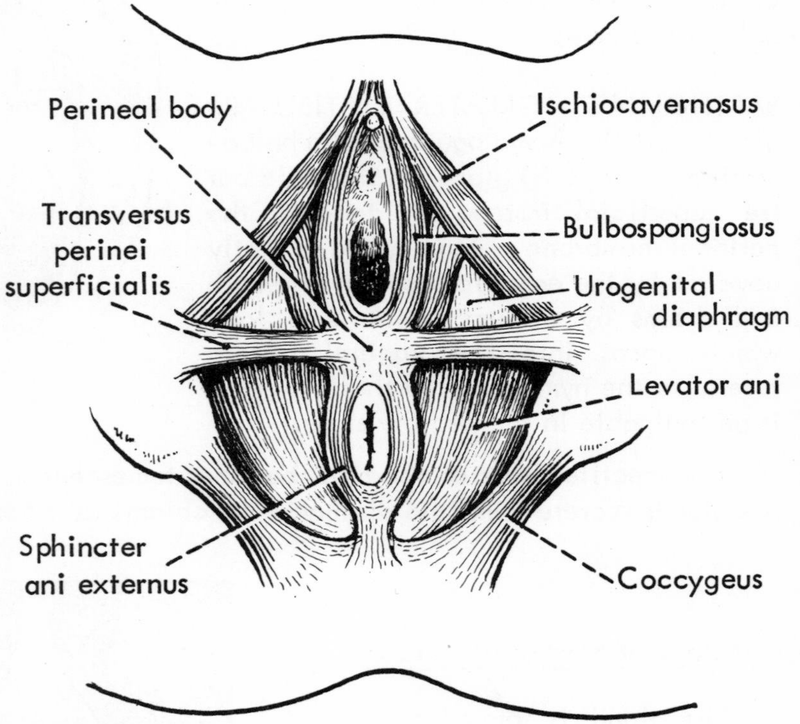

One Sphincter Ani
One Bulbospongiosus
Two Transversi perinei superficiales
Two Transversi perinei profundi (deep: not shown here)
Two Levatores Ani

The whole mass is what gynaecologists mean when they talk about 'the perineum'. If it is damaged during parturition and not properly repaired and healed it will not function properly and the efficiency of the whole pelvic diaphragm may suffer.

THE UROGENITAL DIAPHRAGM

THE UROGENITAL DIAPHRAGM   (Triangular Ligament)

This area of the perineum is more developed and surgically more important in the male. It consists of two sheets of fascia with a layer of muscle in between. It covers the pubic arch and is pierced by the urethra and, in the female, by the vagina.

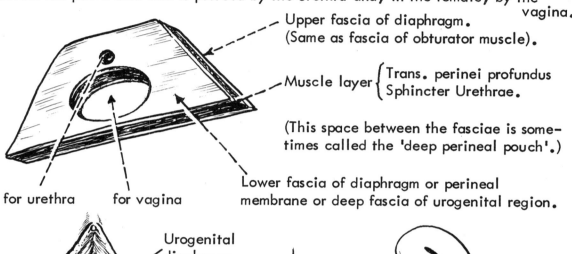

Upper fascia of diaphragm.
(Same as fascia of obturator muscle).

Muscle layer $\begin{cases} \text{Trans. perinei profundus} \\ \text{Sphincter Urethrae.} \end{cases}$

(This space between the fasciae is some-times called the 'deep perineal pouch'.)

for urethra   for vagina

Lower fascia of diaphragm or perineal membrane or deep fascia of urogenital region.

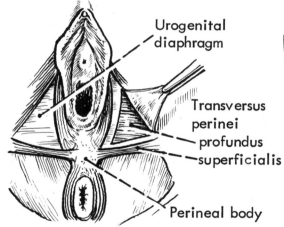

Urogenital diaphragm

Transversus perinei
- profundus
- superficialis

Perineal body

All the perineal muscles lie super-ficial to the perineal membrane except the transversus perinei profundus which helps to fix the perineal body.

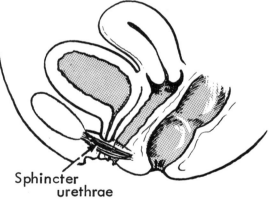

Sphincter urethrae

The sphincter urethrae is app-lied to the lower end of the urethra which it fixes.   (This is the equi-valent of the 'membranous urethra in the male.)

The transversus perinei profundus and sphincter urethrae together form a mass of muscle in the same plane.

ANATOMY OF THE PELVIS

ISCHIORECTAL FOSSA

A wedge-shaped space between the ischial tuberosity and the anus, filled with fat and crossed by vessels and nerves.

Boundaries:-
Laterally the obturator fascia and ischial tuberosity.
Posteriorly the sacrotuberous ligament.
Anteriorly the urogenital diaphragm.
Medially the sphincter ani, and levator (anal) fascia.

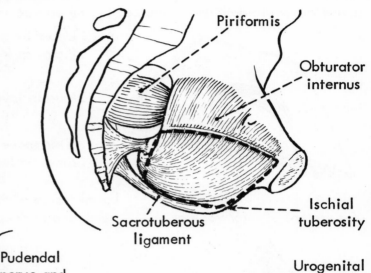

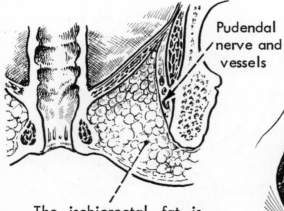

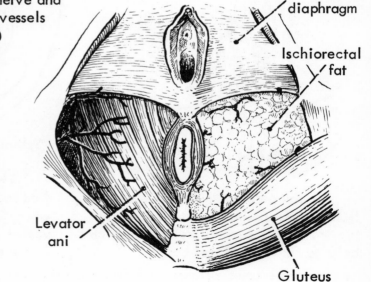

The ischiorectal fat is traversed by the pudendal vessels and nerves and some small perineal branches of sacral nerves.

This pad of fat supports the anal canal and pelvic diaphragm.

MUSCLES OF THE PELVIS

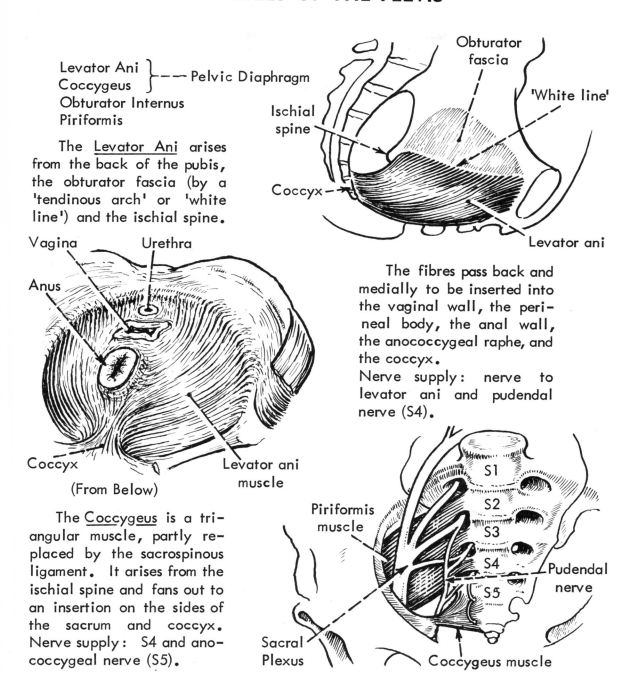

Levator Ani }
Coccygeus   } — — Pelvic Diaphragm
Obturator Internus
Piriformis

The <u>Levator Ani</u> arises from the back of the pubis, the obturator fascia (by a 'tendinous arch' or 'white line') and the ischial spine.

Obturator fascia

'White line'

Ischial spine

Coccyx

Levator ani

Vagina   Urethra

Anus

Coccyx

Levator ani muscle

(From Below)

The fibres pass back and medially to be inserted into the vaginal wall, the perineal body, the anal wall, the anococcygeal raphe, and the coccyx.

Nerve supply: nerve to levator ani and pudendal nerve (S4).

The <u>Coccygeus</u> is a triangular muscle, partly replaced by the sacrospinous ligament. It arises from the ischial spine and fans out to an insertion on the sides of the sacrum and coccyx. Nerve supply: S4 and anococcygeal nerve (S5).

Piriformis muscle

S1
S2
S3
S4
S5

Pudendal nerve

Sacral Plexus

Coccygeus muscle

23

PELVIC DIAPHRAGM

Obturator Internus arises from the anterolateral wall of the pelvis (and obturator membrane) and passes backwards through the lesser sciatic foramen to be inserted into the trochanter of the femur. (L 5, S 1 and 2)

Piriformis arises from the front of the sacrum and passes through the greater sciatic foramen to be inserted into the trochanter of the femur. (S 1 and 2)

These muscles are primarily lateral rotators of the hip and postural muscles.

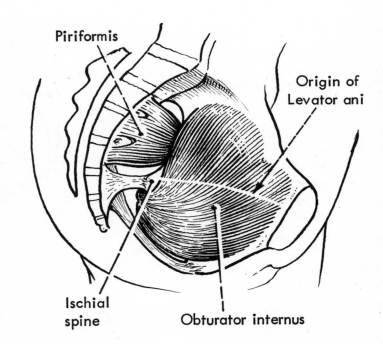

FUNCTIONS OF THE PELVIC DIAPHRAGM

Apart from helping to fix the perineal body and assist the vaginal and anal sphincters, the main function of the pelvic diaphragm is to support the pelvic viscera.

The muscles used to be named:

pubococcygeus ⎫
iliococcygeus ⎬ = levator ani

ischiococcygeus = coccygeus

and in the lower animals their function is to move the tail (the coccyx). In man they have to meet the requirements of the erect position and resist the strain imposed by any increase in intra-abdominal pressure such as laughing, coughing, straining at stool etc. In addition a complete relaxation of the muscles should be possible during parturition so that the vaginal foramen may enlarge almost to the size of the bony pelvic outlet.

PELVIC FASCIA

THE PELVIC FASCIA

Parietal Layer

The aponeuroses and fascial sheaths of the pelvic muscles (the 'wallpaper' of the pelvis).

Visceral Layer

The fascial sheaths of the organs and the fatty tissue filling the space between them (the 'stuffing' of the pelvis).

In certain areas this stuffing is condensed and strengthened by plain muscle fibres and elastic tissue to form the ligaments of the uterus (pages 33,34).

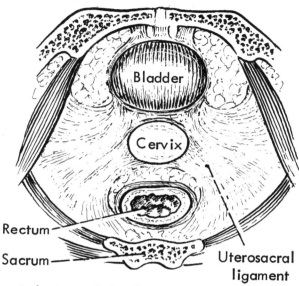

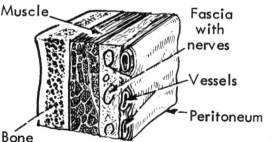

These fascial prolongations on structures leaving the pelvis form points at which pus may track from a pelvic abscess to point in the buttock or groin or above the inguinal ligament.

(The greater sciatic notch is not shown.)

Relations of the Fascia

The nerve trunks, which leave the pelvis may be described as 'outside' the fascia which gives them fascial sheaths. The vessels are 'inside' and lie between fascia and peritoneum.

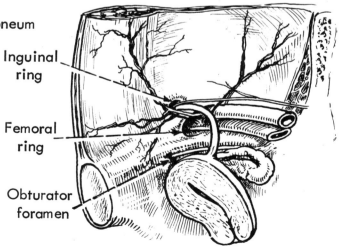

THE VAGINA

A canal of plain muscle extending from the vestibule to the uterus.

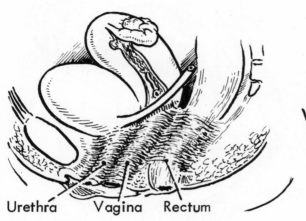

Urethra   Vagina   Rectum

<u>Lateral View</u>. Note the close re-
lationship to urethra, bladder and
rectum.

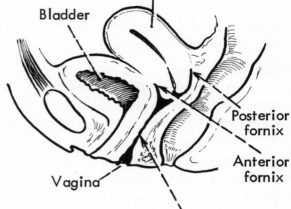

Uterus

Bladder

Posterior
fornix

Anterior
fornix

Vagina

<u>Sagittal Section</u>. Note anterior
and posterior walls normally in
contact, also anterior and posterior
fornices.

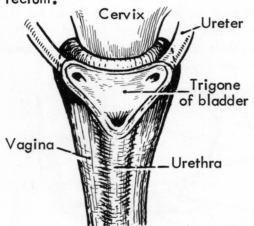

Cervix

Ureter

Trigone
of bladder

Vagina

Urethra

<u>Anterior View</u> shows the very in-
timate relationship with the bladder
base and ureters.

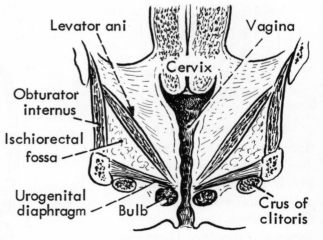

Levator ani

Vagina

Cervix

Obturator
internus

Ischiorectal
fossa

Urogenital
diaphragm

Bulb

Crus of
clitoris

<u>Coronal section</u> shows the relation-
ship of vagina and pelvic floor.

THE VAGINA

In the nulliparous adult the vagina is H-shaped in section and marked by longitudinal furrows – the columns of the vagina – and numerous transverse ridges or rugae. This configuration permits great distension during parturition; and is much less marked in the parous woman.

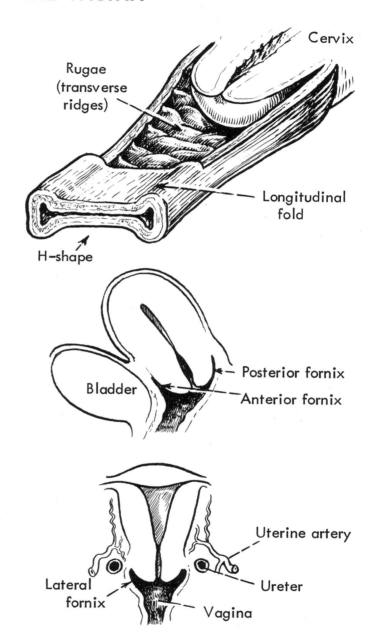

Vaginal Fornices

These are gutters at the top of the vagina, surrounding the cervix.

Anterior Fornix – related to the bladder base and the utero-vesical fossa.

Posterior Fornix – related to peritoneum of the Pouch of Douglas. This fornix is deeper than the anterior one because of the angle the cervix makes with the vagina. The male's ejaculate is deposited in the posterior fornix during coitus, where it is in close contact with the cervical os.

Lateral Fornices – related to the ureters and the uterine vessels.

THE VAGINA

HISTOLOGY

Its length is about 9cm along the posterior wall and 7.5cm along its anterior. The width gradually increases from below upwards.

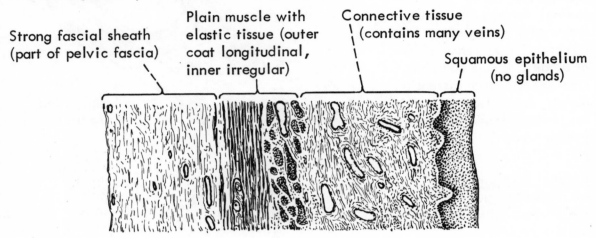

Strong fascial sheath (part of pelvic fascia)

Plain muscle with elastic tissue (outer coat longitudinal, inner irregular)

Connective tissue (contains many veins)

Squamous epithelium (no glands)

The vagina pierces the urogenital diaphragm and is encircled at its lower end by the voluntary bulbospongiosus which has some sphincteric action, although the levator ani muscle is more effective.

Vaginal secretion

This is composed of alkaline cervical secretion, desquamated epithelial cells and bacteria. The epithelium is rich in glycogen which is converted by Doderlein's bacillus into lactic acid. The vaginal pH is about 4.5 and provides a fairly effective barrier against infection.

The vaginal epithelium

This is composed of several layers of squamous cells with no keratinisation. It develops papillae which dip into the fibrous corium. It is much thinner in the child and the rugae are absent. This appearance recurs in old age. Cyclic changes are discussed on page 55.

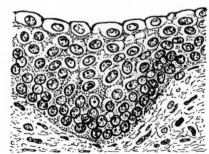

UTERUS

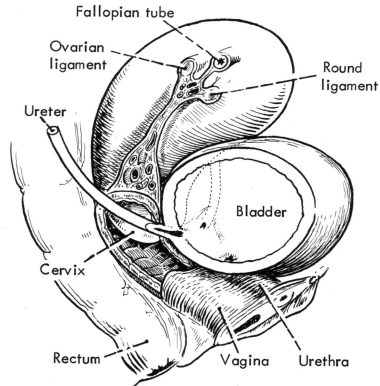

Fallopian tube

Ovarian ligament

Round ligament

Ureter

Bladder

Cervix

Rectum

Vagina

Urethra

The uterus is a hollow viscus composed of plain muscle whose sole function is gestation.

It lies between the rectum and the bladder and is continuous with the vagina.

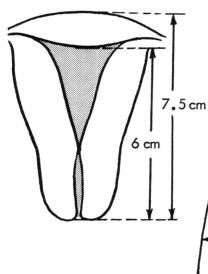

7.5 cm

6 cm

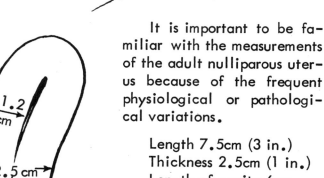

1.2 cm

2.5 cm

It is important to be familiar with the measurements of the adult nulliparous uterus because of the frequent physiological or pathological variations.

Length 7.5cm (3 in.)
Thickness 2.5cm (1 in.)
Length of cavity 6cm
$(2\frac{1}{2}$ in.)
Thickness of muscle wall is about 1.2cm $(\frac{1}{2}$ in.)

29

UTERUS

CORPUS and CERVIX

The upper two-thirds of the uterus are called the corpus or body, and the lower third the cervix or neck. They are quite distinct in function and therefore in structure as well, although the transition from muscle to fibrous tissue is gradual.

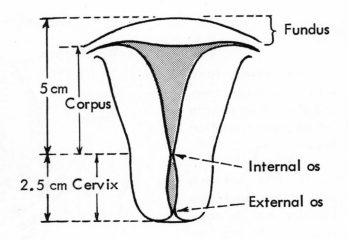

CORPUS

Its function is to provide a mucous membrane (endometrium) suitable for implantation, and thereafter to contain the growing foetus until it is mature. It is composed mainly of unstriped muscle.

CERVIX

Its function is to provide an alkaline secretion favourable to sperm penetration, and once the uterus is gravid, to act as a sphincter. It is composed mainly of fibro-elastic tissue.

ISTHMUS UTERI. This name is sometimes given to the upper few millimetres of the cervical canal below the internal os, an area to which the specific function of developing into the lower segment has been ascribed. The epithelium is intermediate between corpus and cervix; but if it were not for the importance of the lower segment in the modern theory of the physiology of pregnancy, it is unlikely that anatomists would have provided either an identity or a name for the isthmus uteri.

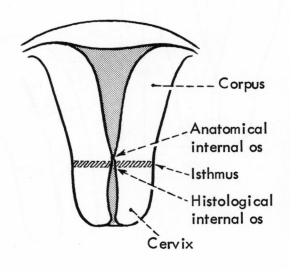

UTERUS

CAVITY OF THE CORPUS

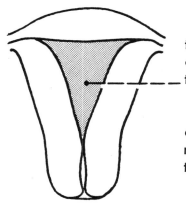

The anterior and posterior walls are almost in contact but in coronal plane the cavity is triangular.

The muscle wall at each cornu is pierced by the very narrow interstitial portion of the fallopian tube.

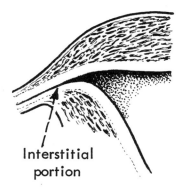

Interstitial portion

CERVIX

The external os is small before parturition and is sometimes called the os tincae (mouth of a small fish). After the birth of a child it becomes a transverse slit – 'the parous os'.

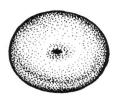

Nulliparous os

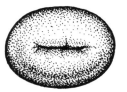

Parous os

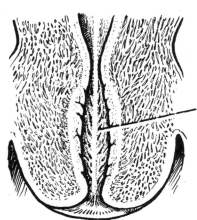

The cervical canal is fusiform and marked by curious folds called the 'arbor vitae'.

The cervix is divided into supra- and infravaginal portions by the attachments of the vagina. The infravaginal part is also called the 'portio vaginalis'.

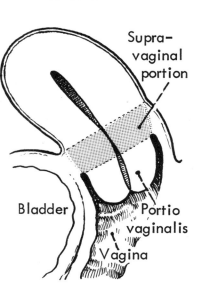

Supra-vaginal portion

Bladder

Portio vaginalis

Vagina

UTERUS

RELATIONSHIP OF UTERUS AND URETER

The ureter is directly related to the uterine artery and the vaginal vault but is not in direct contact with the uterus.

This picture shows the ureter passing under the uterine artery on its course to the bladder.

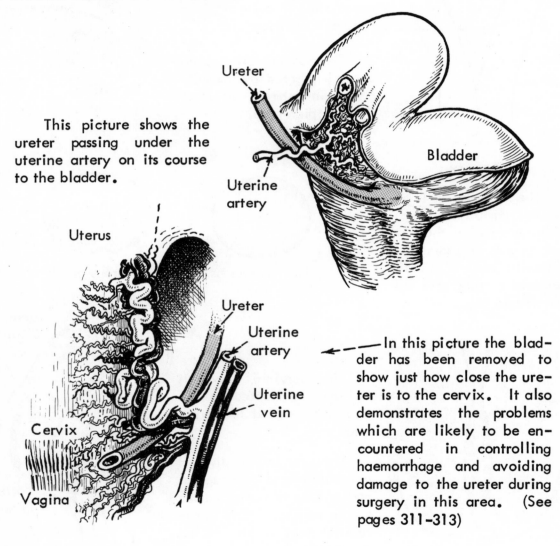

In this picture the bladder has been removed to show just how close the ureter is to the cervix. It also demonstrates the problems which are likely to be encountered in controlling haemorrhage and avoiding damage to the ureter during surgery in this area. (See pages 311–313)

UTERUS

LIGAMENTS OF THE UTERUS

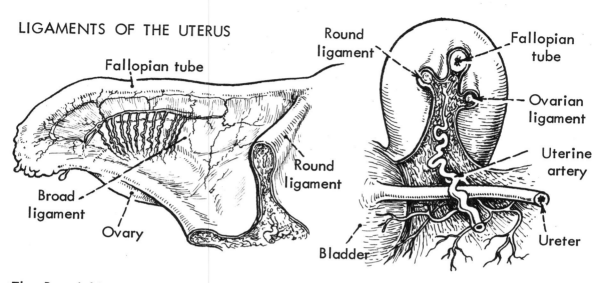

The <u>Broad Ligament</u> is a fold of peritoneum passing from the uterus to the side wall of the pelvis. It contains the fallopian tube, the round and ovarian ligaments, the mesonephric remnants, the ovario-uterine anastomosis and in its base the ureter.

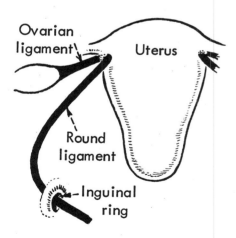

The ovarian and round ligaments are the vestigial gubernaculum. The round ligament ends in the inguinal ring.

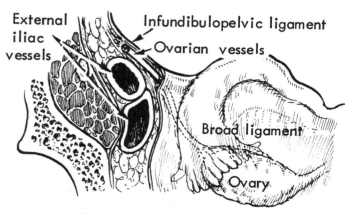

The part of the broad ligament between infundibulum and pelvic wall is called the infundibulopelvic ligament and contains the ovarian vessels and nerves. Note proximity of external iliac vessels.

UTERUS

LIGAMENTS OF THE UTERUS – Continued

The main supports of the uterus are the fibromuscular condensations of tissue in the pelvic fascia (page 25).

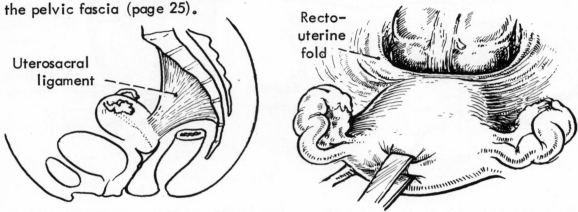

The <u>Uterosacral Ligaments</u> pass from the back of the uterus to the front of the sacrum and are easily identified by the covering recto-uterine fold of peritoneum. These ligaments maintain the anteverted position of the uterus, and they are accompanied by uterine vessels and nerves.

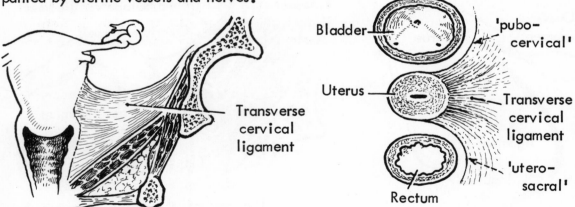

The <u>Transverse Cervical Ligaments</u> (Mackenrodt's, Cardinal ligaments) pass from uterus and vagina to a wide insertion in the lateral pelvic wall.   They lie below the broad ligament and contain vessels and nerves.   The uterosacral ligament may be regarded as the posterior edge of the transverse cervical; its anterior edge is sometimes called the pubocervical but this is not well defined.

UTERUS

HISTOLOGY

The uterus has an incomplete peritoneal coat which is very adherent.   The anterior bare area is to allow movement of the bladder. There is a complete fascial sheath continuous with the vagina and the body is made of plain muscle interspersed with fibro-elastic tissue. There is a reversion of the ratio of muscle to connective tissue as the cervix is approached;   and the cervix is nearly all fibrous.

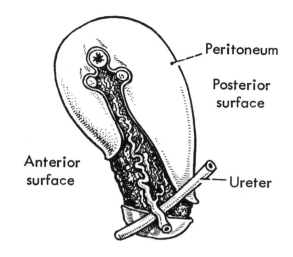

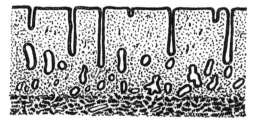

Endometrium   (low power)

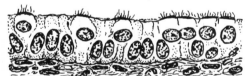

Uterine gland   (high power)

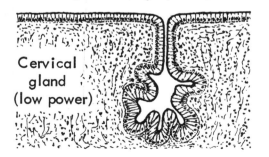

Cervical gland (low power)

The epithelium of the cavity is called endometrium and consists of a single layer of cuboid or columnar ciliated cells on a cellular stroma.   The stroma is deeply pierced by invaginations of the epithelium called uterine glands which secrete a small amount of mucus to maintain moistness.

For cyclical changes in the endometrium see page 54.

The cervix is lined by a single layer of high columnar ciliated epithelium which covers the folds of the arbor vitae (p 31) and lines the cervical glands.   The glands secrete an alkaline mucus which is favourable to the activity of spermatozoa.

FALLOPIAN TUBE

The tube extends from the cornu of the uterus into the peritoneal cavity and is about 10cm long. The two tubes are twice the width of the pelvis and they do more than just provide a passage for the ovum into the uterus. They must be sufficiently mobile to assist the ovum onwards by peristalsis; and sufficiently long to allow the ovum time for maturation after it has been fertilised in the ampulla and before it is ready for implantation in the uterus. The tube and ovary together are called the adnexae ("partes adnexae" - parts attached) of the uterus.

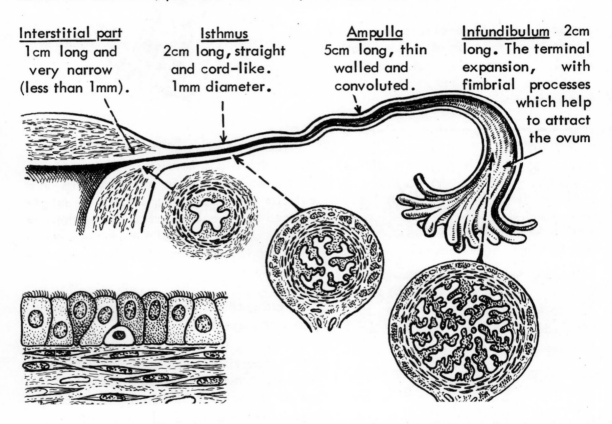

Interstitial part
1cm long and very narrow (less than 1mm).

Isthmus
2cm long, straight and cord-like. 1mm diameter.

Ampulla
5cm long, thin walled and convoluted.

Infundibulum 2cm long. The terminal expansion, with fimbrial processes which help to attract the ovum

The tube has a lining of ciliated cells interspersed with non-ciliated secretory cells ('peg' cells). There is little or no submucosa. The epithelium is arranged in a complex pattern of plications which becomes more marked as the outer end is approached. (For cyclic changes see page 55.)

BROAD LIGAMENT

Blood Vessels

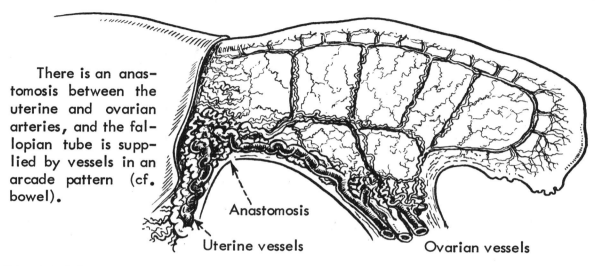

There is an anastomosis between the uterine and ovarian arteries, and the fallopian tube is supplied by vessels in an arcade pattern (cf. bowel).

Anastomosis

Uterine vessels

Ovarian vessels

Vestigial Structures

The epoophoron and the paroophoron are remnants of the mesonephros, and the duct (Gartner's duct) is the vestige of the mesonephric duct which passes into the uterine muscle about the level of the internal os and continues downwards in the vaginal wall.

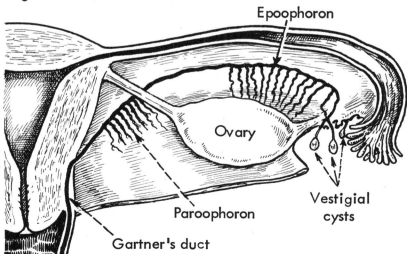

Epoophoron

Ovary

Paroophoron

Gartner's duct

Vestigial cysts

These structures may give rise to cysts (Hydatids of Morgagni, Kobelt's tubules, fimbrial cysts) whose embryonic derivation is uncertain. They are probably mesonephric and can be grouped together as 'vestigial cysts'.

OVARY

The ovary is about 3cm long and 1.5cm wide, roughly the size and shape of a date. It has its own mesentery, the mesovarium from the posterior leaf of the broad ligament and is attached to the cornu of the uterus by the ovarian ligament which is continuous with the round ligament, the vestigial gubernaculum.

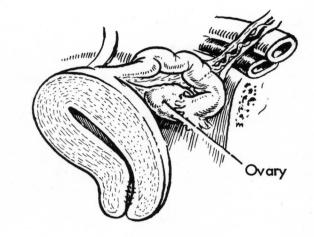

Ovary

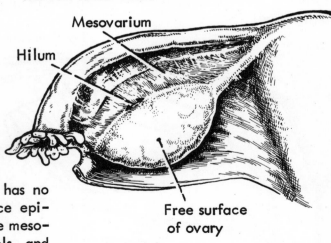

Left renal vein

Abdominal aorta

The ovary is developmentally an abdominal organ and its blood supply is from the abdominal aorta. The ovarian vessels lie in the infundibulopelvic ligaments. Note: The left ovarian vein empties into the left renal vein.

Mesovarium

Hilum

Free surface of ovary

The free surface of the ovary has no peritoneal covering, only a surface epithelium. The part attached to the mesovarium through which all vessels and nerves pass, is called the hilum.

OVARY

HISTOLOGY

Cross-section shows the ovary to be roughly divided into a vascular medulla and a cortex.

The cortex is composed of a specialised ovarian stroma with a cuboidal surface epithelium which like the tubal ostium is intraperitoneal.

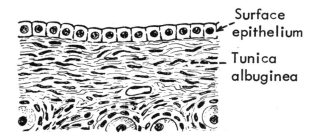

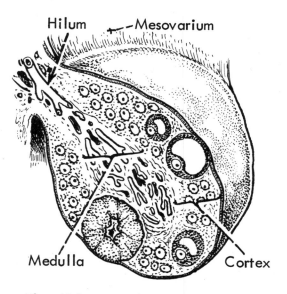

Note the condensed layer of stroma under the surface epithelium, called the tunica albuginea.

Ova are very numerous in the infant and child (at least over 100,000) but much less so in the adult.

The Hilum is characterised by the presence of paroophoron tubules which are of plain muscle lined with ciliated epithelium; and by vestigial remnants of the sex cords called the rete ovarii, the analogue of the seminiferous tubules. These tissues are one reason for the extraordinary variety of ovarian tumours which can develop.

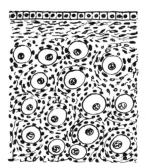

Cortex in an infant.

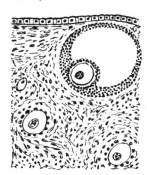

Cortex in an adult.

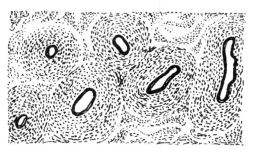

The hilum, showing cross-section of paroophoron tubules.

OVARY

THE CORPUS LUTEUM ('Yellow body': carotene gives the mature corpus luteum a yellow colour.) During growth the Graafian follicle gradually approaches the surface of the ovary and eventually extrudes the ovum through the stigma, into the waiting fimbriae of the tube. The follicle cells then quickly become luteinised by the retention of fluid to form the corpus luteum whose function is to secrete progestins and prepare the organism for implantation of the fertilised ovum.

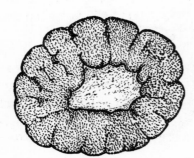

Corpus luteum (low power)

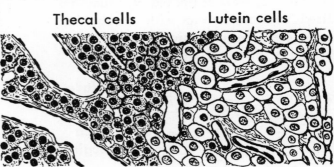

Thecal cells   Lutein cells

Corpus luteum (high power)

The growing corpus luteum is supplied with capillaries from the ovarian stromal vessels, and both theca and granulosa lutein cells secrete all the hormones – oestrogens, progestins (predominantly) and androgens.

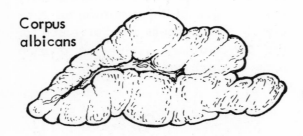

Corpus albicans

As the physiological cycle proceeds degeneration gradually occurs, and eventually the corpus luteum is hyalinised – a corpus albicans – and is absorbed in about a year. This scarring accounts for the irregular surface of the ovary in the more mature woman.

Follicular Atresia

More than half the oocytes present at birth are absorbed before puberty and all are gone at the menopause. Only about 400 can ever become mature follicles, but at each cycle and probably during childhood several follicles may start to develop and for a time produce hormones. This abortive attempt ends in atresia and the atretic follicle is absorbed; but the process may account for anovular cycles and for the oestrogens produced by young pre-pubertal girls whose breasts are beginning to develop.

CHANGES IN THE GENITAL TRACT WITH AGE

Apart from normal growth the appearances of the genital tract depend entirely on the supply of oestrogens.

The Vulva

This is only a cleft in the perineum before puberty. Then the labia minora become more prominent and the fat of the mons and the labia majora is increased. Apart from the effects of coitus and parturition (page 18) the most obvious sign of ageing is the gradual increase in size of the labia minora compared with the labia majora.

The Vagina

The rugae are absent before puberty and gradually (over several years) disappear after the menopause. In old women the vagina is thin, atrophic and completely smooth.

The Ovary

This is at its largest during the reproductive stage and shrinks thereafter. All the oocytes are gone by the time of the menopause and the cortex consists of fibrous tissue.

The Uterus

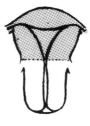

Infantile: the cervix is longer than the corpus and there is no flexion.

Pubertal: with the gradual increase in oestrogens the corpus grows in relation to the cervix.

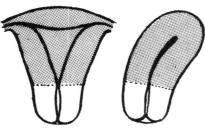

Adult: the corpus is now twice as long as the cervix and the normal degree of flexion has appeared.

After the menopause the uterus gradually atrophies and in an old woman the cavity may be less than 5cm and the cervix simply an aperture in the senile vaginal vault.

The senile endometrium is thin and fibrotic.

BLOOD SUPPLY OF THE PELVIS

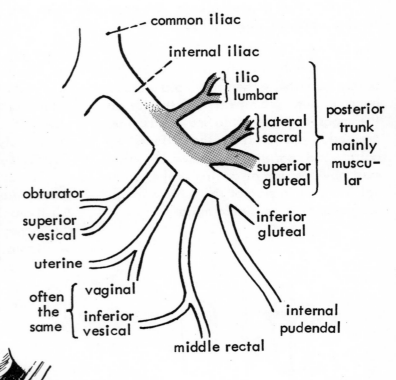

The common iliac artery bifurcates at the level of the sacrovertebral junction into external and internal iliac arteries. The internal iliac runs for about 4cm and divides into an anterior and posterior trunk which are the main pelvic supply. The branches are subject to great variation.

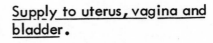

<u>Supply to uterus, vagina and bladder.</u>

This picture shows an arrangement often met with.

BLOOD SUPPLY OF THE PELVIS

The vessels of the uterus and vagina are much coiled to provide extra length during pregnancy. (Cf. the coiled telephone flex.) Note the nearness of the ureter.

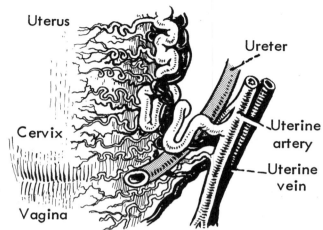

Uterus

Ureter

Cervix

Uterine artery

Uterine vein

Vagina

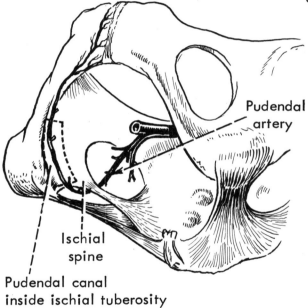

This picture shows the course of the pudendal artery passing behind the ischial spine and along the pudendal canal to the perineum.

Pudendal artery

Ischial spine

Pudendal canal inside ischial tuberosity

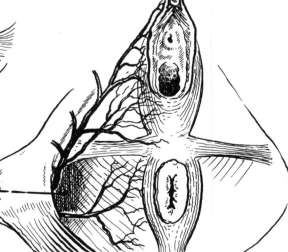

In the ischiorectal fossa the artery divides into inferior rectal and perineal branches.

BLOOD SUPPLY OF THE PELVIS

COLLATERAL BLOOD SUPPLY

If the internal iliac artery has to be ligated, the collateral circulation should be adequate. It depends on anastomoses with the abdominal aorta, external iliac and femoral arteries.

Abdominal aorta

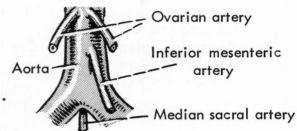

1. Ovarian artery → uterine artery.
2. Inferior mesenteric → superior rectal → inferior rectal (pudendal).
3. Median sacral → lateral sacral.

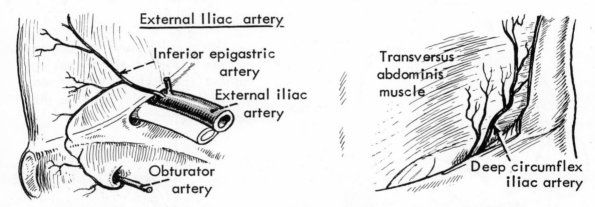

External Iliac artery

The inferior epigastric anastomoses with the obturator; the deep circumflex iliac with the iliolumbar and lumbar arteries.

The Femoral Artery

The deep external pudendal anastomoses with the internal pudendal

The superior and inferior gluteal arteries anastomose with the perforating and circumflex branches of the femoral and profunda femoris. (This is the 'cruciate' anastomosis.)

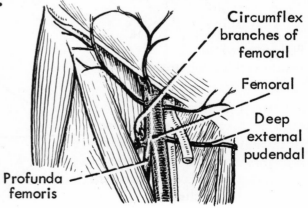

LYMPHATIC DRAINAGE OF THE GENITAL TRACT

The lymphatic plexuses accompany the blood vessels and drain into groups of glands which are constant in position and are given names.

It will be seen that while the uterus is likely to drain into the external iliac group on the lateral wall of the pelvis, the vagina drains into the internal iliac group and the ovary drains direct to the aortic glands.

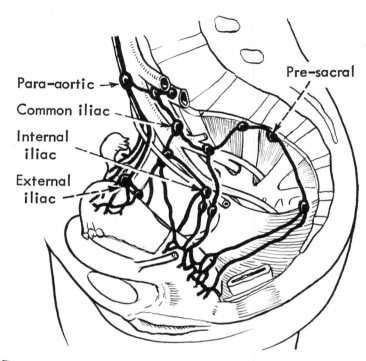

Para-aortic →

Common iliac

Internal iliac

External iliac

Pre-sacral

The superficial inguinal glands also receive lymph drainage from vulva and the lower vagina. (But these structures may also drain via the pudendal vessel channels into the internal iliac group.)

Because lymphatic plexuses and glands are the path of metastatic spread of cancer, treatment either by irradiation or surgery must involve an attack on the area of lymphatic drainage of the organs concerned. But the lymphatic network is so widespread and the metastatic paths are not always the same; and it is now recognised that the chance of cure is much reduced once the spread to the glands has occurred, whatever treatment is given.

NERVES OF THE PELVIS

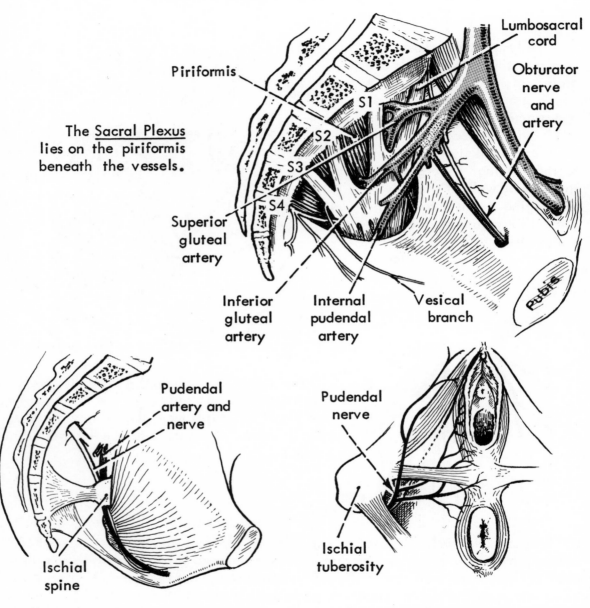

Piriformis

Lumbosacral cord

Obturator nerve and artery

S1

S2

S3

S4

The <u>Sacral Plexus</u> lies on the piriformis beneath the vessels.

Superior gluteal artery

Inferior gluteal artery

Internal pudendal artery

Vesical branch

Pubis

Pudendal artery and nerve

Pudendal nerve

Ischial spine

Ischial tuberosity

The pudendal artery and nerve pass behind the ischial spine to gain the ischiorectal fossa.

The pudendal nerve crosses the ischiorectal fossa to supply the vulva and perineum.

AUTONOMIC NERVE SUPPLY OF THE PELVIS

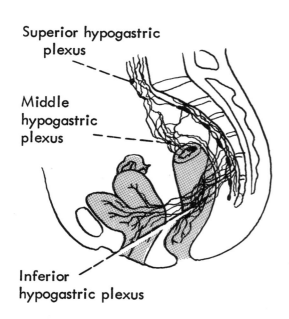

Superior hypogastric plexus

Middle hypogastric plexus

Inferior hypogastric plexus

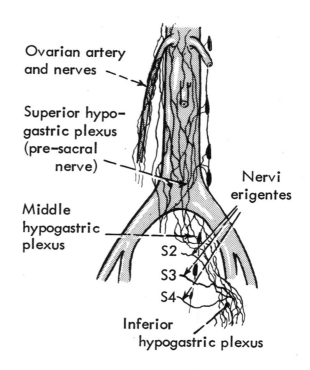

Ovarian artery and nerves

Superior hypogastric plexus (pre-sacral nerve)

Middle hypogastric plexus

Nervi erigentes

S2

S3

S4

Inferior hypogastric plexus

Sympathetic fibres enter via the lumbosacral chain and the mesenteric nerves. These are called the presacral nerve at the bifurcation of the aorta. They pass forward in the uterosacral ligaments to reach the viscera and are known there as the hypogastric plexus or plexus of Frankenhauser.

Parasympathetic nerves ('nervi erigentes) join the hypogastric plexuses from sacral roots 2, 3, 4.

There is an additional sympathetic supply by the nerves accompanying the ovarian vessels.

Function of the autonomic nerves is not understood. In practice it is possible to cauterise the cervix causing only a sensation of heat. The cervix or vagina may be grasped by forceps with only a momentary pricking sensation, and a sound in the uterine cavity causes a vague 'visceral' discomfort. Yet cervical dilatation must be done under anaesthesia, and even then it has been known to cause a severe vasovagal collapse. The relief of pelvic pain by partial cordotomy has to be done well above the pelvis to be effective, and the level of choice is T.2 (see page 231).

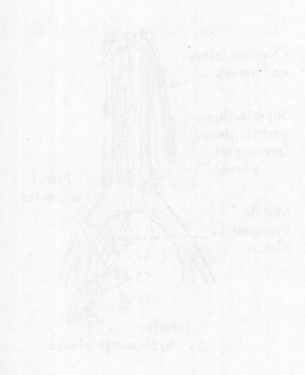

Superior hypogastric plexus

Middle hypogastric plexus

Inferior hypogastric plexus

Ovarian artery and nerves

Superior hypogastric plexus (pre-sacral nerves)

Middle hypogastric plexus

Inferior hypogastric plexus

Pelvic splanchnic nerves

Sympathetic fibres enter via the lumbosacral chain and the mesenteric nerves. These are called the presacral nerve at the bifurcation of the aorta. They pass forward in the uterosacral ligaments to reach the viscera and are known there as the hypogastric plexus or plexus of Frankenhauser.

Parasympathetic nerves (nervi erigentes) join this hypogastric plexus from sacral roots 2, 3, 4.

These is an additional sympathetic supply by the nerves accompanying the ovarian vessels.

Function of the autonomic nerve is not understood. In practice it is possible to sustitute the cervix causing only a sensation of tension. The cervix or vagina can be grasped by forceps with only a momentary pricking sensation, and crushed in the uterine cavity causes a vague visceral discomfort. Yet general dilatation requires to be done under anaesthesia, and even then it has been known to cause a severe vasovagal collapse. The relief of pelvic pain by partial sympathectomy has to be done well above the pelvis to be effective, and the level of choice is T12 (see page 236).

CHAPTER 3
PHYSIOLOGY OF THE REPRODUCTIVE TRACT

OVULATION

FEMALE REPRODUCTIVE PHYSIOLOGY

The dominant process which appears to govern the physiology of the female genital organs during reproductive life is the cyclical growth and maturation of ovarian follicles.

The ovary is covered by a cuboidal "germinal" epithelium which at the hilum is continuous with that lining the peritoneal cavity. This is supported by a thin layer of fibrous tissue beneath which is the true cortex. The latter consists of a specialised stroma or parenchyma embedded in which are the primordial follicles.

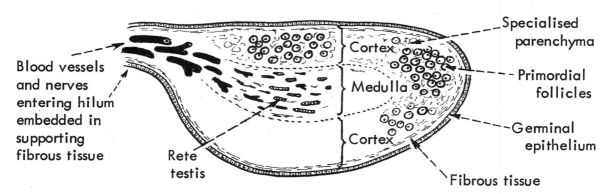

The primordial follicle consists of a primary oocyte surrounded by a single layer of flattened cells, the pre-granulosa, said to be derived from the cells of the sex cords.

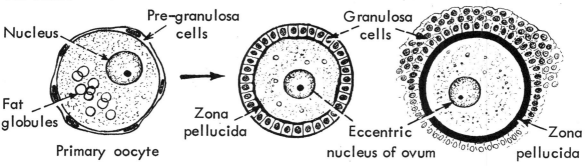

The pre-granulosa cells become cuboidal and proliferate to form a shell several layers thick. At this stage a hyaline membrane is formed immediately around the ovum – the zona pellucida.

OVULATION

The granulosa cells continue to proliferate until the follicle is approximately 200μ in diameter. Fluid spaces now appear between the granulosa cells. They coalesce to form a cavity, the antrum, pushing the ovum to one side. The granulosa cells immediately surrounding the ovum are now known as the corona radiata and the whole mass of cells in this situation is termed the cumulus.

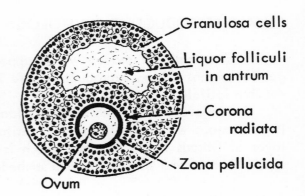

Granulosa cells

Liquor folliculi in antrum

Corona radiata

Zona pellucida

Ovum

At the same time the surrounding parenchymal cells arrange themselves concentrically around the follicle and opposite the site of the ovum some become smaller and epithelial in appearance. As the follicle increases in size this epithelial change spreads to the parenchymal cells around the circumference of the follicle. This band of cells constitutes the theca interna. The cells are surrounded by sinusoidal capillaries thus making a structure like an endocrine gland. External to this band the parenchymal cells are also arranged concentrically but retain their fusiform shape.

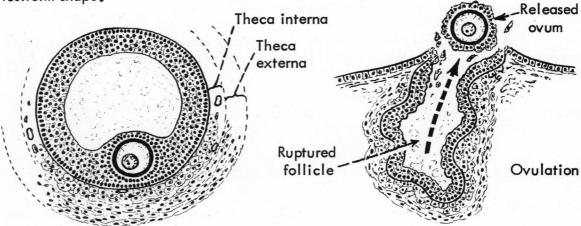

Theca interna

Theca externa

Released ovum

Ruptured follicle

Ovulation

The follicle continues to grow until it reaches a size of 10-12mm. Approximately 5-10 follicles may attain this size at the same time and project on the surface of the ovaries. One of these follicles ruptures on the surface, releasing the ovum surrounded by some of the granulosa cells.

OVULATION

Following the rupture blood vessels quickly invade the granulosa layer, the cells of which become large and polyhedral – lutein cells. The point of rupture is sealed by blood clot which becomes organised. These changes take place in 48-72 hours and the follicle now filled with blood clot and lined by the lutein cells has become a corpus luteum. The theca interna cells form a thin layer externally and are now known as paralutein cells.

The corpus luteum persists for several days but by the 10th day following ovulation, that is the 22nd of the cycle, degeneration has begun and the lutein cells are gradually replaced by a hyaline substance and a white corpus albicans is formed. Meanwhile the other follicles which have enlarged undergo atrophy – termed atresia, the liquor folliculi is absorbed and they disappear.

In the normal female ovulation takes place once every 28 days and the sequence of ovarian events is accompanied by cyclical changes in the secondary sex organs particularly the endometrium. This is due to the secretion of oestrogen and progesterone by the ovary.

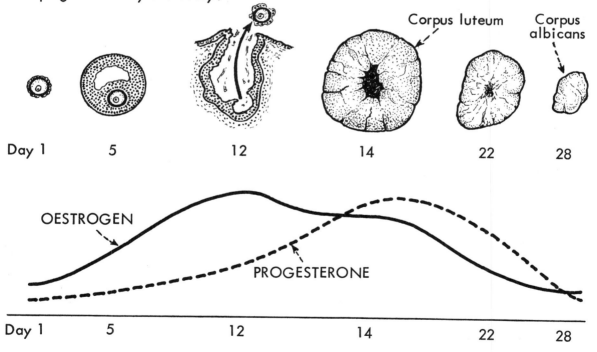

ENDOMETRIAL CYCLE

By the 5th day of this ovarian cycle the endometrium shows proliferation of its stroma and glands, the latter elongating. The cells lining the glands are cuboidal with definite limiting membranes and the stromal cells are thin and spindly – early proliferative phase.

In a week's time (12th day) the glands are very large and are now dilated – late proliferative phase. The blood vessels are also more prominent and capillaries are dilated.

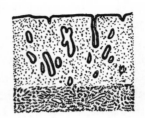 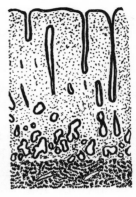

Early proliferative phase

Late proliferative phase

These proliferative changes are due to the influence of oestrogen secreted by the ovary at this time.

Following ovulation the corpus luteum produces large quantities of progesterone which induce secretory changes in the glands and swelling of the stromal cells. There is a rich blood supply and the capillaries become sinusoidal.

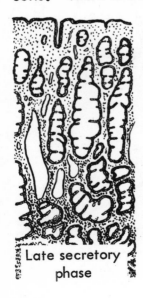 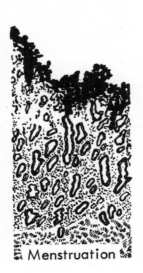

Late secretory phase

Menstruation

Towards the end of the 28 day cycle the stroma becomes even more vascular and oedematous, small haemorrhages and thrombi appear and the endometrium ultimately breaks down due to withdrawal of the hormonal support.

The superficial layers of endometrium together with blood and leucocytes are shed and discharged – menstruation. Within a day or two the raw surface is healed over by epithelium proliferating from the basal portions of glands.

CYCLIC CHANGES IN VAGINA AND TUBE

Changes also occur in other parts of the genital tract.

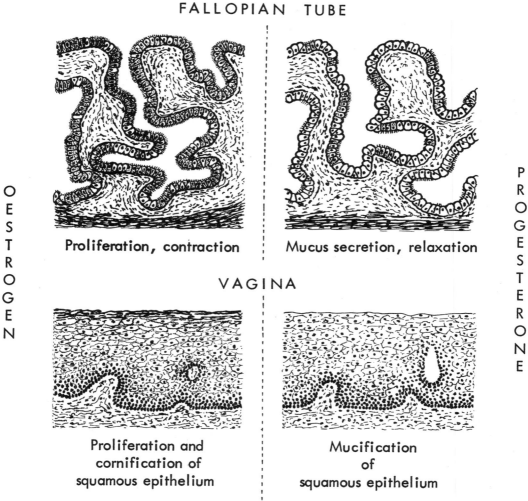

FALLOPIAN TUBE

O E S T R O G E N

P R O G E S T E R O N E

Proliferation, contraction

Mucus secretion, relaxation

VAGINA

Proliferation and
cornification of
squamous epithelium

Mucification
of
squamous epithelium

It is generally considered that a primordial follicle reaches the stage of ovulation in the first 12 days of a menstrual cycle but it is possible that this is not true and that it requires more than one cycle to reach maturity. The important factor however is the increase in hormonal production during the cycle.

CYCLIC OVARIAN HORMONAL CHANGES

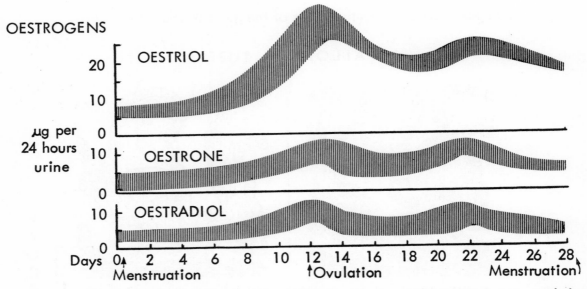

OESTROGENS

OESTRIOL

OESTRONE

OESTRADIOL

µg per 24 hours urine

Days
Menstruation   †Ovulation   Menstruation

Levels of all oestrogens are low during menstruation and it is not until the 7th–8th day of the cycle that any significant rise is noted. Maximum readings are found around the 12th day – this is the ovulation peak. A rapid fall occurs within 24 hours to be followed by a further rise a week later. This peak probably indicates the maximum phase of corpus luteum activity. Oestrone and oestradiol always show a ratio of 2/1 but oestriol output bears no strict mathematical relationship to either of the others.

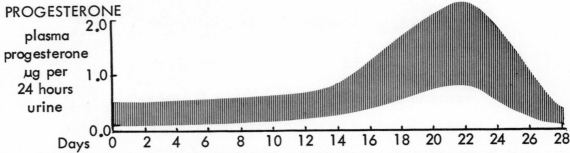

PROGESTERONE

plasma progesterone µg per 24 hours urine

Days

Progesterone is almost absent from the plasma in the early stages of the menstrual cycle. At the time of ovulation there is a steep rise and a maximum value is achieved around 20th–22nd day. Thereafter a steep fall occurs.

CONTROL OF OVULATION

The ovarian changes are controlled by the pituitary which in turn appears to be under the influence of a centre of centres in the hypothalamus, thought to be near the median eminence.

The pituitary produces at least two gonadotrophins, follicle stimulating hormone (FSH) and luteinising hormone (LH) and a third in certain other animals, the luteotrophic hormone (LTH).

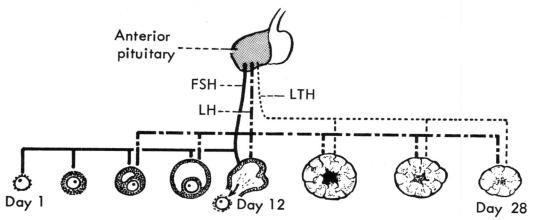

The quantities of these hormones secreted during the cycle are not yet clearly established but it is accepted that there is an "ovulation" peak of LH around the 12th day of the cycle.

GONADOTROPHIC EXCRETION

Human menopausal gonadotrophin (HMG) units per 24 hours

	Menstruation	Follicular phase	Ovulation	Luteal phase
NON PAROUS	8.4	9.2	12.7	8.9
PAROUS	14.9	15.0	26.7	11.2

CONTROL OF OVULATION

The changes may be represented diagrammatically as follows (the curves for ovarian steroids are shown for comparison):-

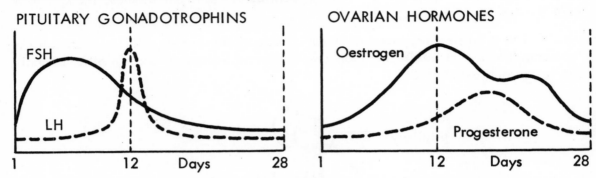

There is an inverse relationship between ovarian and pituitary hormones and this indicates a feed back system of control. At the beginning of the cycle the blood oestrogen level is low and this stimulates FSH secretion. As a result follicles mature and large quantities of oestrogens are secreted. These progressively inhibit FSH secretion and initiate LH secretion, producing ovulation and corpus luteum formation. Progesterone and oestrogen are both produced by the luteal cells. Pituitary LTH is produced by some animals to maintain the corpus luteum. If fertilisation of the ovum does not occur the corpus luteum regresses, oestrogen and progesterone production diminishes, menstruation occurs and FSH secretion is stimulated.

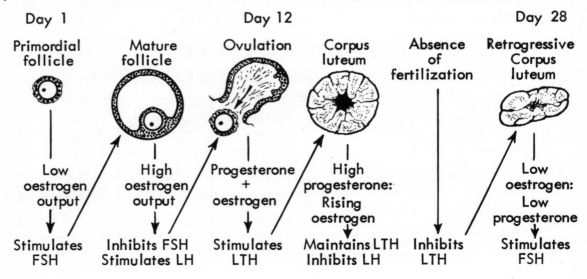

CONTROL OF OVULATION

The feed-back influence of the ovarian steroids is indirect. Anterior pituitary hormone secretion is under the influence of another group of substances produced in the hypothalamus near the medial eminence. These are known as FSH and LH releasing substances, and their secretion is controlled by the levels of the ovarian steroids in the blood. The presence of these centres in the brain helps to explain the influence of emotion on ovarian functions.

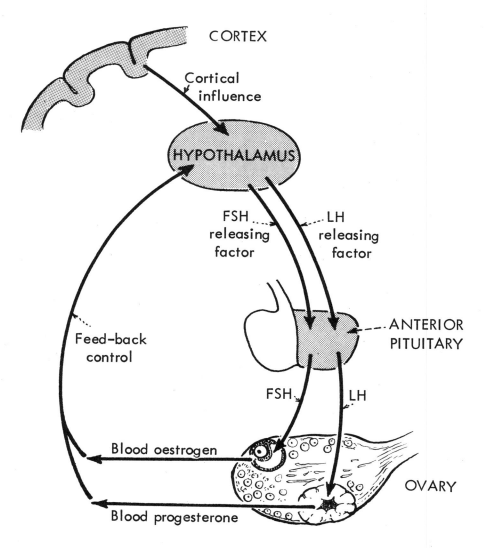

ACTION OF OVARIAN HORMONES

<u>OESTROGEN</u>   <u>PROGESTERONE</u>

Proliferation of stroma and glands – – UTERUS – – – Enlargement of cells of stroma
                                                                          and glands
                                                            Increase of endometrial glycogen

Proliferation of glands – – – – – – CERVIX – – – Increase in mucus secretion
Secretion of salt–rich fluid..
..giving fern crystals when dried

Proliferation of epithelium with – – –VAGINA – – Mucification with polymorpho-
increased cornification and   nuclear leucocytes
deposition of mucopolysaccharides

Diminished output of urine – – – – –KIDNEYS – – Increase of intra-cellular water
Retention of NaCl and water   Corrective diuresis
     in interstitial tissue

Growth of ducts – – – – – – – BREASTS – – – – – Growth of alveoli
Pigmentation of nipple skin

Vasodilatation – – – – –CARDIOVASCULAR – – – Relaxation of smooth
                                    SYSTEM   muscle
                                                              Drop in blood pressure

Retention of calcium in bones – – – BONES

OVARIAN HORMONES AND THE VAGINAL SMEAR

Due to the action of oestrogens and progesterone, cyclical changes occur in the vaginal mucosa which can be identified by examining a stained smear. In turn, such smears can to some extent be used as a rough guide to the hormonal status of the patient.

Post-menstrual phase
The cells are mainly of pre-cornified type and by Papanicolaou's method the cytoplasm is stained blue-green.

Proliferative phase
The rising concentration of oestrogen increases cornification and causes glycogen to appear in the cells. Brown deposits of glycogen appear in the pink cytoplasm. The nuclei are small and pyknotic.

Secretory phase
Cornified cells diminish in number. Pre-cornified cells with folded edges make their appearance and many polymorphs are seen.

Pre-menstrual-menstrual phase
The cells are clumped and degenerate. Debris and leucocytes are present giving a "dirty" appearance to the smear.

Salt crystals and vaginal fluid
During the proliferative phase the vaginal fluid is rich in sodium chloride. If a smear of the fluid is allowed to dry typical salt crystals are formed. These are an indication of oestrogen activity. The advent of the secretory phase due to progesterone action results in a disappearance of these crystals.

Spinnbarkeit (stringiness)
During the secretory phase the vaginal fluid becomes more mucoid and sticky. If a probe or forceps is used to lift the mucus from a slide, the height to which the string of mucus can be raised before it snaps is an indication of progesterone activity. The test is of limited value since the results are altered by such complicating factors as vaginal discharge.

THE MENOPAUSE

This means the cessation of menstruation.   The period during which the woman experiences the physical and psychological changes associated with ovarian failure is properly called the <u>climacteric</u> (Gk. klimakter: a critical phase); but 'menopause' is often used to mean the whole process.

<u>Mechanism of the Menopause</u>.   (This is not yet fully understood.)

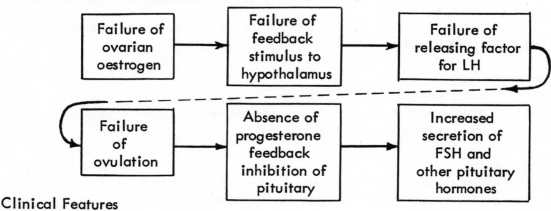

Clinical Features

The menopause now occurs between 45–50 years in British women. The symptoms vary and may be attributed to one of two groups.

Oestrogen Deficiency

1. Cessation of menstruation.
2. Vasomotor disturbances ('Hot flushes').
3. Atrophy of breasts and genital tract.
4. Backache and joint pains due to osteoporosis (a decrease in bone matrix, not a failure of calcium metabolism.)
5. Vascular disease due to atherosclerosis.

Pituitary Overactivity

1. Increased adrenocortical stimulation may lead to obesity, hypertension, virilism (cf. Cushing's syndrome).
2. Increased somatotrophin may lead to a degree of acromegaly, perhaps diabetes.
3. There may be symptoms of hyperthyroidism.

<u>Psychological Changes</u> include depression, emotional instability, fatigue, palpitations, loss or increase of libido.

THE MENOPAUSE

Treatment required at the Menopause

Cessation of Menstruation

This may take place over a year or so, and bleeding will perhaps recur after 6 months' amenorrhoea. In such cases it is advisable to curette the uterus to exclude organic disease. It must be remembered that therapeutic oestrogen in any form will reactivate atrophic endometrium and may produce bleeding.

Vasomotor Disturbances

These are controlled by oestrogens. If severe (some women experience most distressing flushes followed by drenching sweats) stilboestrol 1mg thrice daily will reduce the incidence and severity.

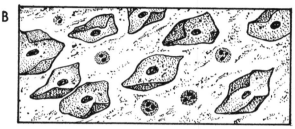

Vaginal smear from atrophic endometrium before (A) and after (B) oestrogen treatment.

Senile Vaginitis

Decrease in vaginal vascularity allows an increase in coliform and streptococcal organisms, which cause irritation. This condition responds well to dienoestrol cream.

Psychological Symptoms

Mild anxiety is helped by small doses of phenobarbitone, but depression may become suicidal in unstable women suffering stress of the menopause.

- -

Long-term Oestrogen Treatment

This is based on the contention that postmenopausal existence is due only to scientific and social advances and must be supported by scientific means i.e. the indefinite consumption of oestrogens to protect the woman against osteoporosis etc. Most doctors however will prescribe oestrogens only as a temporary measure until postmenopausal stability has been achieved.

CHAPTER 4
EXAMINATION OF THE PATIENT

TAKING THE HISTORY

The ancient Greeks believed that the behaviour pattern of hysteria was related to disease of the womb (Gk: hystera, uterus). A woman discussing some condition related to her genital tract is bound to show signs of stress – embarrassment, fear, shame. The gynaecological patient must have...

...PRIVACY

The consultation should ideally be held in a closed room with no-one else present.

...TIME

She should be allowed to tell her own story, before any attempt is made to isolate specific symptoms.

...SYMPATHY

The doctor's manner must be one of interest and understanding.

Once a rapport is established, the usual essential information must be obtained: age, parity, menstrual history, past history with special reference to previous gynaecological treatment.

OBSTETRIC HISTORY

Note the year of each pregnancy, and the type of delivery. Enquire into any history of trauma or excessively long labour.

Puerperal Infection? This may be the origin of a chronic pelvic inflammation.

Infertility? If so, is it voluntary or involuntary? Methods of contraception should be asked about.

Abortions? The degree of haemorrhage should be established, and whether curettage was done. There is a tendency to attribute any irregular and unexplained bleeding to 'a very early miscarriage'.

GENERAL HISTORY

The gynaecologist should know if his patient has ever suffered from tuberculosis, cardiac, renal or blood disease, and whether she has ever had any operation. The existence of previous psychiatric history should be established.

GYNAECOLOGICAL HISTORY

Previous gynaecological treatment is best learnt about from clinical records if obtainable. Gynaecological pathology and terminology are mysterious to most women.

NORMAL MENSTRUAL HISTORY

This can vary very much from patient to patient and still be within normal limits. Vague complaints are unlikely to be due to gynaecological disease, and symptoms (i.e. departures from the normal) if present, are definite.

Menarche

This is the age of onset of menstruation and varies between 10 and 16.

Rhythm of Cycle and Duration of Flow

These are conveniently expressed together as a numerical fraction. Thus 5/28 means that the patient menstruates for 5 days every 28 days. The normal cycle lasts between 21 and 30 days and the bleeding lasts for between 3 and 9 days. No woman is absolutely regular, but some show a surprising uncertainty of recall, giving rise to fractions such as 5 - 10 / 21 - 35. If the patient keeps a diary she should be asked to produce it.

Menopause

The cessation of menstruation.
It usually occurs between 45 and 50. Menorrhagia at this time is not normal. The patient should be asked about the extent of vasomotor disturbance ('hot flushes').

Volume of Blood Loss

This can vary between 1 and 7 ounces (30 and 200ml). Blood should be liquid, but parous women may pass small clots. Large clots mean that the loss is abnormal and the fibrinolytic system cannot break down all the blood that is shed.

15g haemoglobin represents 50mg elemental iron, so a menstrual loss of say 80ml. would mean a loss of about 40mg iron. About a dozen internal tampons might be used for one menstruation; but the patient's estimate of loss may be unreliable, especially if she uses phrases like 'torrential' or 'welling up'.

Menstrual Molimina

(Lat: molimen, great exertion) These are the secondary effects of the menstrual cycle. Some discomfort is normal, and there may be irritability, depression, breast discomfort, backache, pelvic pain. These symptoms should stop short of pre-menstrual tension (p 121) and the pain should not be so severe as to keep the patient off her work.

ABNORMAL MENSTRUAL HISTORY

IRREGULAR BLEEDING

This can be caused by ovulation, hormonal fluctuation or organic disease, and the history is in fact often misleading.

Bleeding after intercourse (post-coital bleeding) and post-menopausal bleeding are always taken to suggest the possibility of malignant disease: yet the cause is more often benign.

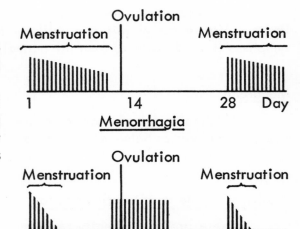

Menstruation — Ovulation — Menstruation

1   14   28   Day

Menorrhagia

Menstruation — Ovulation — Menstruation

1   5   14   28   Day

Metrorrhagia

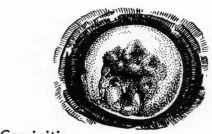

Cervicitis:
The commonest cause of discharge.

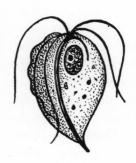

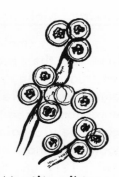

Trichomonas: A very common protozoan infection.

Monilia albicans (Candida albicans): A common yeast infection.

DISCHARGE

Normal discharge is white, made up of coagulated cervical secretion and epithelial cells (smegma). It is normally increased before menstruation.

Leucorrhoea means an increase in this normal discharge.

Yellow purulent discharge suggests cervical and vaginal infection.

Greenish irritant vacuolated discharge suggests trichomonal infection.

White curdy irritant discharge suggests monilial infection.

Bloodstained discharge must raise the question of cancer, but it is more often due to cervicitis or vaginitis.

COMPLAINTS OF PAIN

PAIN

The patient is asked where pain is felt, and whether it is intermittent, related to the period or continuous. The 'ordinary' period pain is felt in the back, lower abdomen and down the thighs. It must be distinguished from other abdominal causes of pain such as appendicitis.

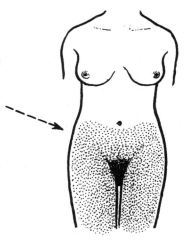

Areas of referred pain during menstruation

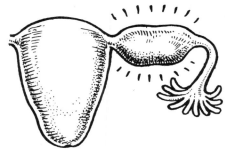

The backache of period pain ('like a steel plate pressing inwards') is referred to the sacral area and should be distinguished from the loin pain of renal disease which can be exacerbated by the congestion of menstruation.

Renal pain

Period pain

Pain associated with intercourse (dyspareunia) may not be mentioned spontaneously, and the doctor should ask of any pain, whether it is aggravated by coitus.

The severity of pain can be judged to some extent by its effect on the patient's behaviour. She should not have to go off her work for 'normal' dysmenorrhoea: if it is so severe as to cause fainting or nausea, tubal pregnancy must be considered. A neurotic patient will employ colourful imagery like 'red-hot drill'.

Tubal pregnancy

EXAMINATION OF THE BREASTS

This should be undertaken if circumstances permit. Signs of pregnancy or lactation may be seen, or a lump may be felt.

The examination can be made with the patient lying on her back. The breast is gently but thoroughly palpated with the fingers, and the axilla is also palpated.

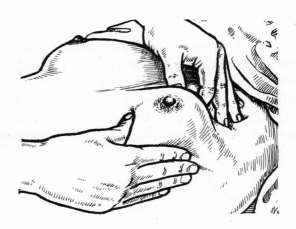

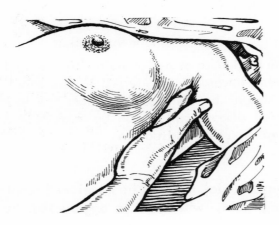

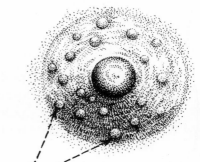

Montgomery's Tubercles, a reliable sign of early pregnancy.

Method of testing for colostrum or milk. The hands gently squeeze the whole breast. - - - →

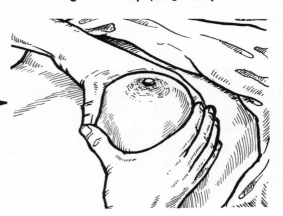

ABDOMINAL EXAMINATION

This must never be omitted, whatever the patient's complaint. Many gynaecological tumours form large swellings which leave the pelvis altogether; and an undisclosed pregnancy may be present.

Ovarian cysts often have long pedicles. This ovarian cyst is completely abdominal, and would not be palpable on bimanual pelvic examination.

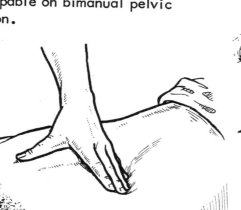

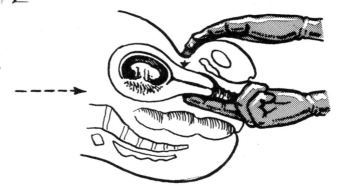

The characteristic swelling of the 16 week pregnancy may not be seen but can always be felt by pressing with the flat of the hand. The bladder must not be full.

Pelvic examination alone might not reveal this pregnancy if the unsuspecting examiner were inadvertently to palpate the soft and elongated cervix without feeling the enlarged corpus (cf. Hegar's sign).

ABDOMINAL EXAMINATION

All the classical techniques of inspection, palpation, and auscultation (for a foetal heart) may be required, but the most important is gentle palpation with the flat of the hand to detect solid or semi-solid tumours.

The examiner must bear in mind the various intra-abdominal structures which may give rise to swellings.

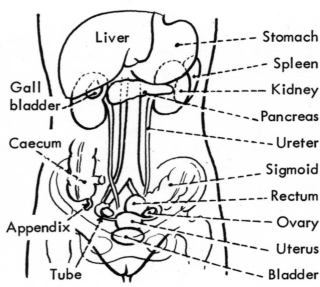

Liver — Stomach
— Spleen
Gall bladder — Kidney
— Pancreas
Caecum — Ureter
— Sigmoid
— Rectum
Appendix — Ovary
— Uterus
Tube — Bladder

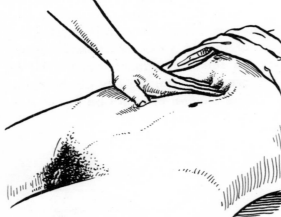

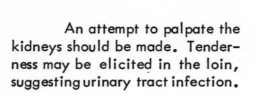

The hypochondria should be examined to exclude liver and spleen enlargement or gall-bladder tenderness, before palpating the lower abdomen.

An attempt to palpate the kidneys should be made. Tenderness may be elicited in the loin, suggesting urinary tract infection.

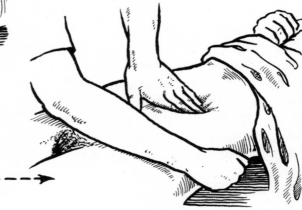

ABDOMINAL EXAMINATION

Inspection may show the characteristic shape of an ovarian cyst. The outline is crescentic and uniform, the skin is stretched, and a fluid thrill may be elicited.

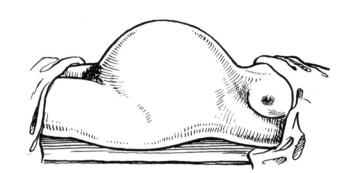

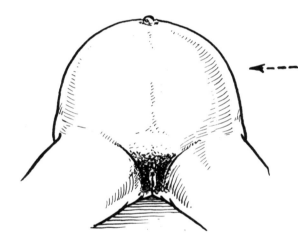

If ascites is present (and this means that the cyst is probably malignant) the outline tends to be cylindrical, with some flattening at the top. The umbilicus is everted and the percussion note is dull in the flanks but tympanitic above because of the upward floating of the intestines.

The very fat abdomen is not uncommon in gynaecology. Palpation is extremely difficult and examination under anaesthesia and more elaborate investigations will be necessary (laparoscopy, X-rays, ultrasonography).

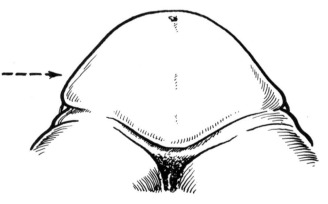

EXAMINATION OF THE VULVA

The dorsal position is most convenient for patient and doctor although some prefer the patient to be in the lateral position. During palpation, the condition of the labia, clitoris, anus and surrounding skin should be noted. Thus excoriation suggests irritating discharge and pruritus, purplish discoloration might be a sign of diabetes.

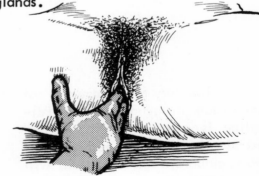

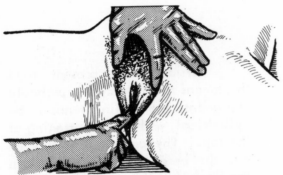

1. A single finger presses on the perineum, avoiding the sensitive vestibule, and accustoming the patient to the examiner's touch.

2. Urethral meatus and vestibule are exposed. Pressure from the finger will squeeze any pus from the peri-urethral glands.

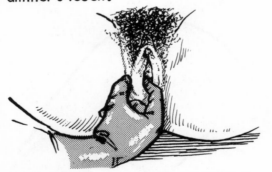

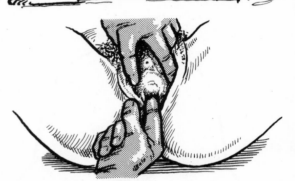

3. Bartholin's gland is palpated (on both sides). It is difficult to feel the normal gland.

4. If there is room, a second finger is inserted and the perineal floor is palpated by stretching.

BIMANUAL PELVIC EXAMINATION

This technique needs practice. The external hand is the more important and supplies more information. It is customary to use two fingers in the vagina, but an adequate outpatient examination may be made with only one finger. Very little information is gained if the patient finds the examination painful. In a virgin or a child only rectal examination should be carried out.

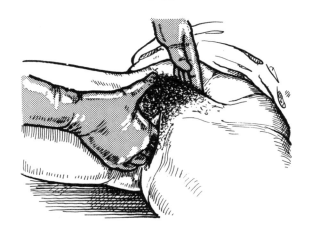

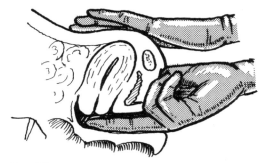

1. The cervix is palpated and any hardness or irregularity noted.

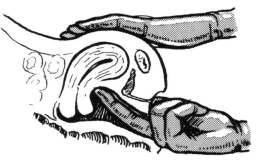

2. The whole uterus is identified, and size, shape, position, mobility and tenderness are noted.

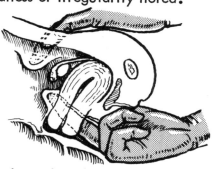

3. The lateral pelvis is palpated and any swelling noted. Normal adnexae are difficult to feel unless the ovary contains a corpus luteum.

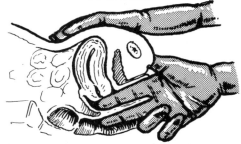

4. Sometimes rectovaginal examination is helpful, if the vagina admits only one finger or if the rectovaginal septum is to be examined.

SPECULUM EXAMINATION

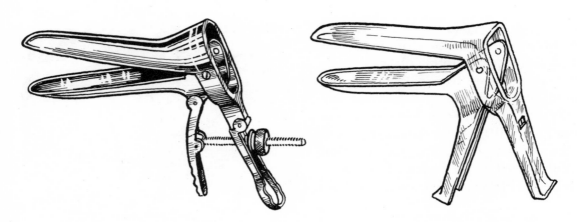

The bi-valve speculum is the most useful (Cusco's pattern is shown here). It is made either of steel or perspex (disposable) and is designed to open after insertion so that the cervix can be seen. The steel speculum has a screw for retaining it in the open position.

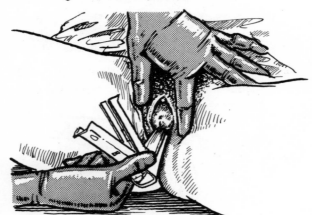

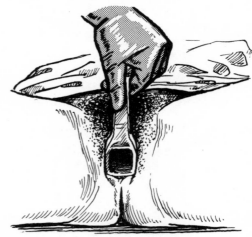

1. The speculum is applied to the vulva at an angle of 45 degrees from the vertical. This allows the easiest insertion.

2. Once in the vagina it is gently opened out and held in position with the cervix between the blades. A good light is needed for inspection.

SPECULUM EXAMINATION

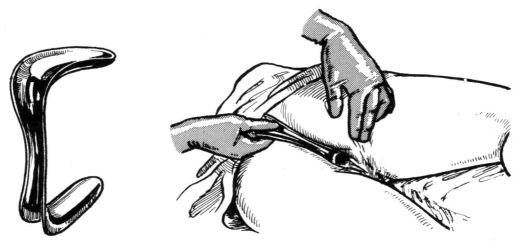

SIMS' SPECULUM (the duck-bill speculum) is designed to hold back the posterior vaginal wall so that air enters and the anterior wall and cervix are exposed.

In this picture the patient is in Sims' position (semi-prone) which is useful if the anterior wall is to be studied (e.g. if fistula is suspected).

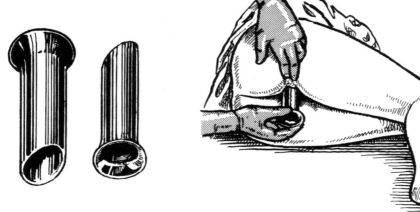

FERGUSON'S SPECULUM is essentially a metal tube, and although old fashioned is useful in cases of marked vaginal prolapse when the bi-valve speculum cannot contain the vaginal wall sufficiently to allow a view of the cervix. In this picture the patient is in the lateral position, which is sometimes used if the cervix cannot be seen in the dorsal position.

LAPAROSCOPY

Inspection of the pelvic cavity through an endoscope passed through the abdominal wall. This investigation is now very frequently performed, but it does carry a risk to the patient and its place in gynaecology is still a matter for discussion.

Technique

The patient is anaesthetised, the bladder emptied, the uterus curetted and a cannula and forceps fixed to the cervix. This allows the uterus to be moved about once the endoscope is passed, and dye can be injected through the cannula to test the patency of the tubes.

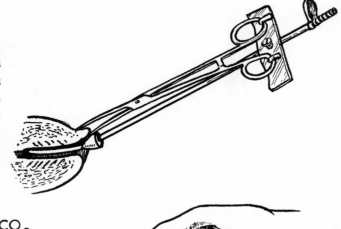

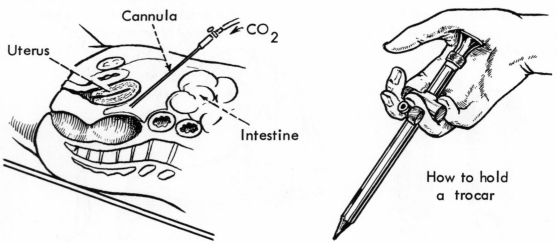

How to hold a trocar

The table is tilted to encourage the intestines to fall away from the pelvis and about 4 litres of CO_2 injected through a thin cannula. A small incision is made through skin, fat and rectus sheath just below the umbilicus and a trocar and cannula large enough to accommodate the endoscope is forced through abdominal wall which should by now be distended away from the viscera.

LAPAROSCOPY

The coldlight endoscope is passed through the cannula and the inspection made.   An assistant or the operator himself can move the uterus about by means of the forceps on the cervix.

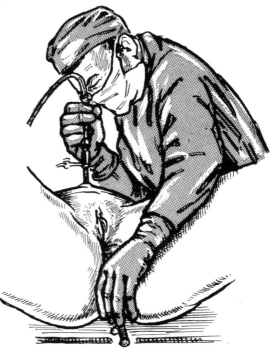

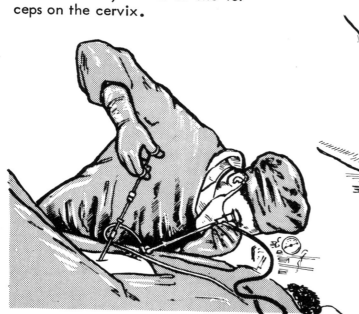

A special biopsy forceps can be passed through another cannula and used to lift up any tissue that may be obstructing the view and take ovarian biopsies. This forceps can also be used as a diathermy electrode to cauterise the fallopian tubes.

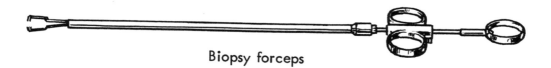

Biopsy forceps

LAPAROSCOPY

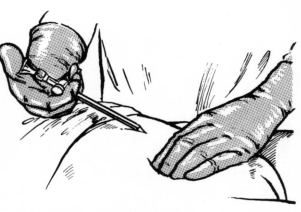

Complications

1. Perforation of a viscus especially adherent bowel.
2. Damage to great vessels especially in the vicinity of the sacral promontory.
3. Infection. This hardly ever occurs as a result of passing the endoscope, but when cautery is being used unnoticed damage to the bowel may occur, or the extensive cauterisation of the tubes may set up a pelvic inflammation.

Indications

1. Suspected pelvic disease (e.g. inflammation, tubal pregnancy.)
2. Infertility investigations.
3. Cauterisation of fallopian tubes.

Contraindications

1. Previous abdominal operation. Bowel may be adherent to the underside of the scar. (Caesarean section usually escapes this prohibition.)
2. Where there is danger of perforating a tumour such as an ovarian cyst or a gravid uterus.
3. Very fat women.

CULDOSCOPY

This is an alternative to laparoscopy in which the endoscope is passed through the posterior fornix. It is a longer established technique but has never achieved the same popularity.

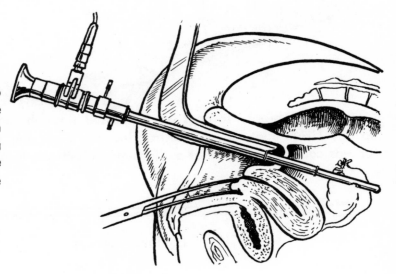

LYMPHOGRAPHY AND GYNAECOGRAPHY

LYMPHOGRAPHY

The X-ray demonstration of lymphatic channels after injection of an iodine contrast medium.

Technique

0.5ml of blue dye injected into a web of the foot will show up the subcutaneous lymphatic network on the dorsum of the foot. The largest channel so displayed is entered by cut-down, and 5ml or more is injected at the rate of 1ml per 10 minutes. To show up both sides of the pelvis both feet must be injected.

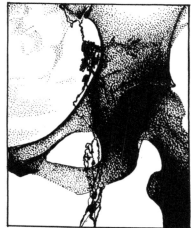

It was hoped that lymphography would demonstrate metastatic spread and that a coloured contrast medium would stain the glands and make their surgical removal an easier matter. Unfortunately the vagaries of lymphatic flow make it impossible to rely on all glands being opacified and nodes containing metastases cannot with certainty be identified.

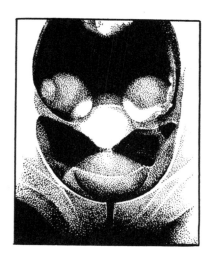

GYNAECOGRAPHY

X-ray demonstration of pelvic organs after injecting gas into the peritoneal cavity. It carries less risk than laparoscopy which has superseded it but is far less informative. The picture shows gynaecographic demonstration of the enlarged ovaries seen in polycystic ovary disease.

CHAPTER 5
ABNORMALITIES OF MENSTRUATION

DYSFUNCTIONAL UTERINE BLEEDING

This means abnormal uterine bleeding due to oestrogen/progesterone aberrations for reasons not known.   This term may only be applied after exclusion of tumour, infection, foreign body, systemic disease.   Bleeding of this type is probably the commonest gynaecological complaint.

Patterns of Dysfunctional Bleeding

1. Normal cycle with excessive loss (menorrhagia). This is usually met with in women over thirty who have had several children. Menstrual loss is naturally greater in the parous woman.

2. Normal menstruation occurring too often (epimenorrhoea). The luteal phase is shortened by too early a degeneration of the corpus luteum.

3. Menstrual bleeding lasting too long. (Irregular shedding: the patient calls it 'stopping and starting'). The corpus luteum degenerates too slowly and the progesterone effect persists. Some secretory endometrium is still present early in the following cycle.

This endometrium was obtained on the 5th day of the cycle.   Note patches of secretory glands among the early proliferative endometrium.

A. Ovulatory

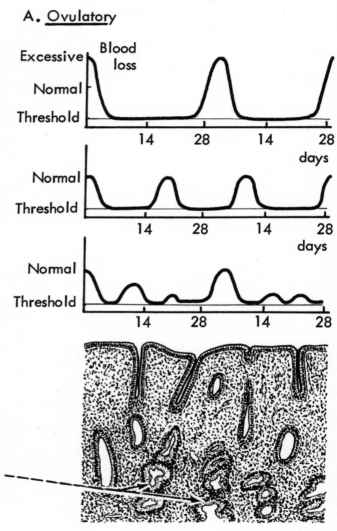

84

DYSFUNCTIONAL UTERINE BLEEDING

4. Prolonged menstrual cycle. The corpus luteum may be slow to develop (irregular ripening) and secretory changes only appear near the end of the cycle. Bleeding occurs before menstruation due to fluctuations in the oestrogen level.

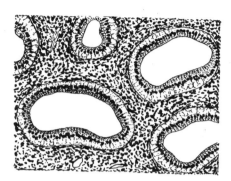

Endometrium 26th day. Note basal vacuoles in the gland cells, an early sign of secretory change.

B. Anovulatory [Irregular bleeding without cyclic pattern (metrorrhagia).]

Too little oestrogen and no progesterone.
("Threshold Bleeding"). This is due to fluctuating oestrogen levels of a low order and is a common complaint. It is met with normally at the time of the menarche and the menopause.

Too much oestrogen and no progesterone (Metropathia Haemorrhagica: Cystic Glandular Hyperplasia.)

In such cases the endometrium becomes hyperplastic from prolonged oestrogen stimulation without any luteal phase and when the oestrogen level falls, the endometrium bleeds. The microscopic pattern shows numerous dilated non-secreting glands, and the patient suffers from bleeding of varying intensity for 6-8 weeks at a time.

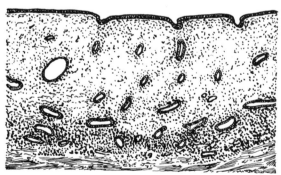

Hypoplastic endometrium associated with low oestrogen levels.

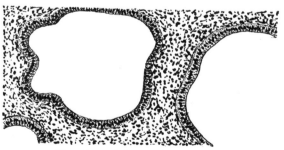

Cystic Glandular Hyperplasia ('Swiss Cheese Pattern'). This endometrium is not pre-malignant.

DYSFUNCTIONAL UTERINE BLEEDING

CLINICAL FEATURES

The patient complains of irregular bleeding or heavy bleeding or both. The menstrual function is fundamental to a woman and any departure from the normal is likely to produce some psychological disturbance and vice versa. The previously normal pattern should be established and an attempt made to estimate the blood loss from the increase in the number of towels used. In this respect some patients will use hysterical words like 'flooding' and 'coming up like a well', giving an impression of blood loss not supported by appearances or by the haemoglobin level. There should be some careful probing of social circumstances to ascertain the degree of stress under which the patient may be living.

Investigations

A general search is made to exclude systemic disease. (Except in the case of young girls at the onset of menstruation who may reasonably be observed for a few months.)

After the usual clinical examination a curettage is advisable. This allows histological inspection of the endometrium and the exclusion of such occult causes as an intra-uterine polyp.

If the ovaries feel enlarged a laparoscopy and ovarian biopsy should be carried out. While the patient is awaiting admission to hospital she should be keeping a written record of her bleedings.

Vacuum Curettage

This new technique allows a sample of endometrium to be obtained by suction without anaesthetising the patient. The method is still experimental but has obvious advantages. It cannot however allow as thorough a search of the uterine cavity as can be made with a conventional curette in the anaesthetised patient.

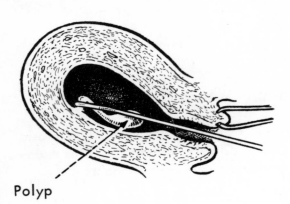

Polyp

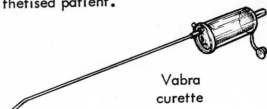

Vabra
curette

DYSFUNCTIONAL UTERINE BLEEDING

TREATMENT

The root cause of dysfunctional bleeding is often psychological and no treatment aimed at the uterus will cure the patient. Also, there is a tendency especially in the younger woman towards a spontaneous return to a normal cycle. Once the diagnosis is certain, it is usual to attempt medical treatment which will improve the condition and allow time for spontaneous cure. If medical treatment fails, hysterectomy or a radiation menopause remain, and the readiness with which one of these is resorted to depends largely on the age of the patient.

Iron Anaemia must be corrected although whether the anaemia itself aggravates the bleeding is doubtful. Total dose infusion of iron-dextran is beneficial in chronic cases.

Thyroid Hormone has been used for many years. It is known that ovarian function is affected by hypothyroidism, but unless there is evidence of this, the use of this hormone for dysfunctional bleeding is empirical; and it is now going out of fashion.

Antifibrinolytic Agents
Endometrium naturally contains plasminogen activators and they have been found in increased concentration in women with menorrhagia. The use of antifibrinolytic agents is based on the assumption that an overactive fibrinolytic system is preventing closure of the basal endometrial arteries by thrombosis. Tranexamic acid 1gm q.i.d. is taken for the duration of the period.

Oestrogens and Progestogens In cyclical treatment an attempt is made to correct the deficiency that is presumed to exist. Thus ethinyl oestradiol 0.05mg might be given daily from the 1st to the 21st day to stop threshold bleeding, and a progestogen - say dydrogesterone 5mg added from the 12th to the 25th day.

Experience with oral contraceptives has clearly demonstrated their regulating and inhibiting effect on endometrium; and combined oestrogen/progestogen tablets are now the best medical treatment of dysfunctional bleeding. A course of treatment should last at least a year.

Androgens have been used in the past for their anti-oestrogenic effects but they carry a risk of virilizing the patient and are little used now.

Gonadotrophins LH is readily available but is of no use in this condition. FSH is a dangerous drug whose only endocrine effect is to increase oestrogen secretion. This is best done by giving oestrogens.

TOTAL HYSTERECTOMY

This is the best treatment for the woman over 45 and is a last resort for the younger patient who has not responded to drug treatment. It puts a stop to the constant blood loss and gets rid of an organ which is a common site of cancer. The disadvantages are:

1. The immediate risks of any abdominal operation – sepsis and thrombo-embolism.

2. The risk to the ureter in total hysterectomy. The operation can present great technical difficulty if the patient is fat and there is some chronic pelvic inflammation.

3. Removal of the uterus may cause depression in a patient who is psychologically unready to lose her childbearing capacity.

<u>Total Hysterectomy</u> (Removal of uterus and cervix)

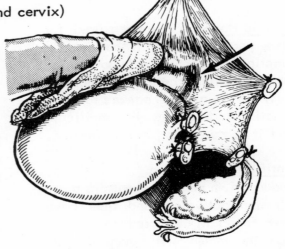

Line of division→

1. Division of adnexae. The ovarian ligament, fallopian tube and round ligament are clamped and divided.

2. Vesico-uterine peritoneum is opened up and bladder is being dissected off cervix. (The 'lateral vesico-uterine ligament' – marked by the arrow, conceals the ureter.)

TOTAL HYSTERECTOMY

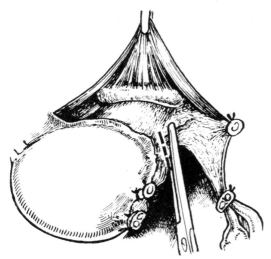

3. Parametrium containing the uterine arteries is clamped and divided.

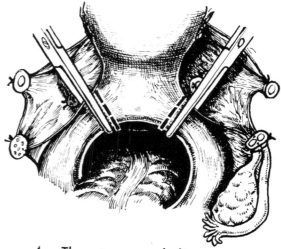

4. The uterosacral ligaments are clamped and divided.

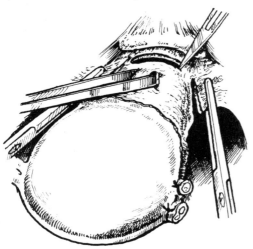

5. The top of the vagina is now clear of bladder and ureters and can be opened to allow excision of uterus and cervix.

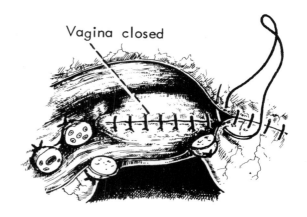

Vagina closed

6. After closing the vagina the raw area is reperitonized.

SUBTOTAL HYSTERECTOMY

Subtotal Hysterectomy – Removal of the body of the uterus only, leaving the cervix.

This operation is easier and safer than total hysterectomy but is little practised today because it does not give protection from the risk of cervical cancer. It would be indicated if the surgeon felt that for technical reasons an attempt at removal of the cervix would be dangerous for the patient.

Excision of the Ovaries

This is an even simpler operation which would cure dysfunctional bleeding quite as well as total

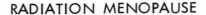

hysterectomy but has no prophylactic value to balance the risk of surgery. It would only be indicated in a patient unfit for anything else.

RADIATION MENOPAUSE

A small amount of external radiation, say 500r in divided doses will in most women put an end to ovarian function.

Advantage
It avoids the risks and discomforts of surgery except for the curettage which must first be done to exclude organic disease of the uterus.

Disadvantages
1. Except in a woman near a natural menopause, the oestrogen withdrawal symptoms are likely to be distressing.
2. It is impossible by this method to exclude an ovarian cause for the bleeding such as a granulosa cell tumour.
3. There is no prophylaxis against uterine cancer.

A radiation menopause is best suited to the woman over 45 who does not wish operation or is unsuitable for it.

ABNORMAL VAGINAL BLEEDING

During the reproductive years 3 forms of abnormal bleeding may be encountered.

1. Mid-cycle bleeding
2. Menorrhagia - excessive menstruation
3. Metrorrhagia - irregular and usually excessive bleeding

Causes

These are multiple and many are common to all three forms of abnormal bleeding.

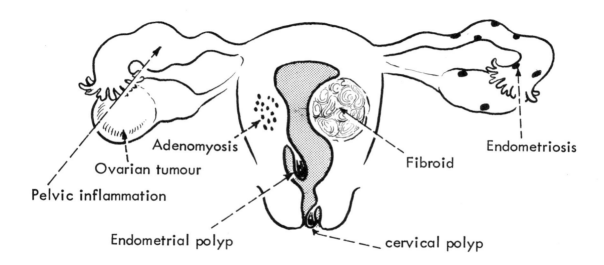

Adenomyosis

Ovarian tumour

Pelvic inflammation

Endometriosis

Fibroid

Endometrial polyp

cervical polyp

Other causes of metrorrhagia are - vaginitis, prolapse, cervicitis, erosion, urethral caruncle, cancer of cervix or uterine body.

In many cases of menorrhagia and metrorrhagia no satisfactory etiology has been found. Metropathia haemorrhagica (or cystic glandular hyperplasia) is a case in point. It appears to be due to excessive or unopposed stimulation of the endometrium by oestrogen but the cause of this has not been clearly defined. It is thought that there is a disturbance in the reciprocal relationships between the pituitary and the ovary.

AMENORRHOEA

Absence of menstrual bleeding during the reproductive years.

Primary Amenorrhoea

Non-occurrence of the menarche. If the patient has not menstruated by the time she is 18, a pathological cause must be assumed.

Secondary Amenorrhoea

Non-occurrence after a period of normal menstruation. By far the commonest cause is pregnancy.

CAUSES

(1) Pregnancy and missed abortion

(2) Psychological
  (a) Stress and emotional disturbance
  (b) Pseudopregnancy
  (c) Anorexia nervosa

The inhibitory chain of events is:-

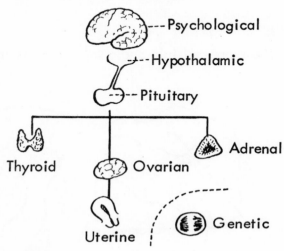

Areas of Activity in which a cause for the amenorrhoea may be found

---Psychological
---Hypothalamic
---Pituitary
Thyroid
Ovarian
Adrenal
Uterine
Genetic

Emotion
Hypothalamus Releasing Factors
Pituitary
Ovary
Uterus

(3) Hypothalamic lesions

AMENORRHOEA

CAUSES

④ Endocrine

Pituitary

Hyperpituitarism (Gigantism, Acromegaly)
Hypopituitarism (Simmonds' Disease and
Sheehan's syndrome)
Tumours

Ovary

Polycystic Disease
Premature ovarian failure
Infection
Tumours

Thyroid

Hypothyroidism
Myxoedema
Tumours

Adrenal

Adrenal failure (Addison's disease)
Adrenal hyperplasia
Virilising tumours

⑤ Systemic Disease

Severe anaemia, tuberculosis

⑥ Congenital malformations of Genital Tract

⑦ Genetic

Gonadal Dysgenesis
(including Turner's syndrome)
Intersex conditions

⑧ Chronic Pelvic Inflammation

⑨ Idiopathic

It will be seen from this list that amenorrhoea must be regarded as a serious symptom until a cause is found. The patient will often explain it to her own satisfaction as a manifestation of pregnancy, an early menopause, a permissable departure from the normal cycle, an hereditary predisposition to 'late starting'; or emotional disturbance and worry. Any of these causes may be the right one, but if the condition is prolonged a systematic search must be made. Some of the conditions associated with amenorrhoea are considered in the following pages.

AMENORRHOEA

INVESTIGATION

The cause must be looked for with determination; but in young girls who appear normal on examination it is usual to wait until the 18th birthday. Similarly mature women who are obviously experiencing some severe psychological disturbance such as the death of a child, should be observed for about 6 months.

History-taking

The usual detailed history is required. If the patient is an embarrassed young girl it is helpful to have the mother present.

The distinction between primary and secondary amenorrhoea should be made; some young women have very infrequent and scanty bleeding which is virtually primary amenorrhoea.

If the patient is experiencing the physical disturbances of menstruation (the molimina) without actually bleeding a cyclical change in hormone levels can be assumed and the cause of the amenorrhoea is likely to be in the genital tract.

Examination

In virgins this is best done under anaesthesia. Bimanual examination will reveal gross congenital anomalies such as cryptomenorrhoea, and the secondary sexual characteristics are inspected. If any endometrium is present it is subjected to histological and bacteriological examination.

Pregnancy

A pregnancy test must be carried out in every case.

Radiology

X-ray examination of the chest (for tuberculosis) and the skull (for opaque tumours in the region of the hypothalamus) are simple investigations which should always be done.

Chromosome Analysis

This will reveal genetic causes.

Laparoscopy

By this means may be detected developmental anomalies (e.g. streak gonads) small ovarian tumours and polycystic disease. Ovarian biopsy will give some information about past ovulation and the possibility of its occurring in the future.

Endocrine Investigations

Estimation of the urinary excretion rate of pituitary, ovarian and adrenal hormones is sometimes helpful; but amenorrhoea due to endocrine disturbance is usually accompanied by other signs and symptoms. Such tests are expensive and have to be repeated several times, but they become essential when no clinical diagnosis can be made.

Vaginal cytology gives a rough guide to oestrogen secretion.

AMENORRHOEA

TREATMENT

The treatment is of the cause, but if no cause is found symptomatic and empirical treatment may be taken.

1. General Measures

These include the removal as far as is possible of any source of psychological or physical stress (including poor diet). Anaemia should be corrected and it used to be fashionable to give small doses of thyroid as a 'tonic'.

2. Weight Reduction

Where the amenorrhoea is associated with obesity it sometimes happens that if the patient can be got to lose weight her periods will return.

3. Cyclical Hormone Therapy

The administration of oestrogens and progestogens over a period of months to simulate normal ovarian secretion.

E.g. ethinyl oestradiol 0.05mg daily from the 5th to the 25th day: norethisterone 5mg from the 18th to the 25th day. If the uterus is capable of responding, bleeding should occur on the 27th-28th day. It is hoped that such treatment may induce ovulation and perhaps after several months initiate a spontaneous hypothalamic rhythm.

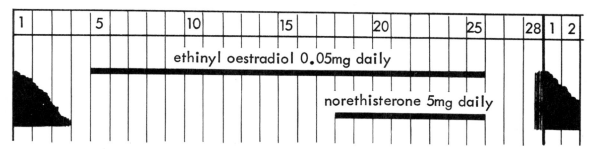

If no cause is found it is probably best to give no treatment unless there is some other objective besides the appearance of menstrual bleeding. A woman wanting a child would be subjected to treatment with drugs designed to produce ovulation which would probably cause menstruation as well; or a girl with a genital hypoplasia might benefit from a prolonged course of oestrogens especially if she were intending marriage.

PRIMARY PITUITARY HYPOFUNCTION

ENDOCRINE CAUSES OF AMENORRHOEA

Patients with obvious stigmata of endocrine disease sometimes present for the first time at the gynaecology clinic.

Primary Pituitary Hypofunction

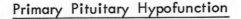

Lack of endocrinotrophic hormones as well as growth hormone.

↓

FROHLICH'S DWARF

Lack of growth hormone (somatotrophin)

PITUITARY DWARF (Lorain-Levi Syndrome or Nansomia pituitaria)

Body proportions and facies of a child
Bones slender and fragile
Lack of genital hair
Normal intelligence

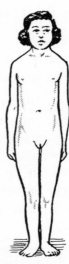

LORAIN DWARF

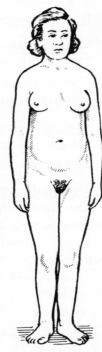

Normal 14 years

Frohlich's Syndrome (Dystrophia Adiposo-genitalis)

Dwarfism, girdle-type obesity, genital hypoplasia and a tendency to drowsiness. In this condition the loss of function is shared by the hypothalamus as well as the pituitary.

SECONDARY PITUITARY HYPOFUNCTION

(Simmonds' Disease means hypopituitarism from any cause; although Simmonds recognised the association with childbirth. Sheehan's syndrome means chronic hypopituitarism caused by postpartum necrosis of the anterior lobe following severe shock and haemorrhage at parturition.

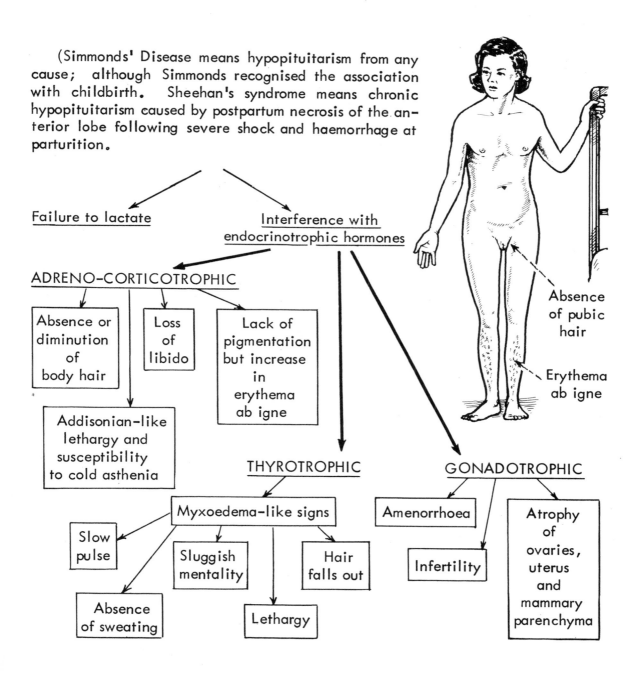

Failure to lactate

Interference with endocrinotrophic hormones

ADRENO-CORTICOTROPHIC

Absence or diminution of body hair

Loss of libido

Lack of pigmentation but increase in erythema ab igne

Addisonian-like lethargy and susceptibility to cold asthenia

Absence of pubic hair

Erythema ab igne

THYROTROPHIC

GONADOTROPHIC

Myxoedema-like signs

Amenorrhoea

Atrophy of ovaries, uterus and mammary parenchyma

Slow pulse

Sluggish mentality

Hair falls out

Infertility

Absence of sweating

Lethargy

ADRENO-GENITAL SYNDROME

(This may be due to hyperplasia or tumour)

INCREASED SECRETION
OF ANDROGENS

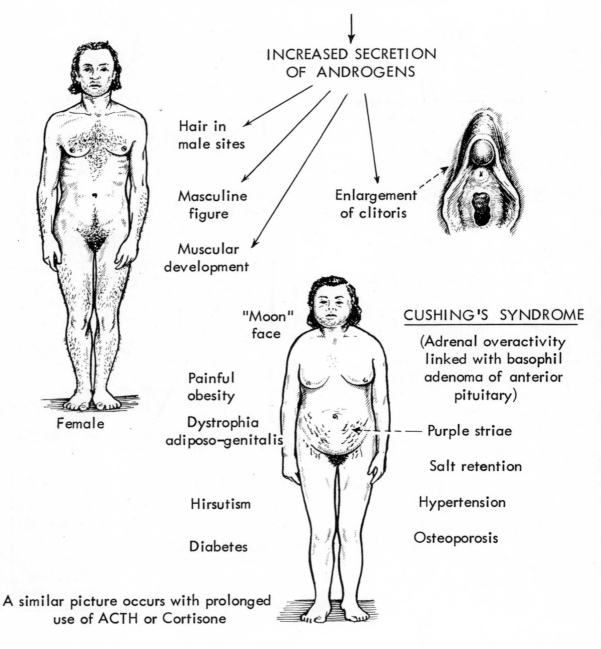

Hair in
male sites

Masculine
figure

Muscular
development

Enlargement
of clitoris

Female

"Moon"
face

Painful
obesity

Dystrophia
adiposo-genitalis

Hirsutism

Diabetes

CUSHING'S SYNDROME

(Adrenal overactivity
linked with basophil
adenoma of anterior
pituitary)

Purple striae

Salt retention

Hypertension

Osteoporosis

A similar picture occurs with prolonged
use of ACTH or Cortisone

ADRENO-GENITAL SYNDROME

The adreno-genital syndrome is important to the gynaecologist not only as a cause of amenorrhoea but because it may be present at birth. Prompt recognition and treatment will allow the baby to survive and grow up as a normal female.

There are several clinical forms of this syndrome but the important one for present purposes is that which gives rise to masculinisation of the female infant. Increased pigmentation of the skin particularly in the genital region is usually present. The labia are fused and resemble a scrotum and at the anterior end of the raphé there is an orifice. This together with an apparent but small penis suggests hypospadias. Testes cannot be palpated in the scrotum.

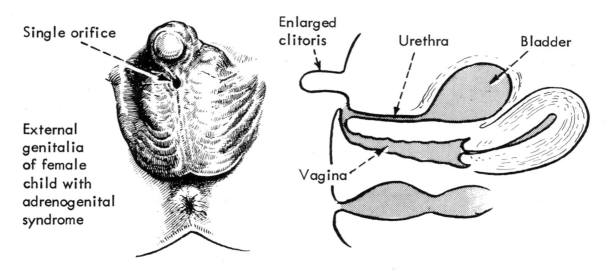

Single orifice

Enlarged clitoris

Urethra

Bladder

External genitalia of female child with adrenogenital syndrome

Vagina

A buccal smear will reveal that the infant is chromatin positive, and the most likely diagnosis is adreno-genital syndrome. Biochemical investigations may help to clinch the diagnosis but the results may be equivocal because the levels tend to vary during the first few days of life. The primary defect in this syndrome is a deficiency in the enzyme 21 hydroxylase which converts 17 hydroxyprogesterone to cortisol.

ADRENO-GENITAL SYNDROME

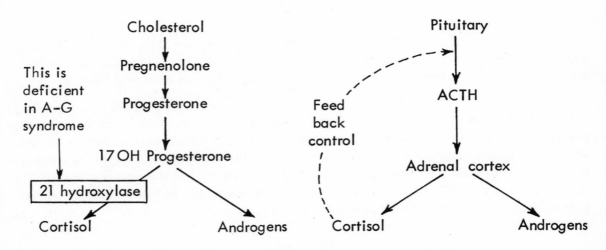

The blood cortisol is low and the feed back mechanism controlling the secretion of ACTH is absent. The pituitary continues to secrete ACTH, causing the adrenal cortex to enlarge and the production of 17 hydroxyprogesterone is greatly increased. Cortisol cannot be formed and the alternative pathway to androgens is favoured with resulting effect on the foetus and infant. 17 hydroxyprogesterone is present in excess in the blood and some is excreted as pregnanetriol, while the metabolic products of androgens, the 17 keto-steroids, are also excreted in increased amounts. This is the basis for the biochemical tests which are as follows :-

1. Urinary 17 keto-steroids greater than 1mg. per 24 hours.
2. Urinary pregnanetriol greater than 0.5mg. per 24 hours.
3. 11/oxy/11 deoxy ratio greater than 0.4.
4. Plasma pregnanetriol over 80μg/100ml.

Satisfactory estimations can rarely be achieved until the infant is at least a week old. Usually health is maintained during this time but an Addisonian crisis may supervene at any time. The baby becomes ill, fluid intake falls, and weight gain ceases. This is followed by vomiting, weight loss, lethargy and hypotonia. The blood urea and potassium rise and the sodium falls. Treatment must be given even if the biochemical results are not available and consists in giving those substances which will suppress the pituitary and thus avoid over-stimulation of the adrenal cortex. Salt will also be required to cancel the low blood sodium.

Addison's disease, due to its effect on general metabolism, is usually associated with amenorrhoea.

LACTATION-AMENORRHOEA SYNDROME
(CHIARI-FROMMEL SYNDROME)

Galactorrhoea, amenorrhoea, uterine and ovarian atrophy following pregnancy. The cause is unknown, but probably due to pituitary-hypothalamic dysfunction.

Clinical Features

The condition is rarely reported. The patient is a young woman who has recently had a baby, and is now complaining that the breasts continue to secrete and that the periods have not returned. There may have been a little sporadic bleeding, but nothing suggesting ovulation. In most cases the patient has fed her baby at the breast but this probably reflects contemporary practice, and the syndrome has been seen in at least one patient who has suppressed lactation from the start.

Examination

The breasts are full and milk is easily expressed. Pelvic examination reveals a small uterus and the ovaries are impalpable. (This atrophy extends to vagina and vulva in long-standing cases.) The patient is generally healthy and there are no other signs of pituitary dysfunction.

Investigations

Curettage is carried out to exclude local conditions (the atrophic uterus is easily perforated) and an ovarian biopsy can be obtained at laparoscopy.

Differential Diagnosis

This includes other causes of galactorrhoea.

1. Pituitary lesions
   Tumour with or without acromegaly
   Encephalitis, meningitis
   Trauma

   (A condition identical with the Chiari-Frommel syndrome can occur without preceding pregnancy: it is then called the Ahumada–del Castillo syndrome.)

2. Galactorrhoea is also associated with psychoses, and large doses of tranquillisers such as phenothiazines and meprobamate. This is presumably a hypothalamic effect.

Treatment

Spontaneous correction may occur at any time, but the treatment of choice is clomiphene citrate which has a good chance of inducing ovulation and initiating the hypothalamic rhythm.

Endocrine Investigations

Galactorrhoea may be the presenting symptom of a pituitary tumour. If there is doubt about the diagnosis, or if treatment is unsuccessful, the patient must be referred to an endocrinologist.

POLYCYSTIC OVARY DISEASE

POLYCYSTIC OVARY DISEASE
(STEIN-LEVENTHAL SYNDROME
HYPERTHECOSIS) } {
1. Oligomenorrhoea or secondary amenorrhoea.
2. Infertility due to failure of ovulation.
3. Obesity.   4. Hirsutism.

The cause is considered to be excessive production of androgens by the ovary.

Hormone Production in the Ovary

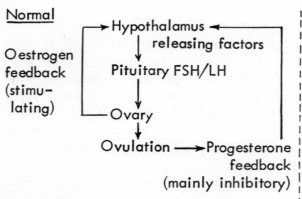

If the enzymes mediating these reactions are altered in amount, the secretion of androgens is increased. Oestrogens may be decreased.

This disturbed synthesis is believed to be a result of failure of cyclical rhythm in the hypothalamus and pituitary. Why this should occur is not known.

Ovarian-Pituitary-Hypothalamus Relationship (Theoretical)

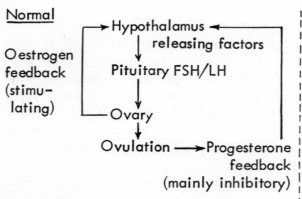

Normal

Oestrogen feedback (stimu-lating)

Hypothalamus ← releasing factors
Pituitary FSH/LH
Ovary
Ovulation → Progesterone feedback (mainly inhibitory)

At a certain level of oestrogen a 'surge' of LH occurs which leads to ovulation and subsequent progesterone inhibition of hypothalamus activity.

In Polycystic Ovary Disease

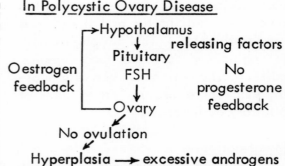

Oestrogen feedback

Hypothalamus
Pituitary FSH
Ovary
releasing factors
No progesterone feedback

No ovulation
Hyperplasia → excessive androgens

There is no LH 'surge' and no ovulation (? hypothalamus failure). Continued gonadotrophic stimulation produces ovarian hyperplasia and androgen secretion.

POLYCYSTIC OVARY DISEASE

Changes in the Ovary

The ovary is enlarged ('oyster' or 'potato' ovary) due to the cortical hyperplasia which is characteristic of the disease. Under the microscope the cortex shows thecal hyperplasia with large numbers of follicles. There are no corpora lutea.

Polycystic ovaries

Hyperplasia of ovarian cortex with multiple follicles

CLINICAL FEATURES

The patient presents as a rule with secondary amenorrhoea and infertility. Hirsutism and obesity are not always present, but the breasts are usually developed.

The uterus is normal; the ovaries may not be palpable, but laparoscopy will show enlargement and an ovarian biopsy should be taken. The endometrium is normal and may show cystic hyperplasia. (There are some claims that this condition may lead to endometrial cancer.)

Urinary 17-ketosteroid excretion may be raised, indicative of increased steroid production, and more refined tests will show an increase in the metabolites of testosterone. Oestrogen excretion is normal or slightly decreased.

The differential diagnosis must include adrenal hyperplasia and adrenal or pituitary tumours.

POLYCYSTIC OVARY DISEASE

TREATMENT

This is not a particularly common condition and spontaneous correction can occur. Medical treatment should always be tried first.

Clomiphene   100mg is given for 5 days, and ovulation often follows within a few days.   Menstruation occurs normally if no conception.

Gonadotrophins should not be used unless their purpose is to treat infertility.   Patients with polycystic ovaries are particularly sensitive to gonadotrophins and the greatest care is required in their use.

Wedge resection of the Ovaries

This means surgical excision of about half the ovarian tissue. This produces a sharp reduction in the secretion of androgens (and of oestrogens) and reduces the feedback stimulus to the hypothalamus. There are conflicting opinions on the rationale and efficacy of this procedure, but it has held its place in the gynaecologist's repertoire for nearly 40 years.   Possible complications are:
(a) Removal of too much ovarian tissue may produce withdrawal symptoms.
(b) Any operation on the ovary tends to produce adhesions which may involve the tubes.

Cyclic Administration of Oestrogens and Progestogens

These hormones have been given in an effort to simulate the physiological cycle, and in particular to introduce a luteal phase. This treatment has never met with much success.

Dexamethasone   This is given to suppress adrenocortical activity, and should not be used unless there is evidence of hyperfunction of this gland.

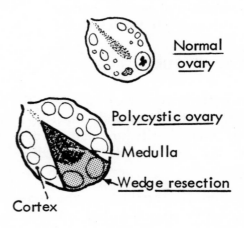

Normal ovary

Polycystic ovary

Medulla

Wedge resection

Cortex

Some cases of secondary amenorrhoea may be due to premature ovarian failure. The possibility of ovarian tumour must always be considered.

GENETIC CAUSES OF AMENORRHOEA

SEX AND GENDER

The sex of cells is genetic and determined at fertilisation, but this does n automatically ensure the subsequent gender of the individual.

Cells of the normal individual possess 46 chromosomes, two of which are s chromosomes, XX in the female, XY in the male. The particular combination determined by the changes during maturation of the ovum and sperm prior fertilisation.

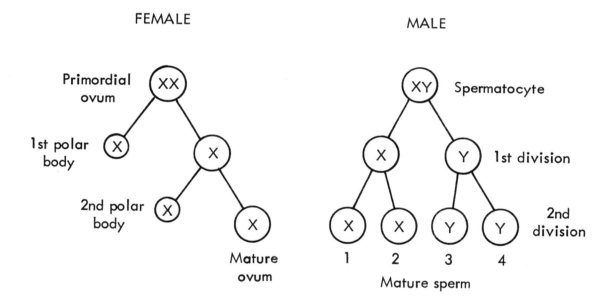

If the ovum is fertilised by either of sperms 1 or 2 the zygote will be female wi an XX sex chromosomal make-up. Sperms 3 and 4 will give rise to a male XY com bination.

GENETIC CAUSES OF AMENORRHOEA

During maturation of the ovum and sperm abnormalities in number and form of the chromosomes may arise by deletion or acquisition of chromosomes or parts of chromosomes. These arise as a result of non-disjunction at first or second meiotic division.

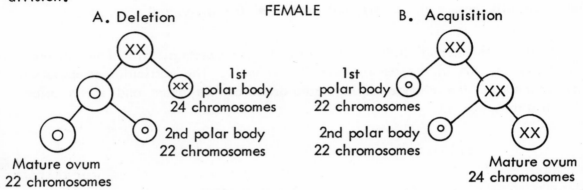

A. Deletion   FEMALE   B. Acquisition

1st polar body 24 chromosomes

2nd polar body 22 chromosomes

Mature ovum 22 chromosomes

1st polar body 22 chromosomes

2nd polar body 22 chromosomes

Mature ovum 24 chromosomes

In the case of A, fertilisation will result in an individual with 45 chromosomes, only one of which is a sex chromosome. In all cases this is an X chromosome, giving an XO make-up. The combination YO is unknown and is probably lethal.

Ovum B when fertilised will have an extra chromosome, 47 in all, with a sex chromosome make-up either XXX or XXY.

A similar change may be found in the MALE

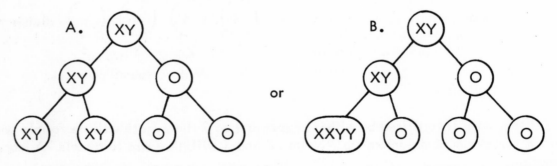

A.   or   B.

Depending on which sperm fertilises an ovum the sex chromosome make-up may be :–
    (a)   XY + X ⟶ XXY with 47 chromosomes
    (b)   O + X ⟶ XO with 45 chromosomes
    (c) XXYY + X ⟶ XXXYY with 49 chromosomes

GENETIC CAUSES OF AMENORRHOEA

PARTIAL DELETION

In this abnormality part of a sex chromosome may not be formed during maturation division.

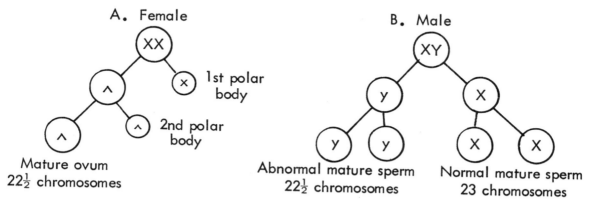

A. Female

1st polar body

2nd polar body

Mature ovum
22½ chromosomes

B. Male

Abnormal mature sperm
22½ chromosomes

Normal mature sperm
23 chromosomes

A.   In this case fertilisation of the ovum will result in an individual with a sex chromosomal make-up either X∧ or Y∧ with 46 chromosomes.

B.   If the abnormal sperm manages to fertilise an ovum the sex chromosome make-up will be Xy, again with 46 chromosomes.

MOSAICS

Abnormalities may also occur during early division of the zygote which give rise to two or more separate "clones" or lines of cells with quite distinct sex chromosome make-up.   These are called mosaics.   The following are examples.

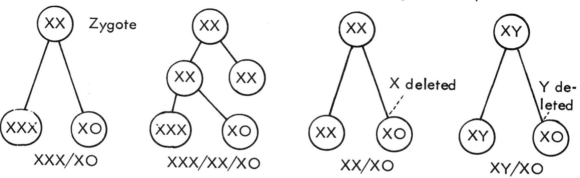

Zygote

XXX/XO

XXX/XX/XO

X deleted

XX/XO

Y de-leted

XY/XO

LABORATORY DETECTION OF GENETIC DEFECTS

BARR BODIES AND DRUMSTICKS

Examination of cells suitably stained from a genetic female will reveal a small pyramidal-shaped mass of chromatin applied to the nuclear membrane. The cells are often referred to as being chromatin positive.

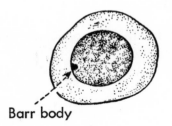

Barr body

The presence of this body indicates that the individual possesses two X chromosomes but it does not necessarily mean that the person is genetically normal. The sex chromosome make-up might be XXY instead of XX. If the individual possesses an extra X i.e. is XXX, there will be two Barr bodies in some nuclei, i.e. there is always one Barr body less than the number of chromosomes.

Absence of the Barr body indicates that the individual has only one X chromosome. The subject is usually a male XY, but may on occasion be an incomplete female XO.

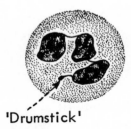

Polymorphonuclear leucocytes in females commonly have a small mass of chromatin projecting from the nucleus in the form of a drumstick.

'Drumstick'

CHROMOSOME ANALYSIS

Blood Analysis

25ml blood is collected in a sterile heparinised bottle. The lymphocytes are cultured in the presence of colchicine which stops mitosis in the metaphase. The separated chromosomes can then be counted and examined.

Fibroblast Culture

A small fragment of fibrous tissue may be cultured in the same way and the chromosomes examined.

TURNER'S SYNDROME

GENETIC ABNORMALITIES

TURNER'S SYNDROME
|
Sex chromosome
deletion

- Normal intelligence
- Webbing of neck
- Coarctation of aorta
- Small stature, poor hip development
- Streak gonad, failure of ovarian development
- Secondary sex characters absent
- Infantile figure of female phenotype

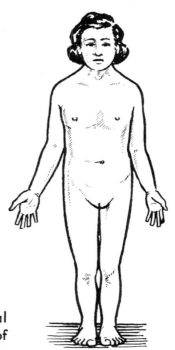

In "typical" Turner's syndrome the chromosomal pattern is 45XO. Some patients may exhibit a few of the stigmata - so-called atypical cases, and in these subjects there is usually partial deletion of an X chromosome, giving an X∧ pattern. Mosaicism, e.g. XO/XX, may result in the appearance of some of the features of Turner's syndrome but the presence of cells with an XX configuration can be associated with perfectly formed ovaries and menstruation may occur.

In males some of the somatic stigmata of Turner's may appear. This may be due to partial deletion of the Y chromosome - Xy, or to mosaicism - XO/XY.

Treatment

It is essential that diagnosis should be established as early as possible. A buccal smear should be examined for Barr bodies in any female child of exceptionally small stature. At the age of 11 or 12 ethinyl oestradiol 0.025 to 0.05mg. should be given daily for 3 to 6 months to stimulate growth of uterus and breasts. Following this it may be given daily for every 3 weeks out of four. This results in a "menstrual" cycle. Occasionally it may be necessary to give anabolic steroids to help breast development.

SEX CHROMOSOME ADDITIONS

Super-female

This is a term sometimes used when the subject possesses extra X chromosomes. The pattern may be XXX, XXXX or even XXXXX. Physically these individuals are normal females but there is usually a degree of mental retardation and the degree of retardation increases with each extra X chromosome. Diagnosis is easily made by examination of a buccal smear which will reveal additional Barr bodies.

Klinefelter's Syndrome – – – – – – – – – →

In this case the individual has at least two X chromosomes but this is nullified by the presence of a Y chromosome. The pattern may be XXY, XXXY, XXXYY or XXXXXY. Due to the presence of the X chromosomes the cells are chromatin positive i.e. possess Barr bodies, but the individual is physically a male. At puberty however, the testes fail to enlarge, facial hair is scanty and the pubic hair has a female distribution. There may be some development of the breasts. The individual is infertile. With increasing numbers of X chromosomes there is increasing mental retardation.

Chromosome Mosaics

Some of these have already been mentioned, XO/XX and XO/XY in relation to Turner's syndrome. The latter mosaic, however, is frequently found in an anatomically normal male. On occasion the gender may be mixed with a testis on one side, a streak gonad on the other, and ambiguous genitalia.

Mosaicism is sometimes associated with hermaphroditism. In such cases the cells are chromatin positive and the chromosomal pattern may be XX/XY, XX/XXY or XX/XXYY. The XX line promotes ovarian formation: the XY testicular.

In such cases there may be a unicornuate uterus with Fallopian tube and ovary on one side, a hemi-scrotum with testis on the other, and a rudimentary penis, but a great variety in the structure of the external genitalia occurs.

TESTICULAR FEMINISATION

This is due to the insensitivity of the foetal tissues to hormones. The chromo-somal pattern is 46XY but although the individual possesses testes he is an apparent female. Androgens are secreted but tissues appear to be insensitive and develop along female lines. Usually the diagnosis is made in early adult life when the patient complains of amenorrhoea.

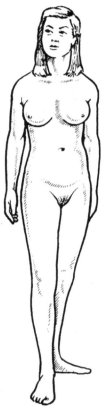

Female phenotype with tendency to eunuchoid proportions

Normal or large breasts with small nipples

Absent or scanty (sometimes normal) pubic hair

Absent or scant axillary hair

Normal external genitalia with blind vagina

Absent or rudimentary internal genitalia

Undescended testes anywhere along course of normal descent (20 % become malignant in 4th decade)

Testes secrete oestrogens and androgens.
Probably Leydig cells produce feminising hormones

Hereditary from mother
$\frac{1}{4}$ of female offspring are carriers.
$\frac{1}{4}$ of male offspring are feminised.
Rest are normal.
Carriers may show scanty pubic and axillary hair and
may have delayed menarche.

Until full growth is achieved no therapy should be attempted. When the epiphyses have fused the gonads should be excised. This is a precautionary measure in view of the increased incidence of tumours in such gonads. Following this treat-ment the patient is liable to have menopausal symptoms and should be given oestro-gen replacement therapy, continuously in the beginning until the vaginal smear is fully oestrogenised and then cyclically.

CRYPTOMENORRHOEA

Obstruction to the menstrual flow by a vaginal septum or an imperforate hymen. Three degrees are recognised.

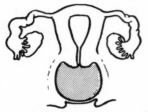 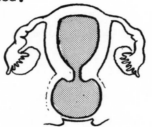 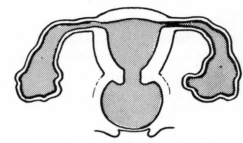

<u>Haematocolpos</u> Only the vagina is distended by altered blood.

<u>Haematometra</u> The uterus is also distended.

<u>Haematosalpinx</u> In longstanding cases the tubes are also involved.

Clinical Features

The patient is usually a girl of seventeen or so, complaining of primary amenorrhoea and pelvic pain of increasing severity. In longstanding cases the pressure of the distended vagina may cause urinary retention. Pregnancy must be excluded.

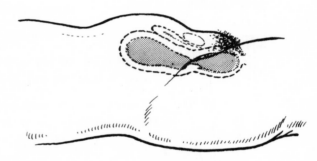

Examination

A pelvic mass is palpated and may even be visible. The vaginal membrane or hymen is bulging.

Treatment

Incision and drainage. Very large amounts of inspissated blood may be released, and if the septum is particularly thick, some form of plastic operation may subsequently be required.

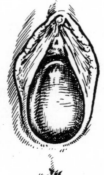 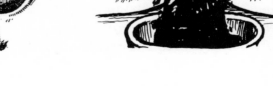

VIRILISM

VIRILISM means signs of excessive androgen stimulation in the muscles, larynx, genitalia and hair. It is always a pathological condition.

Causes of Virilism
1. Ovarian tumour.
2. Adrenal tumour.
3. Delayed onset of adrenal hyperplasia.
4. Hypothalamic or pituitary disease.
5. Chromosomal abnormality (Mosaicism or some cases of testicular feminisation.)

Clinical Features
The affected end-organs vary with the individual, and there is no regular pattern for the appearance of signs. The patient may first notice an increase in hair, or a reduction or cessation of menstruation. The breasts atrophy or fail to develop, the clitoris is enlarged and the voice deepens. In extreme cases a definite male muscular development is apparent and there is marked enlargement of the thyroid cartilage.

Investigations

1. Examination under anaesthesia to allow a full inspection of the genitalia. If a uterus is present an endometrial biopsy is taken. A vaginal smear will give some idea of oestrogen secretion.

2. Laparoscopic inspection and ovarian biopsy are indicated if no mass is palpated.

3. Blood is sent for chromosomal analysis.

4. X-ray investigation may detect a cerebral tumour or adrenal enlargement.

5. Hormone Estimations.
Only a very small excess of testosterone is required to produce signs of virilism, so the 17-ketosteroid excretion rate is unlikely to be raised; but if it is adrenal function tests must be carried out since the adrenal is virtually the only source of 17-ketosteroids in the female. Stimulation of cortisol secretion by dexamethasone, and inhibition by metyrapone is effective in adrenal hyperplasia but not in cases of pituitary tumour.

Most patients suffering from virilism are likely to be seen for the first time at a gynaecological clinic. Because of the association of virilism with tumours, and the irreversibility of voice changes once they have occurred, the gynaecologist must always keep in mind the possibility of encountering a patient with this rare condition.

HIRSUTISM

Increased bodily and facial hair without other signs of virilism. It is unusual for increased androgen secretion to be demonstrated to any degree.

1. Idiopathic (by far the commonest).
   It is believed to be the result of increased sensitivity of the hair follicles.

2. Polycystic Ovary Disease (Stein-Leventhal Syndrome).

Normal Hair Patterns
   These are influenced by race and to some extent by fashion.

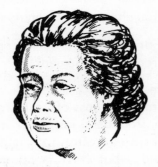

Many women have a slight growth on the upper lip and over the masseters.

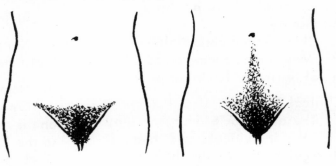

Normal Pubic Patterns. A male escutcheon (hair extending up to the umbilicus) is normal.

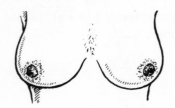

It is normal to have a few hairs over the sternum and round the nipples.

Other normal areas for growth are the axillae, the arms and legs. Hirsutism becomes abnormal if there are heavy growths in normal areas and if hair appears in such places as the shoulders, lumbo-sacral areas, thighs, sacrum.

HIRSUTISM

Investigations

If there is no complaint and the periods are regular no investigation is required, otherwise search for other signs of virilism. This should include examination under anaesthesia and laparoscopic inspection.

Estimation of steroid metabolites depends on laboratory resources. Plasma testosterone may be elevated, but it is known that testosterone may be produced peripherally by the sebaceous glands without entering the circulation.

Treatment

Shaving

This is the best method but has ineradicable associations with virility.

Abrasives

Pads or gloves of fine sandpaper have the same effect as shaving but are as hard on the skin and have no advantage.

Electrolysis

Decomposition of the hair follicle by the passage of an electric current. Low galvanic current is used through a fine electrode. The hair is electrolysed after about 10 seconds and plucked out painlessly.

Diathermy

The follicle is coagulated instantly and the hair pulled out.

Electrical destruction of individual hairs is permanent but prolonged treatment is tedious and expensive.

Depilatory Creams

These are alkaline solutions which dissolve the hairs and allow them to be wiped away. They will injure the skin if left on too long.

Depilatory Waxes

The wax is melted and spread on to the skin. When it sets it is pulled off, plucking the hairs with it. This is painful and leaves the skin tender and reddened.

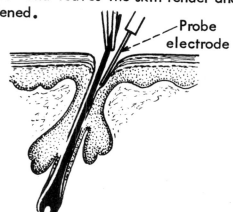

Probe electrode

DYSMENORRHOEA

This is painful menstruation or pain associated with the menstrual cycle.

Most women have some discomfort with menstruation, such as backache and congestive pain in the lower abdomen.

The following questions should be asked:-

1. <u>Timing of the pain.</u>
   (a) Before, after or during the flow?   (b) Mid-cycle?

2. <u>Severity of the pain.</u>
   (a) Does the patient stay off work because of the pain?
   (b) If not off work is she sent home from work or has she to rest at work?
   (c) Is the pain relieved by rest, heat, cold or mild analgesic e.g. aspirin?

3. <u>Character of the pain</u>

PRIMARY, SPASMODIC, ACUTE OR INTRINSIC DYSMENORRHOEA

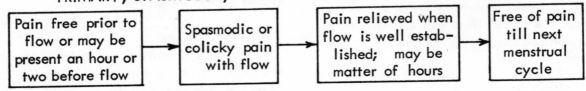

| Pain free prior to flow or may be present an hour or two before flow | → | Spasmodic or colicky pain with flow | → | Pain relieved when flow is well established; may be matter of hours | → | Free of pain till next menstrual cycle |

SECONDARY OR CONGESTIVE DYSMENORRHOEA

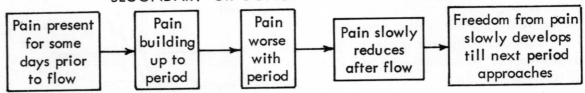

| Pain present for some days prior to flow | → | Pain building up to period | → | Pain worse with period | → | Pain slowly reduces after flow | → | Freedom from pain slowly develops till next period approaches |

MID-CYCLE PAIN (MITTELSCHMERZ)

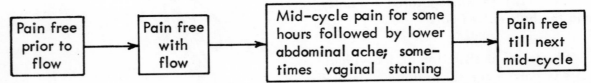

| Pain free prior to flow | → | Pain free with flow | → | Mid-cycle pain for some hours followed by lower abdominal ache; sometimes vaginal staining | → | Pain free till next mid-cycle |

Mid-cycle pain is associated with dehiscence of ovum from follicle.   If it is associated with pelvic inflammatory disease there will also be secondary dysmenorrhoea.

PRIMARY SPASMODIC DYSMENORRHOEA

EXAMINATION and TREATMENT

Commonly from menarche - but not with first periods as these are often anovulatory and painless.

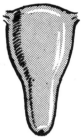

Hypoplastic
uterus

The uterus is often found to be hypoplastic (infantile) with a narrow cervix and a pinhole external os.   Rectal examination only should be carried out on the young girl, but gentle vaginal examination (especially if internal menstrual tampons are used) may be possible in the older girl.

If pain is tolerable or not interfering with work then reassurance, general health measures and analgesics e.g. aspirin, may be sufficient.   This type of pain tends to be relieved as the patient gets older.

If the pain is crippling then oestrogens or progestogens may be exhibited cyclically. These tend to promote uterine growth and reduce the spasmodic element (e.g. Stilboestrol 1.0mg daily from 5th-12th day of cycle and Ethisterone 25mg daily from 13th-25th day).   They may also be used as in the oral contraceptive to give anovulatory menses, but this can only be a temporary treatment.   Oestrogen/androgen mixtures sometimes help.

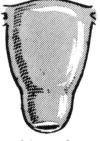

Normal
uterus

If pain is not relieved by these methods then dilatation of the cervix may be resorted to.   Theoretically the fibres of the cervix are disrupted and cannot cause spasm and obstruction. It seldom cures but sometimes gives temporary relief.   The relief may even be psychological.

If crippling pain persists presacral neurectomy may be used. This is a major operation and may substitute complaints of bowel and bladder function instead.

Pregnancy and childbirth usually relieve spasmodic dysmenorrhoea.   There is often associated emotional disturbance which may be helped in some cases by psychotherapy.

SECONDARY CONGESTIVE DYSMENORRHOEA

This is usually associated with pelvic pathology and treatment is that of the cause.

<u>Retroversion</u> (displacement dysmenorrhoea) following childbirth or a fall.

The retroversion should be corrected under anaesthesia if necessary, and the position maintained by a pessary to see if symptoms are relieved. If so then some more permanent method of maintaining the correct position is used (p 258). A fixed retroversion suggests pelvic adhesions.

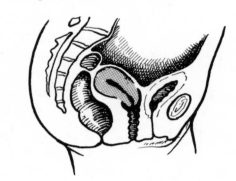

Chronic Salpingo-oophoritis.

This condition follows infection of the genital tract, for example from childbirth or abortion, tuberculosis or venereal disease or following abdominal infection as with appendicitis, diverticulosis or tuberculosis, and may lead to secondary dysmenorrhoea with or without retroversion. No palpable swelling of the tubes and ovaries may be present but there is restricted mobility of the organs and movement causes pain.

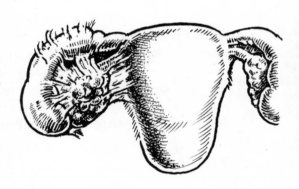

Endometriosis

This is another cause of pain for the bleeding in the ectopic endometrium does not readily escape but is slowly absorbed at the site. The uterus may be fixed and retroverted by the ectopic endometrium.

Chronic salpingo-oophoritis and endometriosis are associated with deep dyspareunia, menorrhagia and infertility.

Laparoscopy (p78-80) is a valuable diagnostic tool in investigation of secondary dysmenorrhoea.

TREATMENT OF DYSMENORRHOEA

Chronic salpingo-oophoritis may be relieved or improved by short wave diathermy. Antibiotics and bed rest may be used in acute and subacute phases. Removal of uterus, tubes and ovaries completely or in part must be considered.

Endometriosis usually requires surgical intervention with removal of the ectopic tissue and cysts or even the ovaries and uterus depending on age and other factors (e.g. extent, fertility). Ovarian suppression for about a year by progestogens may cure the ectopic activity, as will a pregnancy, but will not remove adhesions and the resultant distortion.

Secondary dysmenorrhoea without pelvic distortion, or dyspareunia, but possibly increased menstrual flow suggests a foreign body in the cavity and exploration may then disclose a polyp. (An intra-uterine contraceptive device may cause these symptoms.)

Mid-cycle pain (mittelschmerz) is sometimes accompanied by slight vaginal staining and there is marked tenderness of one ovary. The pelvis is usually palpably normal but signs of chronic salpingo-oophoritis may be present. Pelvic diathermy may relieve the condition

MEMBRANOUS DYSMENORRHOEA.

This is a rare form of painful menstruation. A cast of the uterus is passed with much accompanying pain. Bleeding is minimal till the cast is passed and then is often profuse. Dilatation of the cervix and uterine curettage followed by oestrogen therapy may relieve the condition but hysterectomy might be considered in intractable cases with severe pain.

PRESACRAL NEURECTOMY

Division of the superior hypogastric plexus in order to interrupt afferent pain stimuli from the pelvis.

This is an unreliable and obsolescent operation which might be offered as a last resort to a patient whose dysmenorrhoea was not relieved by any other means.

The superior hypogastric plexus is related to the 5th lumbar vertebra and the left common iliac vein rather than the sacrum and lies in a sheet of fibro-areolar tissue between the peritoneum and the great vessels.

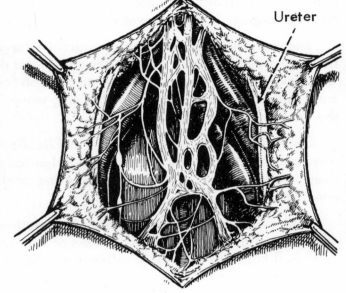

Ureter

Bifurcation of aorta

Peritoneum

Access to the posterior wall of the pelvis may be difficult in a fat woman and there is a risk of haemorrhage and of damage to the left ureter.

Efferent pathways are also divided and there is a transient atonicity of bowel and bladder after the operation and perhaps some heavy uterine bleeding as a result of the vasodilatation.

The picture shows how the tissue containing the plexus is dissected out. It is impossible to be certain of removing all the nerve trunks.

PRE-MENSTRUAL TENSION

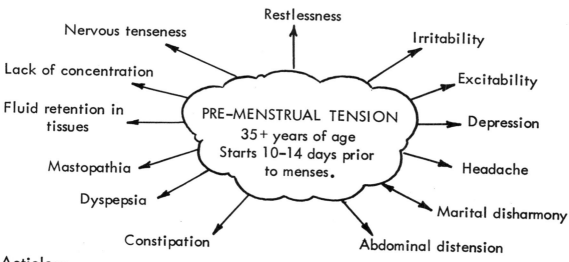

Nervous tenseness

Restlessness

Irritability

Lack of concentration

Excitability

Fluid retention in tissues

PRE-MENSTRUAL TENSION
35+ years of age
Starts 10-14 days prior
to menses.

Depression

Mastopathia

Headache

Dyspepsia

Marital disharmony

Constipation

Abdominal distension

Aetiology

Aetiology is uncertain but is thought to be caused by steroid imbalance due to a defect in luteinising of the follicle. This leads to oestrogen preponderance with sodium retention in the tissues. There is sometimes a psychological upset due to domestic stress.

Examination

Pelvic findings are normal.

Treatment
1. General examination may reveal a degree of anaemia or some chronic infection.
2. Sedation, e.g. barbiturates, promazine, tranquillising drugs. The danger of addiction must be considered.
3. Progestogens – for progestational (anti-oestrogenic) effect (e.g. ethisterone 5mg daily).
4. Androgens – promote well-being and libido (e.g. methyl testosterone 5mg daily).
5. Diuretics – to reduce fluid retention.
6. Psychological support may be required.

CHAPTER 6
CONGENITAL ABNORMALITIES

ABNORMALTIES OF OVARY AND TUBE

These arise from:
1. Incomplete development of the Müllerian ducts.
2. Imperfect development of the gonad.
3. Imperfect development of the cloacal region.
4. Sex chromosome abnormalities.

Many abnormalities in many combinations may be met with, but only those compatible with life and growth are of interest to the gynaecologist. Because of the close relationship between the genital and urinary tracts, intravenous pyelography should always be carried out when a genital abnormality is found.

ABNORMALITIES OF THE OVARY

1. Absence of one ovary may occur in an otherwise normal woman. Before operating on one ovary, always look at the other.

2. Vestigial ('streak') Ovary

This is seen in cases of ovarian dysgenesis (p 109). In place of the ovary there is a strip of whitish connective tissue, continuous with the ovarian ligament.

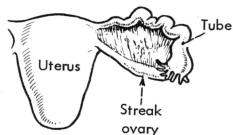

Uterus

Tube

Streak ovary

ABNORMALITIES OF THE FALLOPIAN TUBE

Absence is rare.   The tube may be imperfectly developed or display accessory ostia or diverticula.

This picture shows an accessory ostium and a diverticulum which is probably an undeveloped ostium.

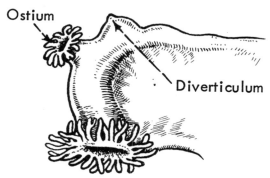

Ostium

Diverticulum

ABNORMALTIES OF TUBE AND UTERUS

ABNORMALITIES OF THE TUBE – Continued

This picture shows a condition in which the proximal half of the left tube has failed to develop. The right adnexae are normal.

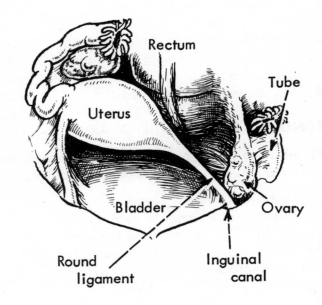

ABNORMALITIES OF THE UTERUS

1. <u>Absent or rudimentary uterus</u>

The uterus is represented by two fleshy nodules connected by a membrane (the 'ribbon' uterus). Note that the ovaries and round ligaments (from the gubernaculum) and even the tubes, are normal.

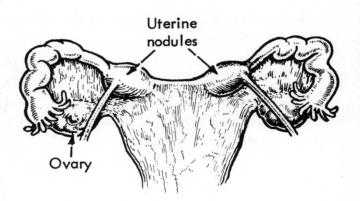

ABNORMALITIES OF THE UTERUS

2. <u>Double Uterus</u> (Bicornuate Uterus)

One or other variant of this condition is the commonest abnormality. It is due to failure of fusion of the Müllerian ducts, or failure of one to develop. A few examples are shown.

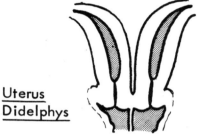

<u>Uterus Didelphys</u>

Double uterus and cervix, usually with double vagina. Some writers call this 'pseudo-didelphys' unless there is also a double vulva.

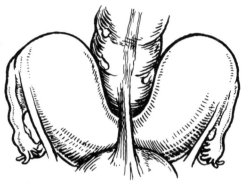

<u>Uterus Bicornis</u>

Note the ligament which usually passes from rectum to bladder.

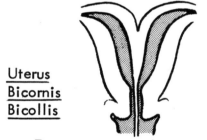

<u>Uterus Bicornis Bicollis</u>

Two corpora, with fused cervices.

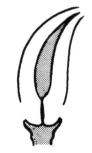

<u>Uterus Unicornis</u>

One duct has failed to develop.

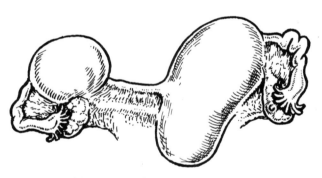

<u>Uterus with accessory horn</u>

The accessory horn has no cervix. If it menstruates cryptomenorrhoea will follow. Spermatozoa can reach the horn by crossing the peritoneal cavity.

ABNORMALITIES OF THE VAGINA

Gynatresia (Occlusion of the genital canal) may be due to complete absence of the vagina, or incomplete development, or the presence of a transverse septum producing the same effect as an imperforate hymen.   There may also be a longitudinal septum producing a double vagina, usually in association with a double uterus.   A few examples are shown.

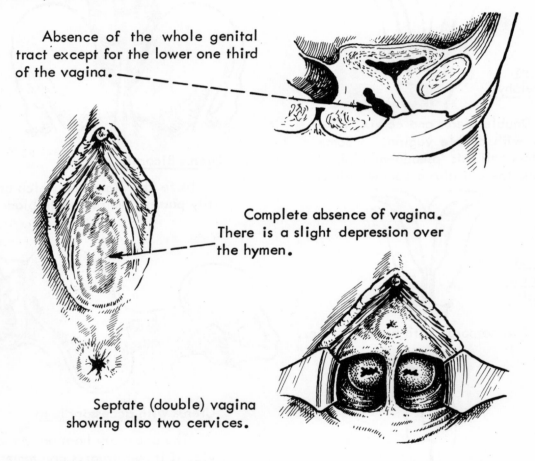

Absence of the whole genital tract except for the lower one third of the vagina.

Complete absence of vagina. There is a slight depression over the hymen.

Septate (double) vagina showing also two cervices.

Vaginal abnormalities can occur alone, but are usually associated with abnormal internal genitalia, and inspection by laparoscopy or laparotomy with gonadal biopsy is called for.

ABNORMALITIES OF THE VULVA

1. Complete absence of the vulva has never been found in a liveborn child. Double vulva is excessively rare, but cases have been reported of complete duplication of the whole genital tract and bladder with normal function.

2. <u>Ectopia Vesicae</u>

This is an extreme defect seen in the newborn, but one which is susceptible to surgical treatment. There is failure of development of the symphysis pubis, mons, lower abdominal wall and anterior wall of bladder. The tissues exposed are the posterior wall of the bladder, the ureteric orifices and the floor of the urethra.

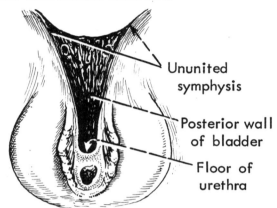

Ununited symphysis

Posterior wall of bladder

Floor of urethra

CONGENITAL ABNORMALITIES OF CLOACAL ORIGIN

These are due to failure of the cloacal septum to divide the cloaca perfectly into hindgut and urogenital sinus. The less serious degrees may persist unnoticed in adults as some form of ectopic anus.

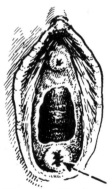

The vestibular anus

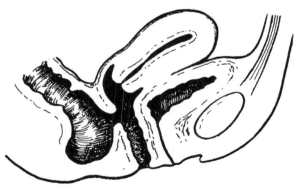

The vaginal anus (very rare)

Patients with these abnormalities can defaecate through vestibule or vagina apparently without suffering from incontinence.

CHAPTER 7
DISEASES OF THE VULVA AND PERINEUM

VULVAL DYSTROPHY—KRAUROSIS

VULVAL DYSTROPHY

Included under this heading are a number of clinical conditions in which the pathology is poorly understood or even unknown. Only a few are reasonably well-defined.

KRAUROSIS

The term means shrinkage and is very descriptive of the condition.

Age Incidence

Most cases occur in the older age groups after the menopause but occasionally it may be seen in younger women of the child-bearing age.

Aetiology

The fundamental cause appears to be lack of oestrogen or in some younger women an insensitivity of the tissues to oestrogen. The condition may therefore occur under the following circumstances :—

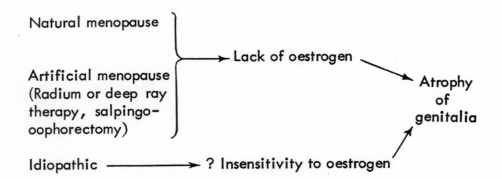

Symptoms

The main complaint is of dyspareunia.
There may be pruritus and pain due to secondary dermatitis.
There is amenorrhoea due to the menopause but in the idiopathic form in young women menstruation may be normal.

KRAUROSIS

Signs

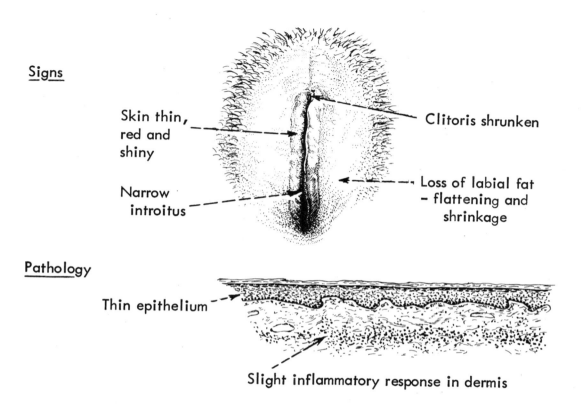

Skin thin, red and shiny

Clitoris shrunken

Narrow introitus

Loss of labial fat – flattening and shrinkage

Pathology

Thin epithelium

Slight inflammatory response in dermis

Infection may supervene causing oedema and pruritus. If this becomes chronic the skin becomes indurated, cracked and fissured. White patches indistinguishable from leukoplakia may form. There is often an associated senile vaginitis.

Treatment

The condition may disappear spontaneously. There is no tendency to malignant change and treatment is entirely palliative. Oestrogens are useful and may be applied locally as creams, or injected as depot oestrogens. Vaginal pessaries can also be employed. Since the tissues appear to be insensitive to oestrogens, all three methods of application may require to be used and even oral oestrogens. Sedative ointments containing benzocaine can give relief from the pain.

When the condition improves it may be possible to enlarge the vaginal orifice surgically if the patient still complains of dyspareunia (see p 398).

LEUKOPLAKIA

This is a descriptive term meaning "white patches". It is still doubtful whether this is a single disease entity with a single aetiology or the end result of a diverse aetiology. It occurs mainly around the menopause.

Symptoms

The characteristic symptom is intractable pruritus causing intense misery. The scratching leads to repeated acute infection superimposed on the chronic changes already present. Coitus may be impossible.

Signs

The raised white plaques are found at the base of the clitoris, on the labia, and in the peri-anal region and perineum. They may involve the whole vulva or be limited to one patch on the labia.

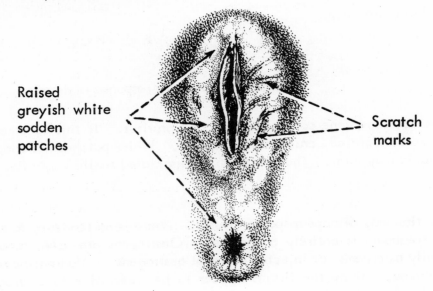

Raised greyish white sodden patches

Scratch marks

At a later stage cracks and fissures appear and considerable pain is experienced.

LEUKOPLAKIA

Pathology

The presence of atypical cells is necessary for the diagnosis.

Hyperkeratosis gives rise to white patches

Hyperplasia of epithelium with downgrowth of papillae

Marked chronic inflammatory reaction

Atypical cells especially in the basal layers

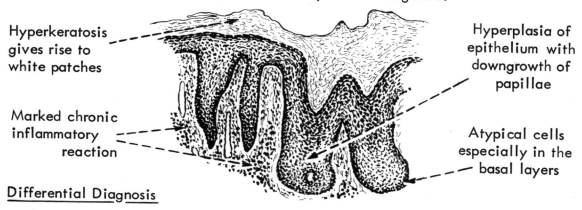

Differential Diagnosis

White patches may appear in this region due to intertrigo, dermatitis and other dermatological conditions and sometimes haemorrhoids. It is possible that leuko-plakia may arise out of these conditions, induced by the constant irritation. Differentiation is only possible by histological examination of a biopsy specimen. The importance lies in the tendency for malignant change to supervene in leuko-plakia. According to some authorities one half of all cases of carcinoma of the vulva follow upon leukoplakia.

Treatment

The diagnosis is difficult both clinically and sometimes even after microscopical examination of a biopsy. In all cases, unless marked cellular atypism is present, conservative treatment should be tried. Sedatives should be given at night when the irritation may interfere with sleep. Oestrogen creams may be helpful but are considered dangerous by some because of the precancerous nature of leukoplakia. Steroid creams, e.g. fluocinolone, give the best result and will restrain the condi-tion as long as they are used.

If dysplastic changes are found in the epithelium of a biopsy, excision of the vulva must be carried out.

LICHEN PLANUS

This is a chronic disease of unknown aetiology.

The patient complains of pruritus of moderate degree. On the labia majora small shiny, reddish brown papules appear. Examination of the vestibule and labia minora reveals irregular stellate white lines.

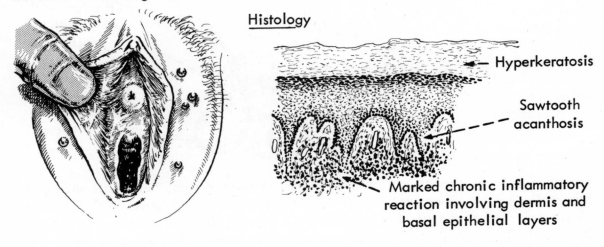

Histology

Hyperkeratosis

Sawtooth acanthosis

Marked chronic inflammatory reaction involving dermis and basal epithelial layers

This first stage may be succeeded by an atrophic phase leading to a kraurotic condition.

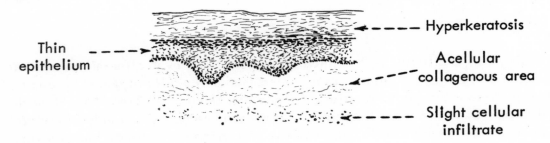

Hyperkeratosis

Thin epithelium

Acellular collagenous area

Slight cellular infiltrate

Treatment

This is wholly palliative to relieve the irritation. Sedative ointments are used at night. Hydrocortisone ointment or creams are useful and may cure the condition but frequently it recurs.

LOCALISED SCLERODERMA AND LICHEN SIMPLEX

LOCALISED SCLERODERMA

This takes the form of rounded or irregular indurated china white depressed patches with reddish brown borders.   The aetiology is unknown.   There may be no symptoms.

Pathology

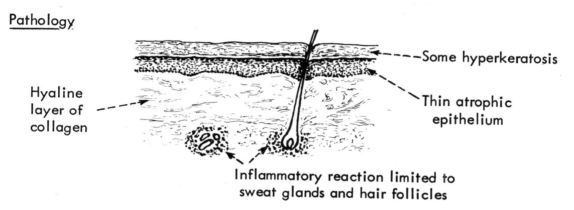

Hyaline layer of collagen

Some hyperkeratosis

Thin atrophic epithelium

Inflammatory reaction limited to sweat glands and hair follicles

The disease is usually self-limiting but recovery is associated with scar formation which may alter the shape and size of the introitus.

LICHEN SIMPLEX

Also known as neurodermatitis.   The patient experiences an intolerable itch localised to a discrete area of the vulval skin.   Constant rubbing and scratching induce a typical shiny reddish lichenified area with papules of varying size.
The lesion is essentially a non-specific chronic inflammation of the dermis with some hyperplasia of the overlying epithelium.
In most cases the patient is approaching the menopause.   Psychological factors are an important element in the aetiology.

Treatment

Locally, soothing salves containing tar are helpful. Stilboestrol may prove useful in menopausal patients. Sedatives are necessary to control the emotional undercurrents.   If possible these emotional factors should be eliminated.

CYST OF BARTHOLIN'S GLAND

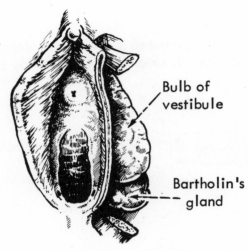

Bulb of
vestibule

Bartholin's
gland

The gland lies partly behind the bulb of the vestibule and is covered by skin and bulbospongiosus muscle. The duct is 2cm long and opens into the vaginal orifice lateral to the hymen.

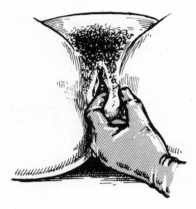

The structures covering the gland are of the same consistency and the gland cannot be palpated in the healthy state.

Cyst and Abscess Formation

This occurs when the duct is blocked and forms a painless cyst occupying the lower half of the labium minus. If infection is present an acute abscess results. The condition is seen during a woman's active sexual life, and any organism including the gonococcus may be responsible.

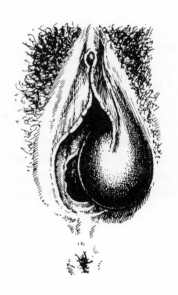

CYST OF BARTHOLIN'S GLAND

Treatment

Marsupialisation (Gk. marsipos, a bag)

The cyst or abscess is widely opened and drained, and its walls sutured to the skin leaving a large orifice which it is hoped will form a new duct orifice and allow conservation of the gland. A ribbon-gauze pack is inserted for 48 hours.

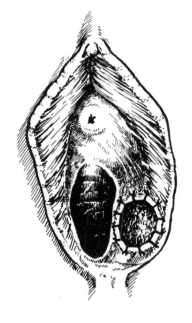

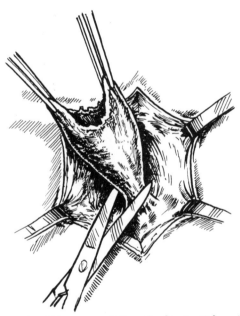

Excision of the Gland

This is done if marsupialisation fails and the condition becomes chronic. Excision is accompanied by very brisk bleeding difficult to control, and often by a postoperative haematoma.

The loss of both Bartholin's glands will lead to some diminution in vaginal moistening during erotic stimulation.

Malignant Disease of Bartholin's Glands

This is exceedingly rare and amounts to carcinoma of the vulva. The treatment is radical vulvectomy. Because of this possibility of cancer, a biopsy should always be taken during operation on an abscess of the gland.

SIMPLE TUMOURS OF THE VULVA

The <u>Complaint</u> is usually of a 'lump' or 'swelling' at the vaginal introitus.

The swelling may be due to extrusion from the vagina of a prolapse – cervix, cystocele or rectocele – and not be a true vulvar tumour.

The commonest simple tumour of the vulva is a <u>Bartholin's Gland cyst</u>.

<u>Endometriosis</u> is uncommon in the labia majora or other parts of the vulva. It enlarges and becomes tender during menstruation. Treatment is by excision.

<u>Lipoma</u> is found rarely. It arises from the subcutaneous tissues of the vulva and usually becomes pedunculated and dependent with growth. Treatment is by excision.

<u>Fibroma</u> is also uncommon but presents as a pedunculated tumour like a lipoma but is firmer. It arises from the fibrous tissue of the round ligament and the vulvar connective tissue. Treatment is by excision. Very rarely it is found to be a myoma. These tumours on occasion become sarcomatous.

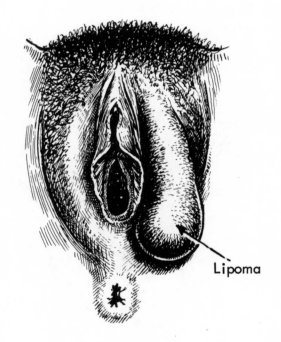

Lipoma

<u>Vulvar haematoma</u> is a result of direct violence or wounding (it is most commonly found with childbirth). The haematoma spreads widely because of the loose tissue structure. Treatment is by incision, evacuation and drainage.

SIMPLE TUMOURS OF THE VULVA

A Cyst or Hydrocele of the Canal of Nuck (an embryonic remnant of a peritoneal pouch which extends along the round ligament).

If causing discomfort the cyst is excised.

An inguinal hernia may cause the patient to believe she has a vulval swelling.

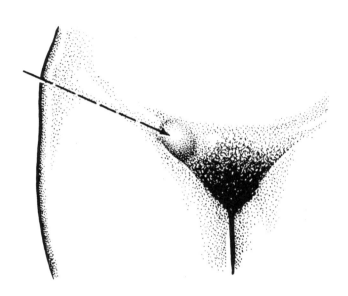

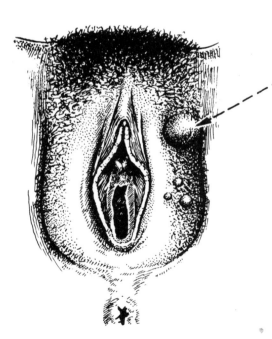

Sebaceous Cyst of the vulva occurs in the hairy region of the labium majus. The cyst may become infected and cause pain. On examination multiple cysts are usually found, mostly small. If painful they can be removed.

Inclusion Cysts are sometimes found in the perineum.

SIMPLE TUMOURS OF THE VULVA

Hidradenoma is a rare tumour of sweat gland origin. It appears as a small nodule on the labium or in the interlabial sulcus. The overlying skin tends to ulcerate and bleed, giving a fungating appearance. The tumour is excised and shows a cystadenomatous structure. It also shows a typical two layer epithelium with some mucous secretion. Intracystic papillary protrusions occur. It may undergo malignant change.

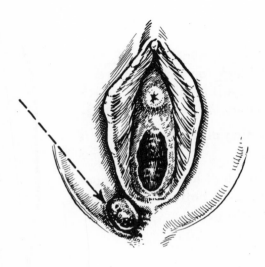

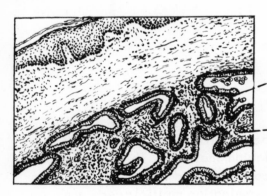

_____ Double layer of cells

_____ Smooth muscle cells

Condylomata Acuminata are due to a viral infection and form a watery mass. Podophyllin ointment usually clears up the condition but cautery or excision may be necessary.

Urethral Caruncle
is dealt with on page 151.

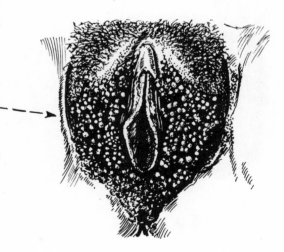

CARCINOMA OF THE VULVA

(Squamous Epithelioma:
                    Invasive Carcinoma)

The most common site is the labium majus followed by the clitoris, but it may arise anywhere including the vestibule when it will involve the urethra. Two or more growths are occasionally seen.

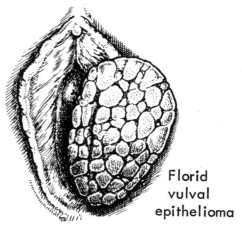

Florid
vulval
epithelioma

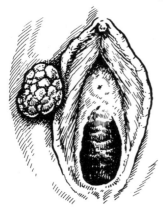

Early epithelioma

<u>Histology</u>.   It is usually a squamous cell carcinoma (p 185).   However any tissue contributing to the vulva may give rise to malignant change.   Rare tumours are melanoma, basal cell carcinoma and sarcoma.

<u>Spread</u>.   The tumour will spread locally if neglected, to involve the whole vulva and will invade the vagina.   Metastatic spread is along the lymphatic system.

<u>Clinical Features</u>.   This is a disease of old women and the average age is over 60.   The patient may have had a pruritus of long standing but quite often the tumour is symptomless except for being palpable, until it ulcerates.   The appearance is often uncharacteristic, and the old descriptive terms ('cauliflower, ulcerated, indurated') are not relevant to diagnosis.   <u>Any lump on the vulva must be histologically examined</u>.

The inguinal glands will often be enlarged, but absence of enlargement does not guarantee absence of lymphatic spread.

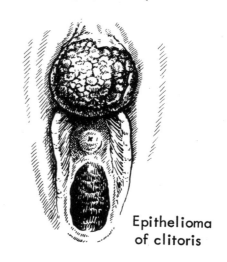

Epithelioma
of clitoris

CARCINOMA OF THE VULVA

LYMPHATIC SPREAD

1. To the superficial inguinal glands which lie along the inguinal ligament and the saphenous vein (vertical group). These nodes lie between the layers of the superficial fascia in relation to numerous superficial vessels.

Drainage may be contralateral i.e. cells from a tumour on the right labium might drain via the left inguinal glands.

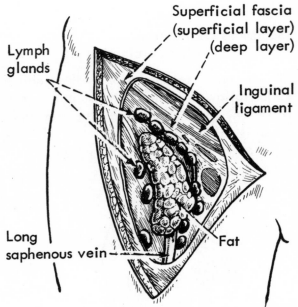

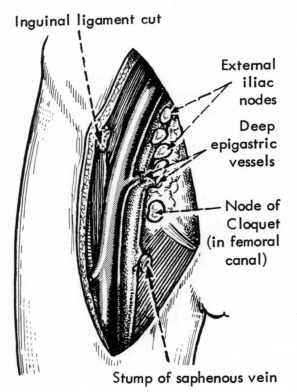

2. Thence to the deep femoral glands represented by the lymph gland of Cloquet which lies in the femoral canal; and from there on to the external iliac, common iliac and para-aortic glands.

3. This path is not invariably followed. The superficial nodes are occasionally bypassed and a tumour near the mid-line might drain via the vesical lymph channels direct to the internal iliac group.

4. Some tumours spread along the lymphatic system more quickly than others and there is no reliable correlation between the size of the tumour and the likelihood of gland involvement.

CARCINOMA OF THE VULVA

TREATMENT

At present, whether the growth is early or advanced, a radical vulvectomy with dissection of the superficial and deep inguinal glands and the external iliac glands is accepted as the ideal treatment. An old and frail patient however might be better served by a more limited dissection which left the deep glands untouched. Indeed if the pelvic glands are involved the prognosis is very poor, and the whole principle of extended node dissection must be examined. No matter how careful and expert the surgeon it is impossible to remove all the lymphatic tissue, and it is perhaps more important to achieve a wide dissection of the surrounding skin and subcutaneous fat, removing if necessary, the anus, the lower vagina and urethra.

The picture shows the area of skin which will be removed along with the subcutaneous fat and lymphatic tissue.

Haemorrhage is brisk and some surgeons use a diathermy knife to reduce blood loss and save time.

The dissection is not so difficult as for example dissection in the deep pelvis, but as the patient is usually old it is better that the operation be kept as short as possible. Because of this and because it is a rare disease, carcinoma of the vulva is better dealt with in centres which specialise in the work.

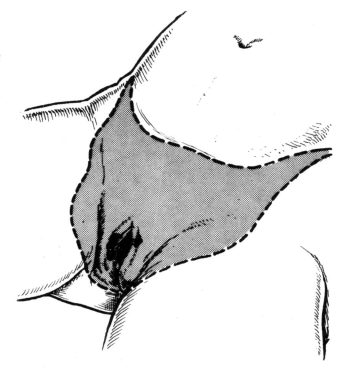

CARCINOMA OF THE VULVA

TREATMENT

The skin and fat are dissected down to the aponeurosis of the external oblique.

Fibro-fatty tissue with lymph nodes

The femoral triangle is cleared of the fibro-fatty tissue containing the lymph glands. Note that about 3 cm of the saphenous vein have been removed.

Saphenous vein

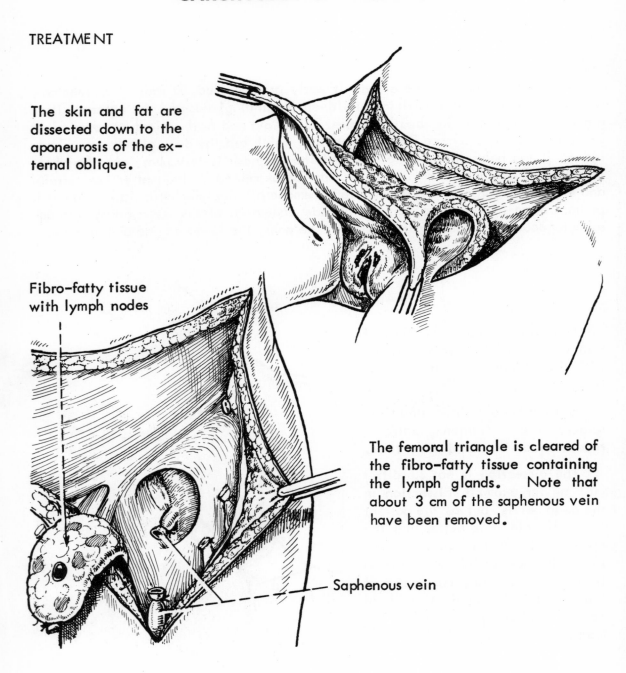

CARCINOMA OF THE VULVA

TREATMENT

The aponeurosis has been opened and the inguinal ligament divided. Peritoneum is retracted medially to expose the external iliac glands.

To achieve this exposure the inferior epigastric vessels must be divided and inconstant vessels may be a cause of haemorrhage.

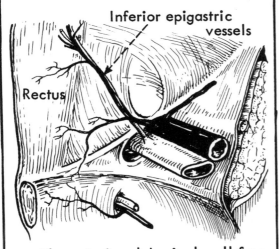

The anterior abdominal wall from inside, showing epigastric vessels.

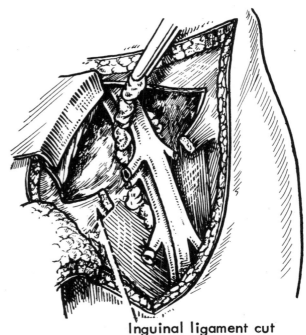

Inguinal ligament cut

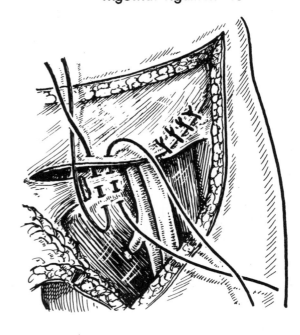

The inguinal ligament is not easily reconstituted and the aponeurosis must be sutured to pectineus muscle and its fascia. Hernia is sometimes a sequel of this operation.

CARCINOMA OF THE VULVA

TREATMENT

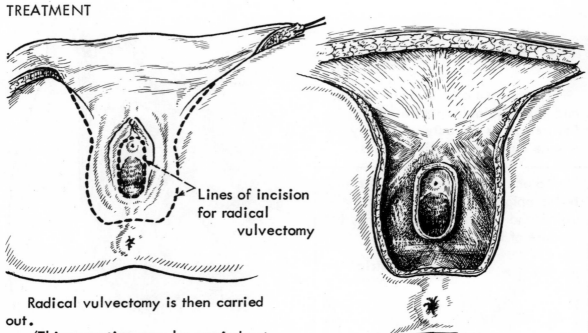

Lines of incision for radical vulvectomy

Radical vulvectomy is then carried out.

(This operation may be carried out in two stages; the vulvectomy first followed a month later by the gland dissection.)

The whole vulva, skin and subcutaneous tissue are excised down to the periosteum.

It will be impossible to clothe the whole area with skin, but the wound should be closed where it can be done without tension. Skin grafting may be required.

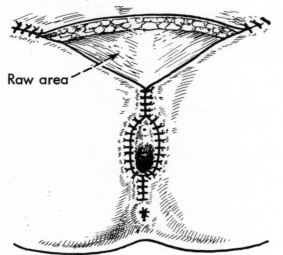

Raw area

CARCINOMA OF THE VULVA

COMPLICATIONS OF RADICAL VULVECTOMY

1. <u>Shock</u>. If the operation is long, and the patient old, this may contribute to the operative mortality.

2. <u>Pulmonary Embolism</u>.

3. <u>Sepsis</u>. The bigger the raw area the greater the risk (cf. extensive burns). Antibiotics and local antiseptics are used routinely and healing may take up to 3 months unless skin grafting is used.

4. <u>Electrolyte imbalance</u>. The prevention of this is well understood today.

5. <u>Chronic oedema of the legs</u>.

6. Hernia and vaginal stenosis are rare. Younger women should be capable of coitus; and vaginal delivery has been reported after this operation.

PROGNOSIS AFTER RADICAL VULVECTOMY

This depends on three factors:

1. <u>Histology</u>. The more differentiated the tumour the better.

2. <u>Lymphatic spread</u>. The more differentiated, the less likely. Lymph node metastases occur in about 50% of patients, and the lateral pelvic nodes are involved in about 15%.

3. <u>The age of the tumour</u>. Elderly women may not immediately recognise a 'small wart' for what it is, or may lack the courage to consult their doctor.

RESULTS

If the nodes are not involved, a 70% 5-year cure rate may be looked for in the best hands. This falls to 40% when the superficial nodes are involved; and below 20% if the disease has reached the pelvic nodes.

RADIOTHERAPY IN THE TREATMENT OF CARCINOMA OF THE VULVA

This has never been successful as a primary treatment because squamous carcinoma is a relatively resistant tumour and the lethal dose required produces a very severe reaction in the vulval skin which is peculiarly sensitive to irradiation. The modern megavoltage machines which are much less limited by skin reaction may be more effective in the future; but at present radiotherapy is restricted to patients too frail for an attempt at cure by surgery, or to reduce the size of a tumour prior to surgery, or for recurrent growths.

SIMPLE VULVECTOMY

Excision of the labia majora, minora and the clitoris.

This is indicated when epithelial dysplasia is found; and vulvectomy does have a place in the treatment of intractable non-malignant conditions although recurrence is possible. The operation is haemorrhagic but not difficult and there is little postoperative disability. The patient continues to be capable of coitus, but as most of the erectile tissue is removed, vaginal gratification is absent.

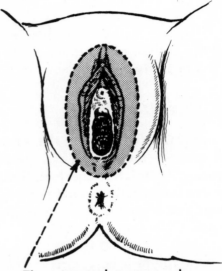

The area to be removed.

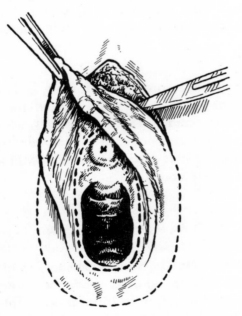

Excision begins with the clitoris. Bleeding must be controlled.

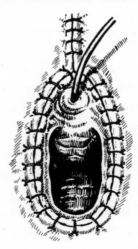

The operation completed. Silk sutures are removed 7 days later.

DISEASES OF THE URETHRA

CARUNCLE

A small tumour arising from the posterior part of the lower end of the urethra. It is composed of a very vascular stroma, almost a haemangioma, usually infected and covered with squamous or transitional epithelium.

Clinical Features   Caruncles are red in colour because of their vascularity, and extremely sensitive.   The patient is usually an elderly woman complaining of dysuria and bleeding.

Treatment   Caruncles should be excised and sent for histological examination although malignant change is rare.   The base of the tumour on the urethral mucosa should be cauterised.

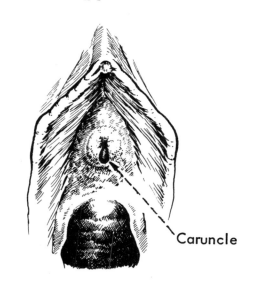

Caruncle

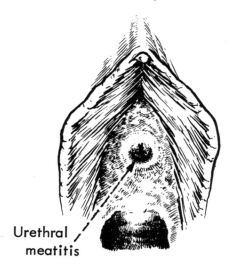

Urethral meatitis

URETHRAL MEATITIS (Granulomatous Caruncle)

Chronic infection of the peri-urethral tissues.   It is often called a caruncle but is not neoplastic and is often symptomless. 'Granulomatous' caruncle is often seen, while the true caruncle is uncommon. Treatment if needed is by cautery and there is a tendency to recurrence. Infection in this area must involve the para-urethral gland network and complete cure is difficult.   A search should be made for a vaginal or bladder source of the infection.

DISEASES OF THE URETHRA

PROLAPSE OF THE URETHRAL MUCOSA

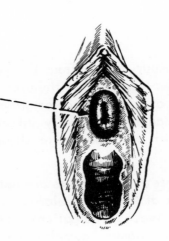

This forms a symmetrical swelling round the meatus and at first
sight looks like a caruncle. If it
causes symptoms the cautery should
be applied. Larger prolapses must
be excised.

CYST OF SKENE'S DUCT

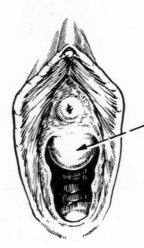

A firm cyst is palpated in the
posterior wall of the urethra. It
may be mistaken for a urethrocele,
but it cannot be reduced by pressure. When it is being dissected
out care must be taken not to create
a urethral fistula.

URETHROCELE

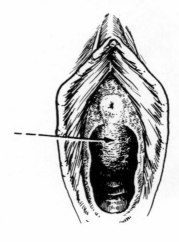

This is a descent of the urethra
from its position under the pubic
arch. It is sometimes a cause of
stress incontinence and may exist
by itself or in company with a cystocele. Treatment is described in
the section on prolapse.

DISEASES OF THE URETHRA

CARCINOMA

This is a rare condition seen in elderly women. The tumour is a transitional or squamous cell epithelioma, and may arise in any part of the urethra.

<u>Clinical Features</u>   The patient complains of local pain, bleeding, dysuria. Inspection will reveal a tumour mass at the meatus, or if the growth is in the proximal urethra, a hard swelling in the vaginal wall. The inguinal glands may be enlarged by infection or metastases, but absence of swelling does not mean absence of spread since the urethra shares the lymphatic drainage of both vulva and bladder and the deep pelvic nodes may be the first affected.

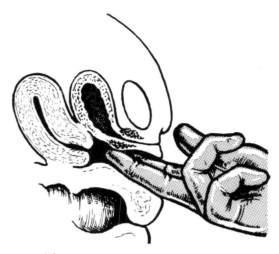

Always palpate
the whole urethra

Treatment

1. The disease is rare and experience of the results of different treatments is restricted.

2. The wide lymphatic drainage means that radical surgery should include removal of vulva, lymph nodes, bladder, uterus and vagina. Such mutilation is difficult to justify when it by no means guarantees a cure.

3. The tumour is not particularly radiosensitive, and large doses of irradiation are needed, which cause an unpleasant local reaction.

Probably the treatment of choice would be the insertion of radium needles round the urethra. This can be preceded by local excision (it is said that half the urethra may be removed without causing stress incontinence) and perhaps followed by lymphadenectomy.

Prognosis is poorer than for carcinoma of the vulva and depends very much on the stage of the disease and whether lymphatic spread has occurred.

OPERATIONS ON THE PERINEUM

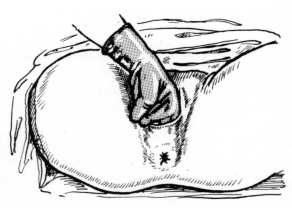

Repair of Deficient Perineum

This condition is due to repeated stretching at parturition and repair is often done to complete an operation for prolapse. The perineal floor is only secondarily responsible for maintaining uterine position, and operation is really only necessary if the patient complains of discomfort or of unsatisfactory coitus.

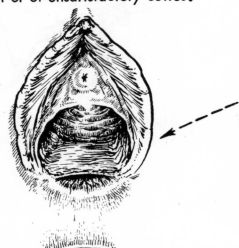

Repair of Complete Tear

The perineal body including anal sphincter and perhaps some rectal wall is completely torn through at parturition. The complaint is usually of faecal incontinence although the patient may be able to prevent this by using her levator ani muscles. Complete tears in gynaecological practice are usually the result of breakdown of a primary repair following delivery.

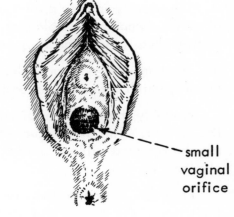

small vaginal orifice

Enlargement of Vaginal Orifice

This is done by dividing the muscles of the perineal body, and it is required when the orifice is too small to allow intromission of the penis. The usual cause is stenosis following a perineal repair, but sometimes the patient may be an older woman with senile shrinkage or, very rarely, a young woman with a congenitally small orifice.

154

REPAIR OF DEFICIENT PERINEUM

The principle is mobilisation and removal of excess vaginal tissue and apposition of levator muscles adjacent to the perineal body.

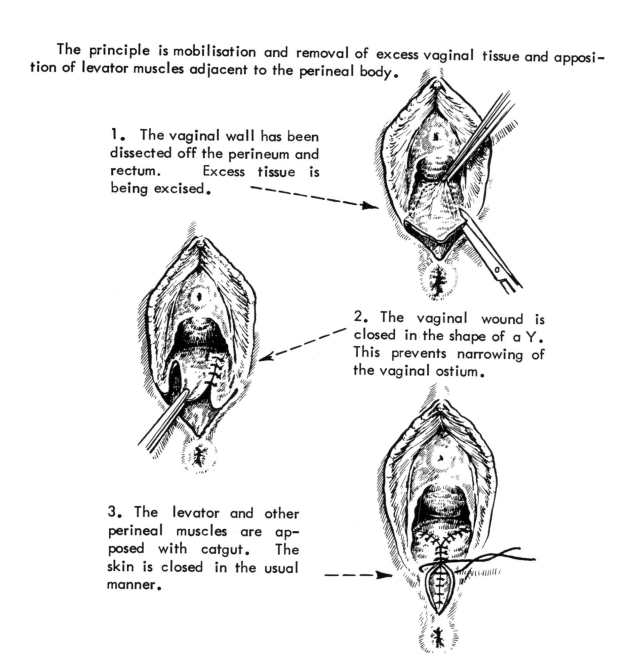

1. The vaginal wall has been dissected off the perineum and rectum.   Excess tissue is being excised.

2. The vaginal wound is closed in the shape of a Y. This prevents narrowing of the vaginal ostium.

3. The levator and other perineal muscles are apposed with catgut. The skin is closed in the usual manner.

REPAIR OF COMPLETE TEAR

Infection must first be dealt with, and 3 months allowed to elapse after breakdown of a primary repair.

1. An H-shaped incision is made which gives access to the rectovaginal space and allows mobilisation of the peri-anal tissues.

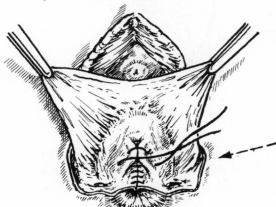

2. The rectal wall is repaired with two layers of sutures.

3. The ends of the anal sphincter are sutured together. (These are often difficult to identify.) The perineum is then repaired in the usual manner.

After the operation the patient's bowels are confined for four days and then laxatives are given.

This sort of reconstituted perineal body looks well on completion but the late results are often disappointing especially in elderly women with atrophic muscles.

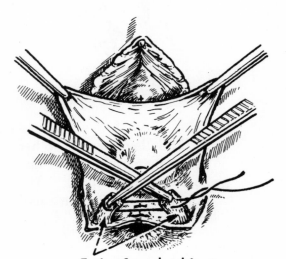

Ends of anal sphincter

OPERATION FOR ENLARGING THE VAGINAL OUTLET

The principle is to divide all the fibres of the perineal body except the anal sphincter.

1. Making the longitudinal incision through skin and muscle. The finger in the rectum allows the surgeon to know how near his knife is to the rectal wall.

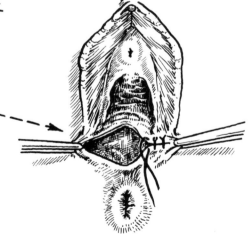

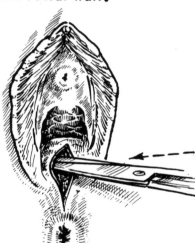

2. The cut muscles retract laterally, and the vaginal wall is further mobilised to allow closure without tension.

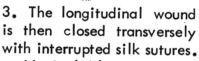

3. The longitudinal wound is then closed transversely with interrupted silk sutures. Vaginal dilators are used once the sutures are removed and continued with for several weeks until all tenderness is gone and coitus can be resumed.

CHAPTER 8
DISEASES OF THE VAGINA

VAGINAL DISCHARGE

Vaginal secretion is normally present in adult life. It is milky or watery and little more than a dampness, but erotic stimulation can increase the quantity.

The normal discharge is the product of the uterine secretions plus the cervical gland exudates, the vaginal transudates, desquamation of the vaginal cells and the secretion of the greater vestibular (Bartholin's) glands.

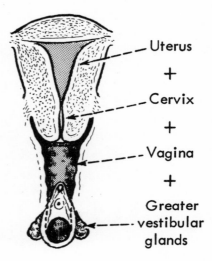

Uterus
+
Cervix
+
Vagina
+
Greater vestibular glands

The discharge is normally acid, pH 3.5-4.5, because of the action of lactogenic (Doderlein) bacilli on glycogen in the vaginal epithelium.

It is increased slightly in the latter part of the menstrual cycle and also for a few days after menstruation.

Before puberty the secretions tend to be alkaline and again in the senile vagina, although the post-menopausal woman at first has an acid secretion.

During pregnancy there is an increase in the physiological discharge, possibly due to oestrogenic stimulation and increased vascularity.

The AMOUNT of discharge considered abnormal varies with the patient's ideas and tolerance, but a discharge requiring frequent change of underclothing or the wearing of an absorbent pad should be regarded as abnormal.

The HISTORY of the discharge is noted. It often dates from a childbirth or abortion or from an illness when antibiotics have been used. It may vary in amount with different phases of the menstrual cycle.

The COLOUR of the discharge may be helpful in diagnosis:-

White or Clear suggests an increased amount of a normal secretion.
Yellow or Green indicates infection with pyogenic bacteria such as the pyocyaneus group.
Brown suggests blood. Normal secretion dries pale brown on white clothing.
Blood - always consider malignancy.

VAGINAL DISCHARGE

The SMELL of the discharge may be significant. Trichomonal vaginitis has a noticably unpleasant smell but not foul or overwhelming. A foul smell may be due to the necrosis of malignancy or a foreign body such as a forgotten tampon.

IRRITATION is often a feature and may be the main complaint.

Yeast infestation (e.g. candida albicans) causes little discharge but much irritation within the vagina and around the labia. It is common after antibiotic therapy.

Glycosuria may be present. Urethral meatal irritation may cause dysuria. Irritation of the perineum may be due to haemorrhoidal tags or intestinal worms.

Irritation of the perineum and upper thighs suggests a very copious discharge; the discomfort is often caused by a secondary intertriginous infection.

DYSPAREUNIA is common when trichomonal or yeast infestations are present and may be associated with penile pruritus in the husband.

EXAMINATION

The vulval region is inspected for general appearance of inflammation, moistness and discharge.

Bearing down is encouraged to see if this produces discharge and to check introital competence.

A speculum with a bland lubricant is introduced.

The colour of the mucosa is noted and also the presence and characteristics of any discharge. Discharge is usually most abundant in the posterior fornix.

A trichomonal discharge sometimes shows tiny vacuoles and a granular appearance of the mucosa, and small petechial haemorrhages.

Bacterial smears are taken for warm slide examination and culture.

A cytological smear of the cervix may show the presence of yeasts or trichomonas when a bacterial smear is negative.

Evidence of chronic cervicitis is sought.

Yeast infection shows white patches adherent to the mucosa of vagina, cervix and labia minora.

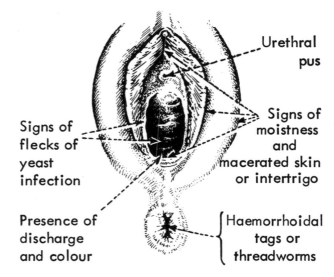

Urethral pus

Signs of moistness and macerated skin or intertrigo

Signs of flecks of yeast infection

Presence of discharge and colour

Haemorrhoidal tags or threadworms

VAGINAL DISCHARGE

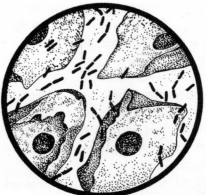

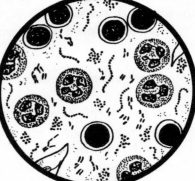

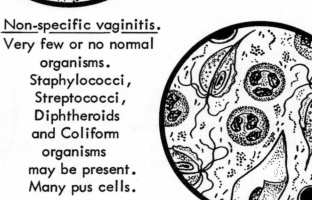

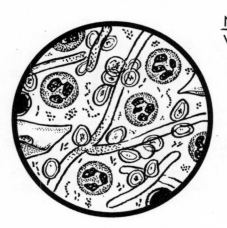

Normal vaginal flora. Desquamated cells. Organisms are nearly all lactobacillus.

Normal and abnormal flora. A mixture of organisms and an occasional pus cell as well as desquamated cells.

Non-specific vaginitis. Very few or no normal organisms. Staphylococci, Streptococci, Diphtheroids and Coliform organisms may be present. Many pus cells.

Yeasts mycelia and buds

Trichomonas vaginalis

Note the varied organisms present and also the pus cells.

VAGINAL DISCHARGE

TREATMENT

Treatment is based on three principles :-

1. Elimination of any pathological lesion.
2. Destruction of the abnormal organism.
3. Restoration of the normal flora.

The pathological lesions have been mentioned and their investigation and treatment may be urgent.

Vulvitis and yeast infections should mean the checking of urine for sugar, as glycosuria allows these to flourish.

Destruction of the infesting organisms is difficult as is indicated by the many remedies commercially available.

In the childbearing years the important and common infections are yeasts and trichomonas.

Nystatin is useful in the treatment of monilial vaginitis. Nystatin is used as a vaginal tablet or pessary inserted high in the vagina night and morning for ten or twelve days. In addition a nystatin ointment may be applied locally to the vulva and thighs, and if the infestation follows an antibiotic course then oral nystatin should be given too. Pants should be washed by boiling or, better still, be disposable.

Gentian Violet 1% aqueous solution painted on the mucosa is an effective but messy treatment.

Trichomonal vaginitis is treated with oral metronidazole (e.g. Flagyl), one tablet three times per day for seven days. It should not be used in the first trimester of pregnancy. (There are a number of pessaries available for use in early pregnancy.)

If the infection reappears quickly after treatment then a second course should be given but this time to the husband as well.

Non-specific vaginitis is treated with antiseptic or antibiotic pessaries or
creams.

VAGINAL DISCHARGE

IN THE CHILD

In the very young the pH is high, the oestrogen levels low and the mucosa is thin. Normal organisms found in later life are not present.

Lack of hygiene may allow infection by bowel organisms or even threadworms and foreign bodies may have been introduced by the child.

Local inspection may suggest the cause. In infancy the vaginal mucosa and labia are redder than in the adult and can suggest falsely that vaginitis is present particularly to an anxious mother.

Frequent washing of the region with ordinary soap and water and thorough drying and then application of a talcum powder is usually adequate treatment.

The underclothes should not be pulled tight into the vulva.

If threadworms are noted round the anus they are eliminated by piperazine or its derivatives.

If the discharge persists the vagina should then be explored (under anaesthesia) for a foreign body.

AFTER THE MENOPAUSE

The post-menopausal fall in oestrogens results in a set of circumstances similar to those in the child – the mucosa is thin and the pH is high so that bacterial infection occurs readily. The complaint is also of discomfort or soreness, sometimes dyspareunia and occasionally of blood staining.

On examination the mucosa is reddened, small punctate haemorrhages are visible and there is a thin yellow discharge. This is atrophic or senile vaginitis.

Bacteriological examination of the discharge is made and if there is a history of blood staining curettage should be carried out.

The vaginitis will respond to oestrogens locally or orally for ten days (extended treatment with oestrogens will cause endometrial proliferation and ultimate withdrawal bleeding).

Lactic acid pessaries are a useful adjuvant to treatment of abnormal bacteria.

A ring pessary is sometimes present; it should be removed till the vaginitis has been eliminated, and then replaced.

VAGINAL DISCHARGE

EXAMINATION OF SMALL CHILDREN

Small girls are occasionally brought to a gynaecological clinic by their mothers who complain that the child is always scratching or staining her pants with discharge.

Examination should always be made under an anaesthetic. A neonatal laryngoscope is useful for inspecting the infant vagina.

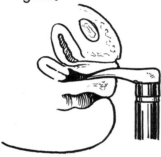

Any foreign body is removed and swabs taken. A specimen of stool should be inspected under water for the presence of threadworms. Occasionally some excoriation and vaginitis are seen but often no clinical signs are present to support the mother's story.

The treatment is of the cause if one can be found. Stilboestrol has been given orally (say 0.2mg daily in a 5 year old child) to encourage growth of a normal vaginal flora. The mother must be warned that the breasts may enlarge temporarily and slight vaginal staining may occur. Stilboestrol should not be given for more than a fortnight.

PRECOCIOUS PUBERTY

Small girls sometimes develop a temporary swelling of the breasts which may persist or disappear after months; and some pubic hair may appear. The child continues to grow at the normal rate and neither sign is necessarily the forerunner of precocious puberty which is diagnosed when menstruation begins before the 8th year. Such patients are best managed by a paediatrician, but the gynaecologist may be the first to see the child and he will be asked to share in the investigation.

1. It is necessary to exclude other causes of vaginal bleeding such as insertion of a foreign body, infection and scratching, tumour, or the mistaken ingestion of oestrogen-containing tablets such as the contraceptive pill.

2. An examination of the genitalia is made under anaesthesia and the pelvis palpated to exclude ovarian tumour.

3. Urinary steroid estimations are carried out to exclude adrenal abnormality; but most cases of precocious puberty in girls are unexplained.

It is usual to prescribe progesterone to suppress menstruation until the child is old enough to accept her condition.

CYSTS OF THE VAGINA

Vaginal cysts are relatively common but rarely large. They are found in the anterior or lateral walls of the lower third of vagina and in the posterior wall of the upper third, seldom larger than a walnut, sometimes multiple, and may be mistaken for a cystocele. These cysts are occasionally a cause of dyspareunia but usually have no symptoms at all.

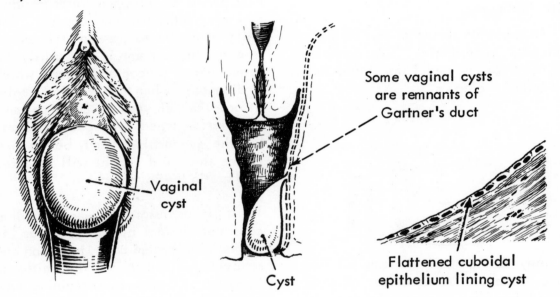

Vaginal cyst

Some vaginal cysts are remnants of Gartner's duct

Cyst

Flattened cuboidal epithelium lining cyst

Treatment is by excision

TRAUMATIC EPITHELIAL CYSTS (inclusion cysts) are found usually in the lower vagina, and are caused by infolding of epithelium at repair operations. If they cause symptoms they should be excised.

CYSTS of KOBELT'S TUBULES, HYDATIDS of MORGAGNI, FIMBRIAL CYSTS

These are names given to small cysts found in the mesosalpinx and around the terminal portion of the fallopian tubes. They are of indeterminate embryonic origin and are of no clinical significance.

CARCINOMA OF THE VAGINA

This is a rare disease and the average gynaecologist will see only one such tumour for every 30 of the cervix.

Secondary growths are more common, especially extension of a cervical cancer. Metastatic deposits may appear from any organ (corpus uteri, ovary, bladder, bowel or breast).

Clinical Features

The patient is usually post-menopausal and complains of bleeding and discharge. If the bladder is involved she will also experience pain and dysuria.

Diagnosis

It must be established by full examination that the primary site is the vagina and not the cervix or bladder or rectum. This may be difficult or even impossible in the case of advanced 'cauliflower' growths. There must be no evidence of a primary growth elsewhere.

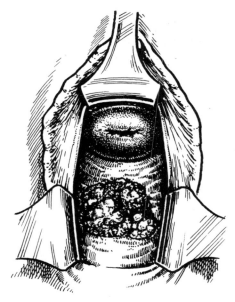

Differential Diagnosis

Endometriosis and infective granulomatous growths must be considered, and biopsy is essential.

Histology

Vaginal cancer is nearly always epidermoid and an adenocarcinoma is very rare.

Survival in relation to Clinical Staging

		5 year Survival Rate
Stage 0	Carcinoma-in-situ	Should be curable
Stage I	Confined to vaginal wall	50%
Stage II	Invading subvaginal tissues	25%
Stage III	Extension to pelvic wall	0
Stage IV	Extension to other viscera	

CARCINOMA OF THE VAGINA

Treatment is by intracavitary radiotherapy. If the bladder or bowel are involved and the patient is young enough, some form of pelvic exenteration may be justified

Factors Affecting Survival

1. The Stage of the Disease

This tumour is not at first painful and unless it appears in a woman who is still practising intercourse it is not likely to be noticed until it has penetrated the vaginal wall. Old women often believe or affect to believe that bleeding from the vagina is due to haemorrhoids.

It is not difficult to miss an early tumour of the vagina at routine gynaecological examination if it is obscured by the blade of the speculum. The whole vagina should always be inspected and cytological smears taken of anything at all unusual.

Tumour obscured by speculum in vagina

2. The degree of radiosensitivity of the tumour

Squamous growths are not particularly sensitive and relatively high dosages are required.

3. Histological differentiation

Poorly differentiated tumours are very sensitive to radiation but unfortunately spread more rapidly.

4. Location of the Tumour in the Vagina

This is important because of the ease with which the vaginal wall is penetrated. A tumour in the fornix has much the same prognosis as a stage II cervical cancer if discovered early enough, while a tumour on the anterior wall is likely to involve the bladder at an early stage.

Upper third: approximately same drainage as cervix.

Middle third: any pelvic lymphatic channel may be involved.

Lower third: approximately same drainage as vulva.

The lymphatic drainage of the vagina is variable and affects spread.

PLASTIC SURGERY OF THE VAGINA

This is required when the patient is prevented from coitus by congenital absence of the vagina or by distortion and contractures due to injury. Such a situation is rare; but various operations have been devised.

The McIndoe-Bannister Operation - using a free skin graft from the thigh.

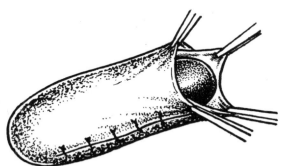

1. A plastic mould is covered with skin from the thigh. (This is done by a plastic surgeon.)

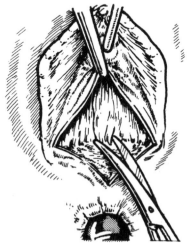

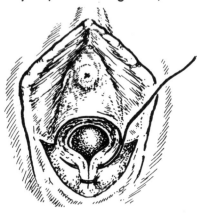

2. The space between urethra/bladder and rectum is opened up. The finger in the anus helps the surgeon to avoid damaging the rectum.

   The mould must be kept in situ for several months and once it is removed the patient should have regular and frequent coitus to prevent contraction of the new vagina.

   The main complications to be avoided are graft failure due to venous oozing or sepsis; and pressure necrosis of bladder or rectal wall from too large a mould.

3. Mould and graft are inserted and kept in place by suturing the split ends of the labia minora. (The vaginal orifice may need enlarging later on.)

PLASTIC SURGERY OF THE VAGINA

Williams' Operation

The formation of a cul-de-sac by suturing the labia majora in two layers. This means that the anterior wall of the new 'vagina' is the vulva. It is a simple operation which seems to provide a satisfying coitus for both parties.

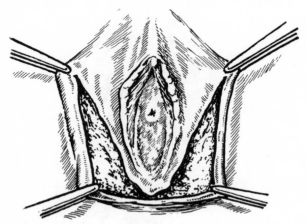

1. The labia majora are split down to the perineal muscles. Bleeding is free.

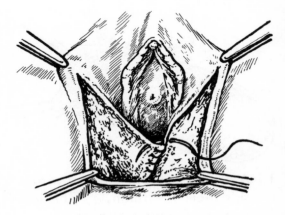

2. The inner margins of the labia are sutured together.

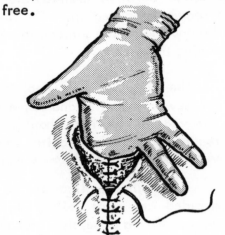

3. The outer margins are sutured. The resulting cavity should accommodate two fingers.

Other methods include the use of pedicle grafts from the labia, and encouraging natural epithelialisation of the dissected cavity without any grafting. There is sometimes a rudimentary vaginal depression already developed which can be enlarged to a functional size by using a pessary to maintain prolonged upward pressure.

CHAPTER 9
DISEASES OF THE CERVIX

CERVICAL EROSION

This is an area of columnar epithelium partly or completely surrounding the external os. It becomes abraded with resulting inflammation of the underlying tissues. The area is bright pink or red, raw-looking and feels "velvety" with a characteristic appearance. It is often limited to the posterior lip, with retroversion of the uterus.

In infancy the ectocervix is covered with columnar epithelium and this may persist in adult life.

In adult life erosion is more commonly the result of cervical catarrh, often following childbirth, and is aggravated by oral contraceptives.

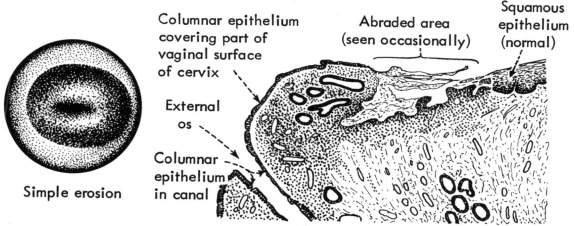

Columnar epithelium covering part of vaginal surface of cervix

External os

Columnar epithelium in canal

Simple erosion

Abraded area (seen occasionally)

Squamous epithelium (normal)

Symptoms and Signs

1. There may be none.
2. Discharge (serous unless infected).
3. Sometimes staining following coitus.
4. Staining or even bleeding from trauma of Ayre's spatula.
5. Raw appearance.

Treatment

If there are no symptoms treatment is unnecessary, otherwise conisation by knife or diathermic cautery – this removes the chronically infected tissue and allows contraction of the cervix and new growth of normal tissue. An acid buffered vaginal pessary is said to help promote the growth of normal vaginal organisms.

ECTROPION OF CERVIX AND TRACHELORRHAPHY

ECTROPION OF CERVIX

This is a turning outwards of the endocervix and is due to laceration of the cervix plus chronic cervicitis (catarrh).

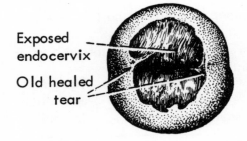

Exposed endocervix

Old healed tear

Symptoms
1. Discharge.
2. Sometimes post-coital staining especially premenstrually.
3. Blood staining with Ayre's spatula.

Treatment

This used to be by a plastic operation (Trachelorrhaphy) but surgery has in the main given place to diathermic cautery.

TRACHELORRHAPHY

Excision of infected tissue from the cervix. This is an old operation now out of fashion, but indicated when the ectropion is very large and ulcerated. The infected tissue is cut out and the raw areas sutured together.

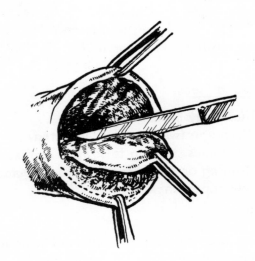

CONISATION OF CERVIX

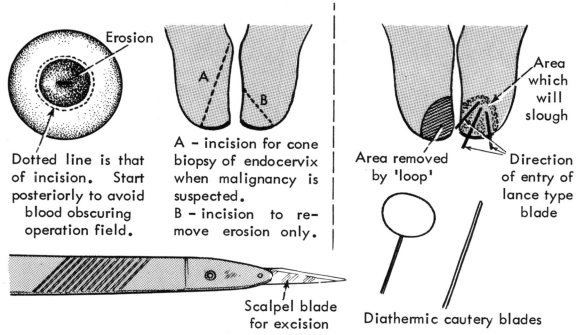

Erosion

Dotted line is that of incision. Start posteriorly to avoid blood obscuring operation field.

A – incision for cone biopsy of endocervix when malignancy is suspected.
B – incision to remove erosion only.

Area which will slough

Area removed by 'loop'

Direction of entry of lance type blade

Scalpel blade for excision

Diathermic cautery blades

The ordinary simple cautery may be used for small erosions with minimal cervicitis.
Diathermy destroys tissue and must never be used for obtaining biopsy material.

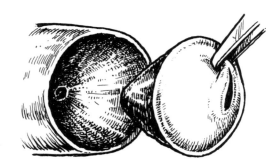

The picture shows the cervix after the cone of tissue has been cut out with a knife. This is the simplest method.

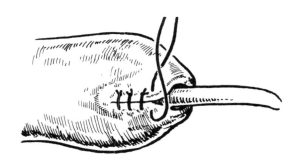

The raw areas are sutured together. A dilator is passed to ensure patency.

175

CERVICAL POLYPS AND CHRONIC CERVICITIS

CERVICAL POLYPS

Cervical polyps are nodular or pedunculated growths from endocervix associated with chronic cervicitis. Polypoid fibroids may present as a cervical polyp (p

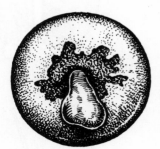

Cervical polyp
with cervicitis

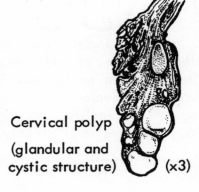

Cervical polyp

(glandular and
cystic structure) (x3)

Symptoms

1. Discharge.
2. Slight irregular bleeding often following trauma (coitus).

Treatment

Avulsion – by grasping with forceps and torsion. The endocervix may be cauterised. With marked cervicitis conisation by knife or diathermic cautery may be carried out.

CHRONIC CERVICITIS

Symptoms. The cervix is bulky, firm, usually with erosion and the surface has a "velvet" feeling; stains with Ayre's spatula but there is not normally a history of bleeding. Discharge is the principal symptom. Chronic cervicitis is associated with small retention cysts in the cervix (Nabothian follicles).

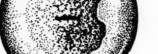

Treatment

Simple cautery, diathermic cautery or conisation depending on bulk of tissue.

SPECIFIC INFECTIONS

CHANCRE OF THE CERVIX

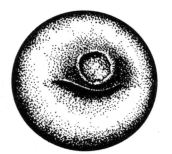

This is very rarely recognised. Secondary infection is uncommon so that the characteristic hard indurated base does not form. A chancre may be papular or ulcerative in which case it looks like an erosion and may be mistaken for carcinoma on palpation.

Herpes simplex of the cervix may look like a chancre.

TUBERCULOSIS OF THE CERVIX

This is rare as an isolated lesion. It is usually secondary to tubal and uterine infections.

It may show (1) a proliferative form – not unlike the appearance of an erosion.
(2) an ulcerative type.

The lesion may give rise to an itch and discharge but usually it is found when investigating complaints associated with chronic pelvic inflammation or infertility. The lesion may be mistaken for carcinoma.

Biopsy and guinea pig inoculation will make the diagnosis.

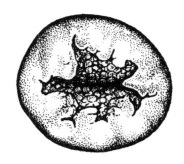

SQUAMOUS METAPLASIA

EPITHELIAL CHANGES

There are three changes in cervical epithelium which seem to form a chain of events leading to invasive carcinoma. The relationship is far from being established and the change from one stage to the other is not inevitable.

1. SQUAMOUS METAPLASIA

This is a benign lesion which is extremely common especially in parous women and of itself is of little significance. There are no typical clinical signs or symptoms and the lesion is discovered accidentally when the cervix is amputated for prolapse or if hysterectomy for some other gynaecological complaint is carried out.

Histology

The earliest change is a proliferation of 'reserve' epithelial cells beneath the columnar mucus-secreting epithelium. This is followed by progressive transformation to a stratified epithelium which is similar to the stratified squamous epithelium of the vagina.

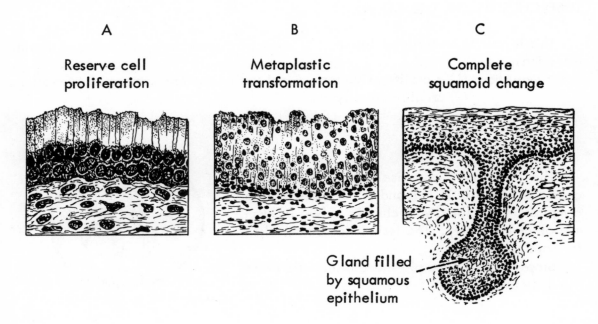

A	B	C
Reserve cell proliferation	Metaplastic transformation	Complete squamoid change

Gland filled by squamous epithelium

DYSPLASIA

2. DYSPLASIA

In a certain number of patients the metaplastic epithelium is 'restless' i.e. active proliferation is constantly observed.

Ultimately the growth becomes disordered or 'dysplastic' and this is thought to be of malign significance.

Clinical Features

There are no distinctive symptoms or signs. Sometimes the change is found in a cervix showing an erosion but in view of the frequency of the latter the association is fortuitous. Leukoplakia may be present and this is of some significance and should alert the observer to the possibility of malignancy. The Schiller test, that is the application of a solution of iodine to the cervix, may be helpful. Normal cervical epithelium stains brown because of its glycogen content. In dysplasia and carcinoma in situ the abnormal epithelium is poor in glycogen and fails to stain. Dysplasia is found during the 3rd and 4th decades of life.

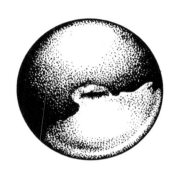

Histology

Stratification of the squamoid epithelium tends to be ill-defined, 'young' cells being found at all levels of the epithelium. Mitotic figures may be present in some of these young cells as well as in the basal layer of epithelium.

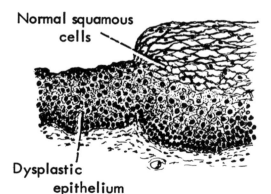

Normal squamous cells

Dysplastic epithelium

The exact significance of dysplasia is unknown. Dysplasia and carcinoma in situ may co-exist in the same cervix suggesting a sequential relationship but in many cases of localised carcinoma in situ there is no evidence of dysplasia in other areas. Nevertheless because of the histological appearance it is regarded as a step on the way to invasive carcinoma and the treatment is as for carcinoma in situ.

3. CARCINOMA IN SITU

This means carcinoma confined to the cervical epithelium and implies lack of stromal invasion. As in dysplasia there are no distinctive symptoms or signs. Erosion or leukoplakia may on occasion be present but frequently the cervix appears normal to the naked eye. Schiller's test is sometimes helpful in alerting suspicion.

Histology

There is complete loss of stratification of the epithelium, the superficial cells being as immature as those in the basal layer. Nuclei are large and hyperchromatic while cytoplasm is reduced in amount, so that the cells are frequently smaller than in normal squamous epithelium. Mitoses may be frequent.

The malignant cells form a thin layer of epithelium which creeps over the cervical surface, dipping down into the crypts and replacing the normal columnar epithelium.

Cytological Examination

This is a useful procedure which is easily carried out at an out-patient gynaecological examination. There are various ways of taking the specimen but the most consistent results are obtained by scraping the cervix with an Ayre's spatula.

A speculum is placed in the vagina so that the cervix is clearly visible. The larger rounded projection of the spatula is placed in the cervical canal and rotated in a complete circle scraping the **squamo-columnar junction**.

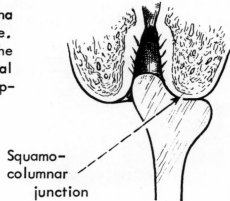

Squamo-
columnar
junction

CARCINOMA IN SITU

Cytological Examination

The material obtained is smeared on slides which are immediately placed in a mixture of equal proportions of 95 per cent ethyl alcohol and ether, for fixation of the cells. The smears are subsequently stained by Papanicolau's method. This consists of three dye solutions (1) haematoxylin, which stains nuclei, (2) orange G and (3) a mixture of Bismark brown, eosin yellowish and light green. The latter two solutions stain the cytoplasm of cells, the more mature cells taking up the orange G and eosin, the less mature cells are stained by light green. Smears from the normal cervix and non-malign lesions show superficial and intermediate squamous cells and frequently some endocervical columnar cells. Inflammation can alter the nuclei and cytoplasm of cells making interpretation difficult and it is frequently advisable to repeat a smear after treatment of the inflammatory process.

Differentiation between dysplasia and carcinoma in situ in smears is extremely difficult and is a matter of experience, the difference in the smears being a matter of degree rather than of quality.

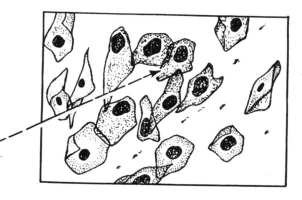

In dysplasia the smears contain a mixture of normal and dyskaryotic cells, the latter having large nuclei with coarse chromatin. The disproportion between cytoplasm and nuclei is not so marked as in carcinoma in situ.

The smear in carcinoma in situ is usually heavily blood stained since the epithelium is easily detached by the spatula exposing the underlying blood vessels. For the same reason the malignant cells tend to occur in clumps. They show a marked disproportion between cytoplasm and nucleus and the chromatin is extremely coarse.

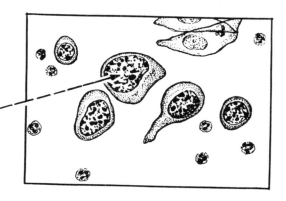

PROGNOSIS IN DYSPLASIA AND CARCINOMA IN SITU

Progress to invasive carcinoma is not inevitable. Some cases treated conservatively have shown regression, but most have resulted in invasion. Growth is relatively slow however, and it would appear that a number of years elapse between the onset of carcinoma in situ and the occurrence of invasion. There is no way of knowing how long the lesion has existed but at least in a proved case of carcinoma in situ, time is available to consider treatment should circumstances warrant delay, e.g. desire for pregnancy.

TREATMENT This varies with the patient and with the attitude of the surgeon.

1. If the patient has completed her family simple hysterectomy is the best treatment. A preliminary cone biopsy could be done to exclude micro-invasion as far as possible; but even if it were present, total hysterectomy is probably an adequate treatment.

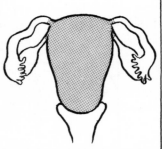

2. 'Radical Treatment' - Total hysterectomy with removal of a cuff of vagina after a ring biopsy of the squamo-columnar junction to exclude invasive carcinoma.

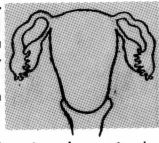

This treatment is based on the maxim that 'cancer is cancer' and one cannot be sure that anything less will remove all the diseased epithelium.

3. If more children are wanted the treatment can be restricted to a full cone biopsy which may eliminate the disease. The patient should be told of the possibility of subsequent abortion and of the need to have a cervical smear examination every year.

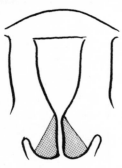

4. If the patient is nulliparous and very anxious for at least one child, a ring biopsy can be taken which excises the squamo-columnar junction but leaves the internal os intact. Cervical smears must be examined every year or more often if necessary.

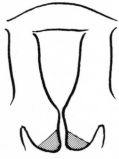

THE POSITIVE SMEAR IN PREGNANCY

Particular difficulty arises when a positive smear is discovered during pregnancy. An opinion may be given as to whether the malignant condition is of an in situ or invasive nature, but this can only be regarded as tentative at the best. Only a biopsy can provide proof. A great deal depends on the stage of the pregnancy. If pregnancy is to continue and a normal delivery achieved, cone biopsy should be avoided. In early pregnancy it is likely to cause abortion and in late pregnancy it may bring on labour and leads to serious haemorrhage. In any case a satisfactory cone biopsy is difficult to achieve. In late pregnancy surgical interference is better delayed until some considerable time after delivery. If anxiety is felt in early pregnancy a ring biopsy of the squamo-columnar junction may be carried out to determine the nature of the lesion. Further treatment will depend on the histological findings.

Microcarcinoma

This is the earliest stage of invasion and can only be diagnosed microscopically. Logically in such a case the treatment should be the same as that for clinical carcinoma of the cervix.

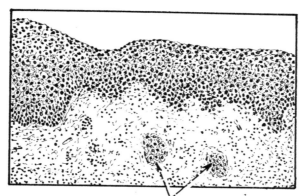

Microcarcinoma. Isolated buds of abnormal epithelium which have invaded the stroma.

CARCINOMA OF THE UTERINE CERVIX

This is the most common malignant tumour of the genital tract.

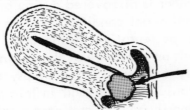 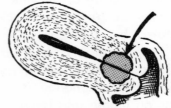

It usually arises in the epithelium of the external os and is called a squamous epithelioma or epidermoid carcinoma.

About one case in twenty arises in the glandular mucosa of the cervical canal and is called an adenocarcinoma.

An endocervical growth is one arising in the cervical canal and may be squamous or glandular: and a glandular growth may begin at the external os. But in most cases the tumour has involved the cervix to such an extent and shows so much variation on histological examination, that it is not possible to be certain of its origin.

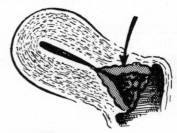

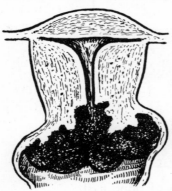 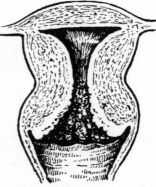

The tumour may form a proliferating growth which protrudes into the vagina – a 'cauliflower', 'exophytic', 'everting' growth. This type bleeds easily and soon becomes ulcerated.

Sometimes the spread is in the substance of the cervix – 'excavating', 'endophytic', 'inverting' growth. The cervix becomes stony hard and enlarged – the 'barrel-shaped' cervix.

HISTOLOGY OF CERVICAL CARCINOMA

<u>Low Power Examination</u>

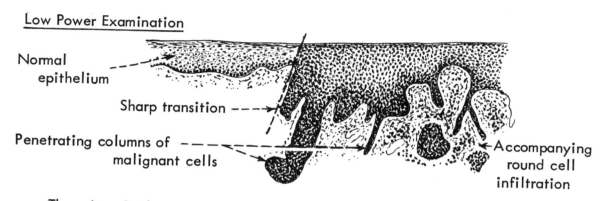

Normal epithelium

Sharp transition - - - →

Penetrating columns of - - - - malignant cells

Accompanying round cell infiltration

There is a fairly sharp transition from normal stratified squamous epithelium to the malignant epithelium. Stratification is lost and columns of malignant cells spread into the underlying connective tissue.

<u>High Power Examination</u>

The rapid cell division produces the increased mitotic activity and cellular denseness seen in all cancers. The cells themselves show varying degrees of meta-plasia and de-differentiation; but three groups are described which may be compared with different layers of cervical epithelium. In most cases however the tumour will exhibit a variety of cell types.

In the spinal cell type the cells are large and plate-like with distinct cell borders, resembling adult squames but with large nuclei.

Spindle cell tumours resemble sarcomata. They vaguely resemble the basal cells of normal squamous epithelium in that they are small and darkly stained with little cytoplasm.

Transitional cells are the commonest type to be → found. They are intermediate in size and superficially give an appearance of uniformity.

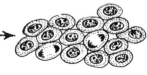

HISTOLOGY OF CERVICAL CARCINOMA

Microscopic Appearances - Adenocarcinoma

This tumour arises from the columnar epithelium of the cervix or cervical glands.

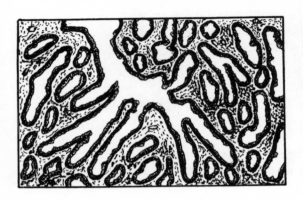

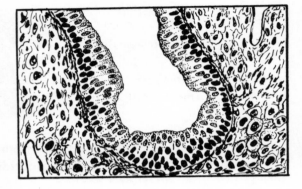

Low Power   Tubular processes spread out from the lumina of the glands. The characteristic pattern is an aggressive adenomatous formation with very little fibrous stroma.

High Power   The cells show the usual malignant features of irregular size and shape and dark-staining nuclei.   The columnar epithelium may show some heaping up of layers.

Many indeterminate patterns are seen on microscopic examination. Sometimes both glandular and squamous malignant cells appear together - adenoacanthoma - and squamous meta-plasia is common.

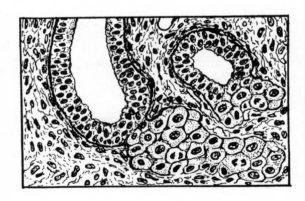

High power appearance of squam-ous epithelium which appears to ori-ginate by metaplasia from columnar epithelium.

AETIOLOGY OF CERVICAL CARCINOMA

One fact is consistently attested to by all investigators: the disease is not found in virgins, or very very seldom. (Rare cases have been reported among nuns.) From this it appears that seminal fluid must be an aetiological factor; and the much higher incidence of the disease among women of the poorest class may be seen as an expression of differing sexual behaviour.

Thus coitus or marriage at an early age is regarded as predisposing: so is parity, especially an early first pregnancy. Male hygiene has also come under suspicion. There is a higher incidence among women married to uncircumcised husbands, (perhaps because of the increase in smegma stored under the prepuce) and cervical cancer is uncommon among Jewesses. It is five times more likely to appear among prostitutes than among the rest of the community.

Cervicitis has for many years been suspected of being in some way premalignant, but this has never been proved. Preinvasive carcinoma is discussed on page 180. The herpes virus has recently been suspected of being carcinogenic.

In clinical practice, it is unusual to encounter a patient with cervical cancer under 40 or over 60, although no age is immune. The woman is nearly always married and has had several children.

Incidence

In the United Kingdom about 16 women per 100,000 develop the disease each year - a total of between two and three thousand. The 'average' gynaecologist might see six cases in a year, so it is a disease more often looked for than found. The incidence varies very much between countries: among South African Bantu it is about 50 per 100,000 while in Israel it is about 6 per 100,000.

SPREAD OF CERVICAL CARCINOMA

<u>Direct spread</u> into related organs usually occurs first

Involvement of the corpus uteri may produce pyometra. Spread into the parametrium produces the signs and symptoms of chronic pelvic inflammation.

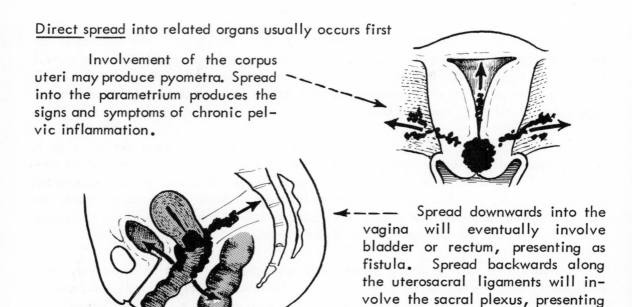

Spread downwards into the vagina will eventually involve bladder or rectum, presenting as fistula. Spread backwards along the uterosacral ligaments will involve the sacral plexus, presenting as sciatic pain.

<u>Lymphatic spread</u> usually follows but may precede direct spread.

The spread is along the network of lymphatic vessels draining the cervix, usually along the paracervical to the external iliac group. Sometimes malignant cells pass backwards to the internal iliac group, and sometimes spread is irregular – for example the pelvic glands may be missed out and there is 'knight's move' involvement of aortic or even neck glands.

Bloodborne dissemination is very rare.

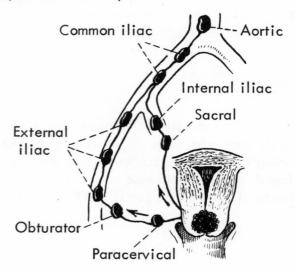

SYMPTOMS OF CERVICAL CARCINOMA

1. <u>Irregular Bleeding</u>, if superimposed on normal menstruation, may be mistaken for menopausal irregularity. <u>Postmenopausal</u> and <u>post-coital</u> bleeding are reported early; but only a minority of such complaints are due to carcinoma.

2. <u>Infection</u>   The growth is soon infected by vaginal organisms, and a foul discharge develops.

<u>Bimanual Examination</u>   Once past the early stage, cervical cancer has a stony hard feeling on palpation, the cervix is fixed by indurated vaginal fornices, and the friable tissue bleeds on touch.

3. <u>Pain</u> is a late symptom, arising when the growth spreads to the pelvic walls and compresses the nerve trunks. Such pain is either local or referred down the thighs.

4. <u>Cachexia</u> is characteristic in advanced cases.   The patient is slightly fevered, shows signs of weight loss and anaemia, and feels ill and frightened. This is a consequence of prolonged infection.

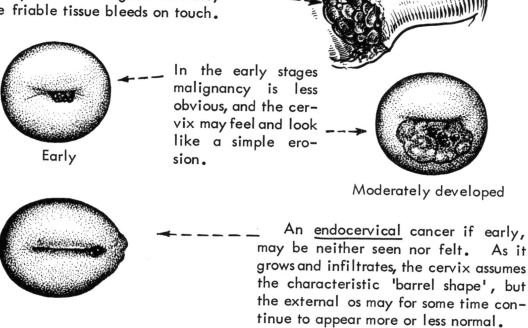

In the early stages malignancy is less obvious, and the cervix may feel and look like a simple erosion.

Early

Moderately developed

An <u>endocervical</u> cancer if early, may be neither seen nor felt.   As it grows and infiltrates, the cervix assumes the characteristic 'barrel shape', but the external os may for some time continue to appear more or less normal.

DIFFERENTIAL DIAGNOSIS OF CERVICAL CARCINOMA

Biopsy is necessary for histological confirmation, but in very few cases is there any doubt. If the growth is early, some normal tissue should be removed as well, and a diagram provided to show the pathologist where the biopsy was taken. It should be no bigger than necessary and cone biopsy is not done in the presence of naked eye evidence of malignant growth. Curettage should also be done if the external os is accessible. (For biopsy techniques see p 175).

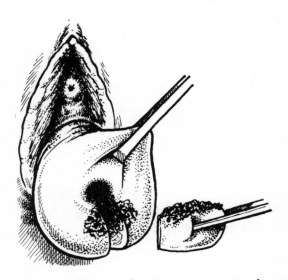

Very occasionally what appears to be a definitely malignant lesion turns out to be benign.

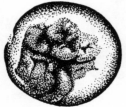

Cervicitis with erosion is the commonest cervical lesion and if florid can be most misleading.

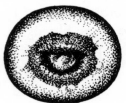

Mucous cervical polyps when infected can present a very suspicious appearance. (But all polyps require examination.)

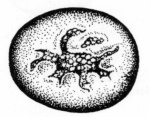

Tuberculosis is rare in the cervix. There is nearly always a history of genital tuberculosis.

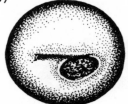

A primary chancre can appear in the cervix: ulcerated hard and indurated. In the United Kingdom it is rare.

CLINICAL STAGING OF CERVICAL CARCINOMA

Each growth is allocated to one of four stages, according to the extent of spread.   This system was first introduced in 1928 to facilitate comparisons between different methods of treatment mainly by irradiation; it has been altered several times, and different centres tend to promulgate their own modifications.   Pre-invasive carcinoma is not staged but is often referred to as 'stage O'.

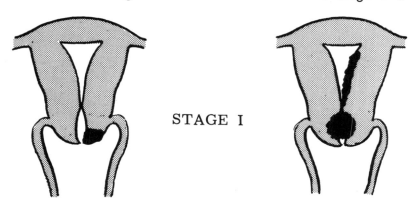

STAGE I

Stage I   The growth is confined to the cervix or uterus. (This includes 'histological finds' not detected clinically.)

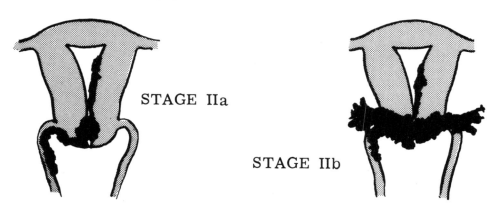

STAGE IIa

STAGE IIb

Stage IIa   Extension to the vagina not beyond the upper two thirds.

Stage IIb   Extension into the parametrium but not as far as the pelvic walls.

CLINICAL STAGING OF CERVICAL CARCINOMA

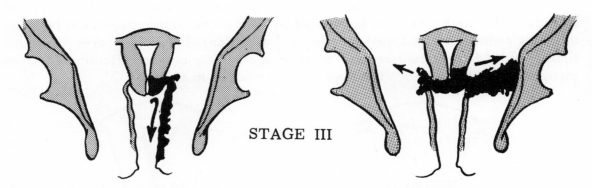

Stage III Extension to lower third of vagina or to pelvic wall.

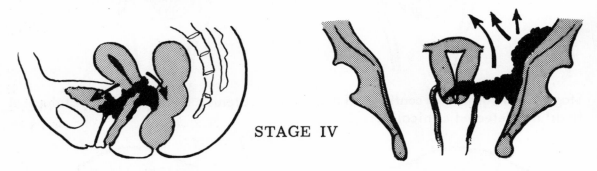

Stage IV Extension through vagina into bladder or rectum or outside pelvis.

Classification is made after vaginal and rectal examination followed by cystoscopy and sigmoidoscopy when indicated, and doubtful cases are placed in the less advanced stage. There are two serious sources of error:

1. It is impossible to distinguish between malignant and inflammatory thickening in an indurated parametrium.

2. Pelvic lymph nodes can be invaded without being enlarged. The incidence of this is put at:

    Stage I, 15%   Stage II, 30%   Stage III, 45%

Surgeons who practice radical surgical treatment tend to classify their cases according to the 'percentage operability' of the total number of patients seen.

TREATMENT OF CERVICAL CARCINOMA

Treatment aimed at cure is by radiotherapy or surgery or some combination of the two. The results seem to be much the same with each method, but radiotherapy is more commonly used.

RADIOTHERAPY

1. Virtually no mortality.

2. Can be applied at any stage of the disease in any patient.

3. Morbidity is decreasing as techniques and apparatus improve.

4. There are specialist radiotherapy units in all main centres.

5. 'Radium cannot get the pelvic glands.' But megavoltage external radiation may do so.

6. Radiotherapy is contraindicated in presence of pelvic abscess.

7. The patient undergoing radiotherapy must nearly always surmise her condition.

8. A few growths are in practice radioresistant.

SURGERY

The mortality rate is in the region of 1 to 3% in the best hands.

Patient must be fit for surgery: the growth must be 'operable' - not fixed to the pelvic wall, not metastatic.

There must always be some interference with ureteric blood supply. The more thorough the clearance the greater the risk of fistula (anything between 1 and 10%).

Only a few gynaecologists are really expert in radical surgery. If it could be made 'a specialty within a specialty' more patients might be treated by surgery.

At the least surgery ensures extirpation of the primary growth and a large part of the drainage area.

Surgery can deal with pelvic abscess at operation.

Surgical patients may be kept in ignorance.

Surgery is the only treatment for radioresistant growths. Surgery may be applicable to some recurrences following radiotherapy.

RESULTS OF TREATMENT

All centres report their results nowadays and 'cure' is usually qualified as 5 year- or 10 year- cure.   The long follow-up that is required slows down the rate at which modifications can be seen to be needed and published results do not necessarily reflect current techniques.   Comparison between surgery and radiotherapy is further clouded by the difference between the radiotherapist's staging, and the surgeon's classification of 'operability' which must depend on his personal judgement once the abdomen is opened.

The following figures may be taken as representing the majority of published experience in this country.   (5 year cure.)

Radiotherapy		Surgery (Combined with radiotherapy)
Stage I	80–90%	Operability rate 50–75%.
II	60–80%	5 year cure rate 70%. This represents a combination of stage I and II growths.
III	20–40%	
IV	negligible	

Over the country as a whole, and taking all stages of the disease, the 5 year cure rate is in the region of 40% irrespective of treatment, a figure which should be improved upon.   Survival depends very much on two factors (assuming competent treatment):-

1. Early diagnosis.

2. Absence of gland involvement.

The first is unfortunately not always a guarantee of the second.

INDICATIONS FOR SURGERY

Because of the availability and relative efficacy of radiotherapy with its very low risk, it has become necessary to justify recourse to surgery.   It can be offered as the sole treatment or as an attempt to improve the results of radiotherapy, but whatever the basis the following conditions should prevail.

1. The gynaecologist must be particularly skilled and experienced in radical surgery and be working in a hospital which supplies high standards of clinical and laboratory support.

2. The patient must be a 'suitable subject' - in good general health, not too fat, not too old.

3. The growth must be 'operable' - not fixed to the pelvic wall.   Operability is finally assessed by the surgeon once the abdomen is opened.

4. The patient should be provided with enough information to allow her to choose between surgery and radiation.   If she is sexually active she should know that radical surgery includes excision of the vagina.

For some patients, an operation of some sort must be done.   These are (a) those in whom the growth has been proved to be radioresistant: and (b) those in whom the growth has invaded the bladder or rectum.

COMBINED RADIOTHERAPY AND SURGERY

There is no completely reliable method of extirpating cancer cells which have passed into the pelvic lymphatics and there is therefore a theoretical advantage to be gained in following radiotherapy with surgery, either a radical hysterectomy and lymphadenectomy, or a lymphadenectomy alone. Some very successful results have been reported; but the survival rates achieved are not so evidently superior as to place combined treatment beyond controversy.

1. The early case does very well with either treatment, and it may be difficult for the gynaecologist to convince both himself and his patient that a mutilating and dangerous operation is going to make more than a statistically marginal difference to her chance of survival.

2. It is known that pelvic glands removed after irradiation often contain apparently unaffected cancer cells; although the primary should be destroyed. A regional lymphadenectomy without hysterectomy does seem a sensible supplementary treatment; but the operation has its risks of haemorrhage and thrombosis and is performed unnecessarily if the glands turn out to be unaffected.

3. Radiotherapy requires a good blood supply to the tumour and tumour bed if it is to have its maximum effect, so the irradiation should be given first. This creates more difficulty for the surgeon who must operate on more fibrotic and avascular tissue with an inevitably greater chance of producing a ureteric fistula. It is usual in this country if combined treatment is being given, to omit the external radiation and operate about 4 weeks after the radium treatment when the increased vascularity has regressed and fibrosis is still minimal.

SCHEME OF TREATMENT OF CERVICAL CARCINOMA

1. It is now accepted that the best results will be obtained if all patients are treated in centres which specialise in the work and are staffed by radiotherapists and gynaecologists working in close co-operation.

2. Since both forms of treatment give equal results in favourable cases, adherence to one or other form becomes a matter of preference or prejudice. In this country the average radiotherapist is more experienced in irradiation techniques than is the average gynaecologist in radical surgery.

Stage I   Radiotherapy.

Stage II   Radiotherapy alone or followed by surgery. (The glands are more likely to be involved.)

Stage III   Radiotherapy alone or followed by surgery.

Stage IV   Radiotherapy alone if distant metastases are present. Pelvic exenteration if bladder or rectum is invaded.

——

CARCINOMA OF THE CERVICAL STUMP

Cervical carcinoma appearing after subtotal hysterectomy is called 'stump carcinoma' and is now a rare occurrence. Its treatment was formerly a subject of controversy; the absent corpus reduced the possible dosage of intracavitary radium, and radical surgery was made more difficult by the pelvic fibrosis and adhesions between bladder, cervical stump and rectum. It is now recognised that treatment by modern radiotherapy offers much the same chance of cure as when the uterus is intact.

X-RAYS

PHYSICAL BASIS OF RADIOTHERAPY

Radiotherapy includes the use of high energy electromagnetic waves to destroy or sterilise cancer cells.   Two types of electromagnetic wave are used, X-rays and gamma rays. They are identical forms of energy but X-rays are obtained artificially by the acceleration of electrons, and gamma rays are emissions from a natural or man-made disintegrating atomic nucleus.

PRODUCTION OF X-RAYS

The device used is an X-ray tube.   In principle this is a vacuum tube with an electrode at either end.

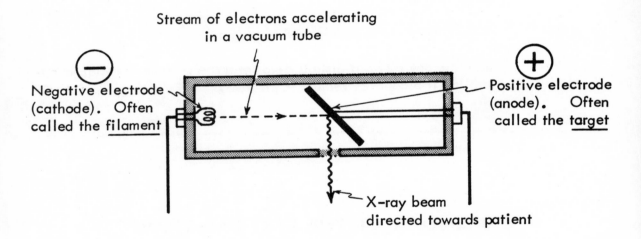

Stream of electrons accelerating in a vacuum tube

Negative electrode (cathode). Often called the filament

Positive electrode (anode).   Often called the target

X-ray beam directed towards patient

The negative electrode, the cathode, is made of a metal filament, usually tungsten.   When this filament is heated by the passage of a low electric current it will, in a vacuum, emit electrons.

The positive electrode, the anode, is a metal plate (the target – often tungsten, gold or platinum) which is maintained at a higher potential than the cathode so that electrons will be attracted (accelerated) towards it.   When these electrons bombard the target atoms, movements of target electrons are produced which cause the emission of energy in the form of X-rays.

X-RAYS

Two types of X-ray are emitted

Characteristic X-rays

(Of characteristic wavelength for each element.) An atom may be thought of as a positively charged nucleus surrounded by a number of electrons in orbit round it. These orbits (or shells) are named K, L, M etc.

The electron in orbit K, nearest the nucleus is more strongly bound to the nucleus than one further away, and is therefore more stable and in a lower state of energy. If an electron is removed from the K shell (by bombardment from cathode electrons) an electron will move from the L shell into its place, from instability to stability, from a higher to a lower state of energy. The surplus energy is discharged as X-rays of characteristic wavelength.

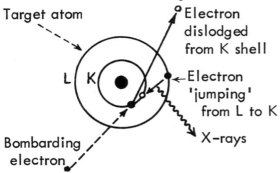

Continuous Spectrum X-rays

These X-rays are emitted continuously as the kinetic energy dissipated by accelerating or decelerating electrons. (Electrons moving at a constant velocity do not emit energy.)

The main contribution is from the deceleration of the electron when it passes near or through the nucleus of a target atom. The course of the electron is deflected and its speed is decelerated by the very powerful electric field of the nucleus.

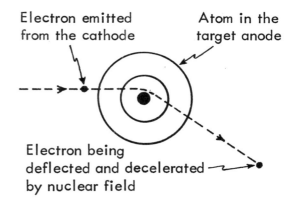

This 'braking' effect on the electron is usually referred to by the German word 'Bremsstrahlung'.

Both braking and characteristic radiation have the same biological effect.

LINEAR ACCELERATOR

TYPES OF X-RAY APPARATUS

'Conventional' X-ray apparatus, using a potential between the electrodes of 200–400KV is now much less used for gynaecological conditions because of the limited capacity of such X-rays for penetrating the skin compared with the high energy X-rays produced by the linear accelerator and the betatron.

The Linear Accelerator

Electrons from the filament are accelerated by the injection into the vacuum tube of electromagnetic waves travelling in the same direction. There is an analogy with a man on a surf board who travels faster and faster as each wave imparts more energy.

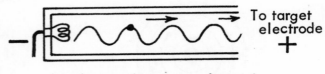

An electron being accelerated by an electromagnetic wave

This gives an acceleration equal to the potential difference of several million volts, and such machines are of practical use in radiotherapy to produce energies of up to 20MeV. (Twenty million electron volts. The electron volt is the work done when an electron is accelerated by a potential of one volt.)

Linear Accelerator

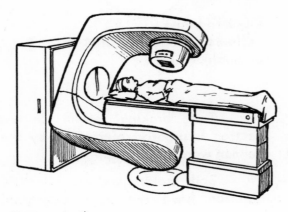

(Sierex Ltd)

Most linear accelerators used in gynaecological work are in the range of 4–6MeV, and although the energy varies directly with the length of the accelerator, modern apparatus is more compact than formerly.

When energies above 20 MeV are required in radiotherapy, a betatron is used.

BETATRON

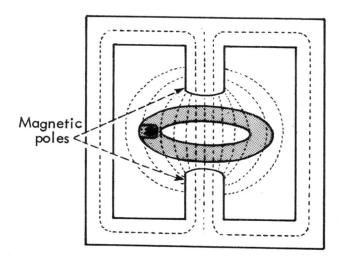

The betatron may be regarded as a machine for accelerating electrons in a spiral instead of along a straight line; so it can be made more compactly than a linear accelerator.

In principle it is a hollow evacuated ring (the 'doughnut') which lies in an electromagnetic field between the poles of a large electromagnet.

Electrons are injected into the doughnut and accelerated by increasing the force of the electromagnetic field.

This field both guides and accelerates the electrons which may make hundreds of thousands of circuits round the doughnut before they reach maximum energy.

They are finally directed to a target electrode and so produce X-radiation.

The 'doughnut' in the electromagnetic field

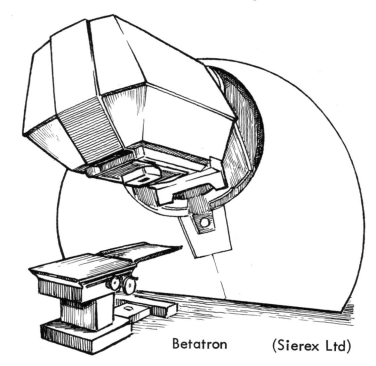

Betatron   (Sierex Ltd)

201

GAMMA RAYS

Gamma Rays

Gamma rays are very short electromagnetic waves emitted by radioactive elements. Radioactivity is due to the disintegration of the atomic nucleus of an unstable element. Each element has its characteristic rate of decay, and each emits one or more of three types of radiation.

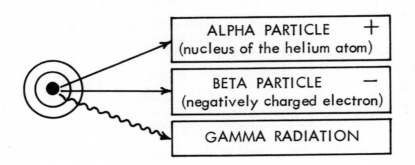

ALPHA PARTICLE   +
(nucleus of the helium atom)

BETA PARTICLE   —
(negatively charged electron)

GAMMA RADIATION

Different elements have different emissions, and those with a high gamma ray activity are most useful in gynaecology.

Alpha Particles

The nucleus is made up of protons carrying a positive charge, and neutrons of slightly greater mass, carrying a neutral charge. These particles move in very complex orbits and also spin on their own axes; and there is a tendency for two opposite-spinning particles to form a pair.

$$N\uparrow \; + \; N\downarrow \longrightarrow N\uparrow \, N\downarrow$$

$$P\uparrow \; + \; P\downarrow \longrightarrow P\uparrow \, P\downarrow$$

The helium nucleus or alpha particle consists of two neutrons and two protons.

$$N\uparrow \, N\downarrow \; + \; P\uparrow \, P\downarrow \quad \text{(atomic weight 4)}$$

which is a very stable grouping

Alpha particles have very little penetrating power and would be stopped by a page of this book. The significance of alpha particle emission is that it reduces the atomic weight and therefore the physical properties of the element; and by reducing the atomic number it changes the nature of the element.

GAMMA RAYS

Beta Particles and Gamma Rays

The symbol for radium is $_{88}Ra^{226}$ which means that the nucleus contains 88 protons – the atomic number – and has an atomic weight of 226, denoting $226-88 = 138$ neutrons. Decay begins with the emission of an alpha particle and a change of element until the gamma-emitting radiums B and C are reached.

Because the neutron has a slightly greater mass than the proton (and therefore more energy) it has a tendency to change into a proton which is a more stable state. When it makes this change it gets rid of its negative charge by emitting an electron (beta particle); and the movement of neutrons and protons causes the emission of energy as gamma rays, very much like the bremsstrahlung phenomenon in the production of X-rays. This increase in the number of protons must of course change the atomic number and the nature of the element.

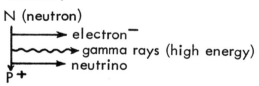

N (neutron)
→ electron⁻
→ gamma rays (high energy)
→ neutrino
P +

(The neutrino is a third particle which at present has no medical significance.)

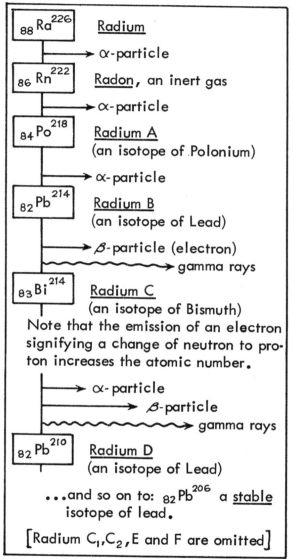

$_{88}Ra^{226}$ Radium
→ α-particle

$_{86}Rn^{222}$ Radon, an inert gas
→ α-particle

$_{84}Po^{218}$ Radium A
(an isotope of Polonium)
→ α-particle

$_{82}Pb^{214}$ Radium B
(an isotope of Lead)
→ β-particle (electron)
→ gamma rays

$_{83}Bi^{214}$ Radium C
(an isotope of Bismuth)

Note that the emission of an electron signifying a change of neutron to proton increases the atomic number.

→ α-particle
→ β-particle
→ gamma rays

$_{82}Pb^{210}$ Radium D
(an isotope of Lead)

...and so on to: $_{82}Pb^{206}$ a stable isotope of lead.

[Radium C_1, C_2, E and F are omitted]

Beta particles have a mass only 1/1800 of protons, but have a velocity approaching that of light. The fastest particles can penetrate 1cm of aluminium and in radiotherapy the tissues are usually shielded from their activity. Gamma rays are the most penetrating of all and the fastest (those with the shortest wavelength) can pass through 15cm of lead.

EFFECTS OF IRRADIATION

Effect of X- and Gamma Rays on Living Tissue

These radiations are used as a means of conveying energy to deep-seated tissues. As they penetrate the body, ionisation occurs and energy is transferred to the liberated electrons. It is these electrons travelling at high speeds which destroy or damage tissue cells in a manner which is still not understood.

Tissue culture experiments suggest that both normal and malignant cells are equally susceptible, but the cell appears to be more vulnerable during mitosis. The actively reproducing and least differentiated cell - bone marrow, spleen, vascular endothelium, intestinal epithelium and fortunately the malignant cell - is often the most easily damaged.

Effect on the Cell

Cell proliferation is immediately inhibited, and the cells either die at once or during the next mitosis. If the dose is not lethal, the cell may differentiate thus becoming sterile.

Importance of Blood Supply

Effect on tumour stroma and tumour bed.

There is at first an inflammatory reaction, and if the dose is very high, there may be widespread necrosis followed by granulation and fibrosis. With usual therapeutic dosage, tissue reorganisation follows, with migration of unaffected cells into the irradiated area, often with complete recovery.

Anoxic cells can withstand a very high level of radiation, and a tumour is more sensitive if its blood supply is not impaired by over-radiation or by previous surgery.

Radiosensitivity and Radioresistance

These are relative descriptions of response to irradiation, and difficult to forecast or demonstrate by cytological examination.

Radiosensitivity

The tumour is destroyed by irradiation, and if it recurs does so in a different part of the body.

Radioresistance

A high dosage is needed to have any effect, and although the growth rate will be slowed down, the tumour will not be completely eradicated.

Various degrees of sensitivity-resistance are met with between these extremes.

RADIOTHERAPY OF CERVICAL CARCINOMA

Cervical carcinoma may spread along the vagina or uterine cavity, or laterally into the parametria, or along the lymphatic system to the lateral pelvic lymph nodes. Such spread is often not detectable by examination; so the whole area must be irradiated. This is best done by using intracavitary sources of radiation placed in the vagina and uterus, and external X-radiation through the skin.

Intracavitary Application

Radium or an artificial isotope is inserted into the uterine cavity and vaginal vault. This should destroy the primary growth and part of any pelvic spread; but the intensity of dosage falls off very quickly; and intracavitary radiation cannot deliver an adequate dose to the lateral pelvis.

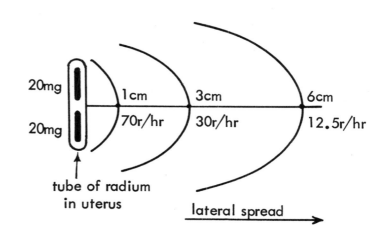

tube of radium
in uterus

lateral spread

'Gammatron'
Cobalt Beam
Applicator

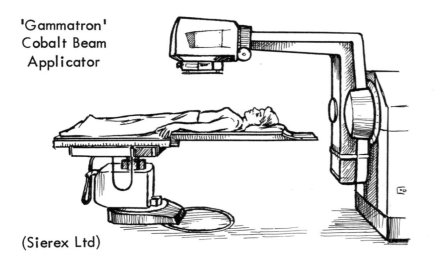

(Sierex Ltd)

External Radiation

This is sometimes called teletherapy. The lateral pelvis is given a series of doses of X-rays usually from a linear accelerator; or gamma rays from a cobalt beam.

205

RADIATION DOSAGE

Distance Factor

The intensity of radiation diminishes inversely as the square of the distance from the source. In the diagram the radiation received by ABCD at 1cm from a point source is so to speak 'diluted' four times when the receiving area is 2cm away. It will be seen that even 1cm of packing placed between radium and tissue, will enormously reduce the dose received.

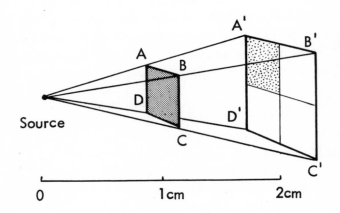

% of radiation transmitted		
through:	γ –rays	β –rays
1mm Silver	95.5	0.04
1mm Platinum	90.5	0.00

Filtration

Beta rays must be filtered out by the screening metal used to contain the radium, and some gamma rays will also be absorbed.

Time Factor and Fractionation of Total Dose

The interval between periods of radiation is ideally the optimum time which allows normal cells but not malignant ones to recover. This fractionation of the total dose is at present based largely on experience.

Röntgens

The röntgen, written 'r', is the administered dose and may be defined as the amount of radiation which produces ionisation carrying one electrostatic unit of electricity in one cubic centimetre of dry air, at normal temperature and pressure.

Rads

The rad (Radiation Absorbed Dose) is the dose absorbed by a particular tissue. It is equal to 100 ergs of energy per gram of tissue.

206

EXTERNAL RADIATION

Metastatic spread to the lateral pelvic lymph nodes can only be determined by surgical biopsy or post-mortem examination. The majority of patients, certainly those with advanced disease are at present treated by radiotherapy; and positive post-mortem findings are not evidence of the existence of metastasis at the time of treatment. Experience suggests that the probability of metastasis increases with the extent of lateral spread; but even growths which appear on examination to be confined to the cervix may have already involved the lateral nodes which are beyond the effective reach of intracavitary radium. Because of this, supplementary X-radiation is nearly always given.

The Lateral Pelvic Nodes

These nodes maintain a more or less constant relationship to the bony pelvis, so that the area which must be irradiated is quite clearly defined.

The use of megavoltage X-rays with great penetrative powers has made it possible to deliver a lethal dose to the deep structures without any major skin reactions at the portals of irradiation.

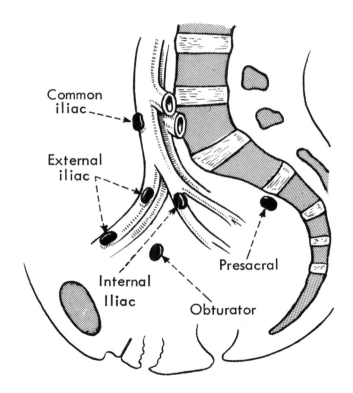

EXTERNAL RADIATION

Treatment is usually through several portals and is designed to give a uniform dose to the whole lateral pelvis. The central pelvis which will already have received a heavy dosage from the intracavitary radium is screened with lead during part or all of this treatment.

Cross section at the level of the cervix. (The black areas show the parts to be irradiated.)

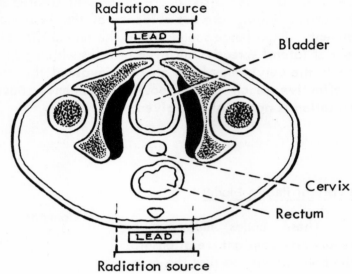

The proportion of external to internal radiation depends on the extent of the local spread and the likelihood of node involvement, but the object is to deliver 5-7000r to the tumour and its field of potential spread over a period of about six weeks. The intracavitary contribution is the more important for a stage I growth, while a stage III growth would receive a higher extracavitary dosage, a part of which might be given first to obtain some local regression in the vagina and simplify internal application.

Intracavitary treatment is essential to control the primary growth but this dosage can be reduced if it is thought that the parametrial spread is better controlled by external radiation.

Some advanced tumours are suitable only for external radiation. Experimental work is at present directed towards treatment entirely by this method, given in an oxygen chamber under 3-4 atmospheres of oxygen to increase radiosensitivity of the anoxic portions of the tumour. Anoxic cells can also be destroyed more easily by neutron irradiation, a technique of the future.

RADIO-ACTIVE ISOTOPES

Radium

Radium, a natural isotope of the uranium series is still the most common source of gamma rays. Its half-life of 1600 years allows it to be used in calculating dosage, as a constant source.

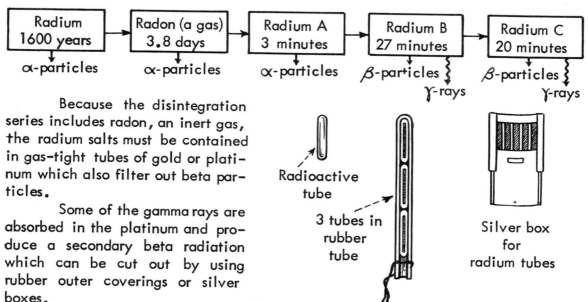

| Radium 1600 years | → | Radon (a gas) 3.8 days | → | Radium A 3 minutes | → | Radium B 27 minutes | → | Radium C 20 minutes |

α-particles   α-particles   α-particles   β-particles } γ-rays   β-particles } γ-rays

Because the disintegration series includes radon, an inert gas, the radium salts must be contained in gas-tight tubes of gold or platinum which also filter out beta particles.

Some of the gamma rays are absorbed in the platinum and produce a secondary beta radiation which can be cut out by using rubber outer coverings or silver boxes.

Radioactive tube

3 tubes in rubber tube

Silver box for radium tubes

Artificial Isotopes

The two gamma-emitters in common use are Cobalt 60 and Caesium 137.

Cobalt 60

This is used for external radiation as a 'cobalt beam' – a cylinder of cobalt about 2 x 2cm, enclosed in a tungsten or lead container. It has the same penetrating power as megavoltage X-rays, but its half-life of 5.25 years requires a monthly dosage correction and of course the material has to be renewed. Cobalt 60 is also available as a ductile wire (55% nickel) which can be inserted into the uterine cavity without the need to disturb the cervix by dilatation.

Caesium 137

This isotope has a half-life of 30 years which makes it more economical than cobalt; but it has a lower gamma-energy with less penetrating power, and its use for external radiation carries a greater risk of injury to skin or bones.

INTRACAVITARY IRRADIATION

Whatever technique is used, certain problems must be faced:-

1. Cervical cancers are not very sensitive tumours and high dosage must be used.

2. The adjacent normal tissues must be protected.   The function of the uterus and ovaries must be sacrificed, but it is often desirable to retain the sexual function of the vagina.   This is destroyed by shrinkage and fibrosis if too high a dosage is given.   In addition the bladder and rectum must be completely protected.

One method of avoiding damage to adjacent structures is to plan the radium dosage with reference to an imaginary point in the pelvis called point A.   (This is the basis of the Manchester method, see page 213).

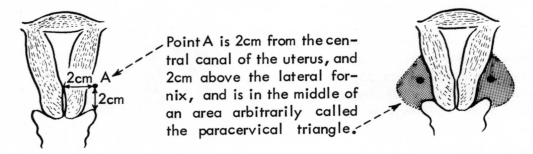

Point A is 2cm from the central canal of the uterus, and 2cm above the lateral fornix, and is in the middle of an area arbitrarily called the paracervical triangle.

Too large a dosage in this very vascular area will cause ischaemia and fibrosis with a risk of subsequent stricture of the ureter.   This is however a very rare complication and the real limiting factor in intracavitary radiation is the sensitivity of the loops of bowel lying in the pelvis.

The size of the tumour and the space available in the uterus and vagina vary from patient to patient.   Sometimes the uterine canal cannot be found because of the invasiveness of the tumour; and the degree of lateral distension of the vaginal vault affects the dosage delivered to the pelvic wall.   The treatment of each patient must therefore be adapted to the conditions found on examination under anaesthesia.

TECHNIQUES OF INTRACAVITARY APPLICATION

The Paris Method

This technique is now more or less obsolete but is still frequently referred to in the literature. It involved the application over long periods of low intensity dosage which was sufficient to sterilise the cancer cells but was well tolerated by the normal tissues. This treatment was continued for five days, the radium being removed daily to allow vaginal douching. This method involved a good deal of handling of radium, and was tedious for the patient.

The radium is in platinum tubes and in the uterus is contained in a rubber tube (the uterine tandem).

The vaginal radium tubes are contained in corks which act as secondary filters.

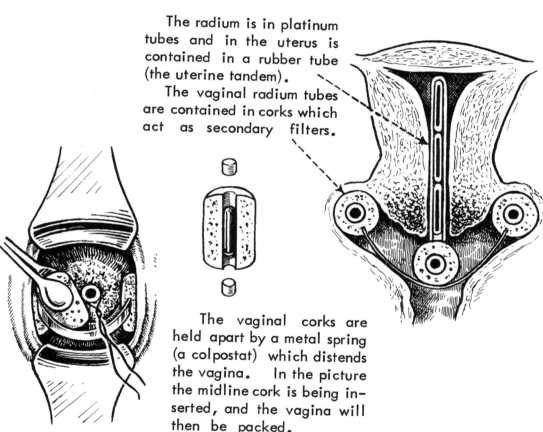

The vaginal corks are held apart by a metal spring (a colpostat) which distends the vagina. In the picture the midline cork is being inserted, and the vagina will then be packed.

THE STOCKHOLM METHOD

This is a system of interrupted dosages of moderately high intensity, such as three twenty-hour treatments at intervals of one and then two weeks. This fractionation of dosage is based partly on the experience of fifty years and partly on the theory that cancer cell death is gradually achieved with successive applications, while the normal tissues recover during the intervals.

The uterine dose is two 25 mg. platinum tubes contained in a rubber tandem. The vaginal applicators are made of silver and are usually flat boxes although various designs and sizes are used for the various situations met with.

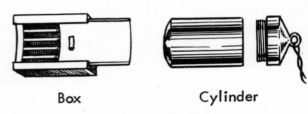

Box   Cylinder

Vaginal Applicators

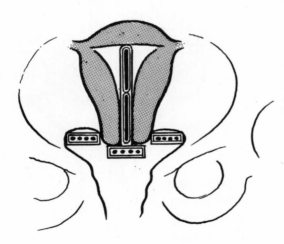

Stockholm application in position. (No packing is shown.)

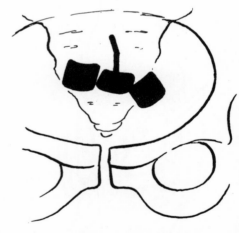

The position of the application is checked by X-ray. In this picture the X-ray beam is at right angles to the cervical canal.

THE MANCHESTER METHOD

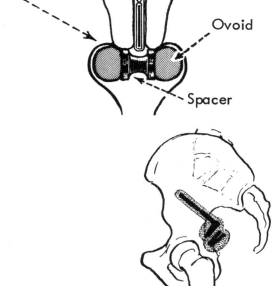

Special vaginal applicators are used called ovoids. The ovoid is a rubber container whose shape follows the isodose curve round a radium tube (p 205) so that the dose from the ovoid is homogeneous round its surface. By varying the amount of radium in the ovoids and the rubber intra-uterine tandem it is possible to estimate by calculation the dose at two reference points - A (see (page 210) and B, which is 5cm lateral to the cervical canal and represents the lateral pelvic nodes. Like the Stockholm method its effectiveness depends on the skill of the radiotherapist.

A Manchester application of radium in position. The ovoids are made in different sizes for different patients and are kept apart by a spacer, a small rubber stud. The dosage is fractionated as for the Stockholm method. The position of the applicators must always be checked by X-ray.

Ovoid

Spacer

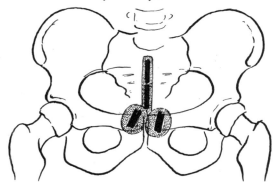

Antero-posterior view of a correct Manchester application.

Lateral view of the same application, shows the degree of anteversion of the uterus not appreciated in the A-P view.

PROTECTION OF NORMAL TISSUE

Whatever the technique used, the operator must make sure that the bladder and bowel are protected and that the radium applicator does not slip. This is achieved by gauze packing and by the use of mechanical colpostats.

Gauze Packing

Once the applicators are in position the vagina is filled with gauze packing. It is particularly important to pack the radium sources up against the tumour and away from the rectum (unless the posterior vaginal wall is invaded). Because of the inverse square law (p 206) one or two cm of packing can change the rectal dose from a potentially dangerous dose to a safe one.

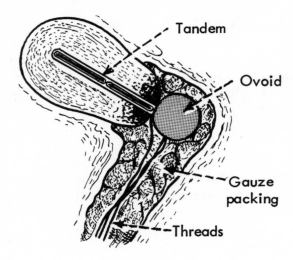

Tandem

Ovoid

Gauze packing

Threads

Colpostats

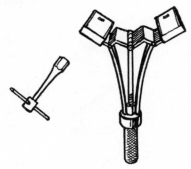

This 'butterfly' pessary can be used to keep boxes in position with the Stockholm method. Packing would be required as well.

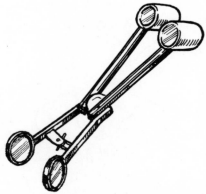

The Fletcher colpostat is a modern design and has been modified to allow after-loading. (See page 216).

DOSAGE TO BLADDER AND RECTUM

As soon as the radium is in place the rectum and bladder are explored by a probe dosimeter, an apparatus which is calibrated in such a way as to indicate the amount of radiation that will be received in röntgens per hour at the position of the point of the probe.

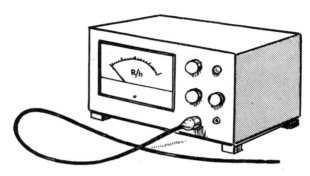

Probe Dosimeter

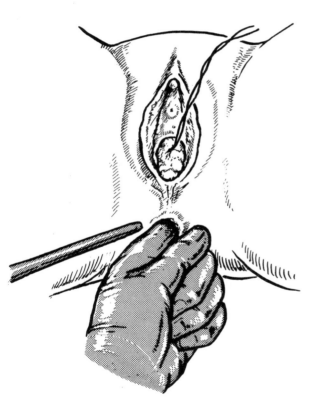

Readings are taken at various points, in the rectum for example at distances up to 10cm from the anal margin. An acceptable reading must depend on the amount of radiation decided on, the time factor, and the degree of involvement of the vaginal wall; but a dose rate of over 40 r/hour would suggest that there was not enough packing between the radium source and the rectum. Bowel is very sensitive to irradiation, and rectal necrosis and fistula are the most notorious complications of this type of radiotherapy, but are becoming rare occurrences as techniques improve. Fistula may also be due to malignant spread; and in a good department the incidence of radiation fistula is about 1 per cent.

AFTERLOADING TECHNIQUE

This means using a special tandem and colpostat which are first of all placed in position in the uterus and vagina and then loaded with radium. The technique has been developed to allow the radiotherapist to take more time and care in inserting and adjusting the applicators without exposing himself to radiation while doing so. It also allows more flexibility in dosage: one applicator can be unloaded, or the amount of radium altered without interrupting treatment.

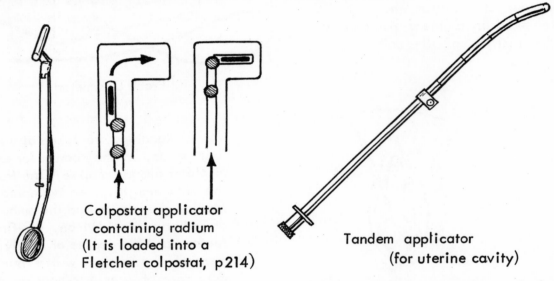

Colpostat applicator
containing radium
(It is loaded into a
Fletcher colpostat, p214)

Tandem applicator
(for uterine cavity)

1. The size and loading of applicators is decided on after examination of the anaesthetised patient.

2. Special micro-dose tubes of radium are loaded into the applicators, (thus 50μg instead of 50mg) and the micro-dose to bladder and rectum ascertained with a special probe dosimeter. The very small quantities of radium involved allow the operator to be as deliberate as he wishes. Position of applicators is checked by X-ray.

3. The micro-dosage tubes are withdrawn and the full dosage ones quickly inserted. This can be done in the ward in the conscious patient. The radium must be transported in a lead container.

PREPARATION FOR RADIOTHERAPY

Physical

1. Any anaemia must be corrected by transfusion. A low haemoglobin level increases the anoxia of the growth and renders it less radiosensitive.

2. Any local infection must be treated. It will be impossible to sterilise a septic fungating growth; and some external whole-pelvis radiation might be given as a preliminary to bring about some regression. Antiseptics and antibiotics both local and systemic may be needed.

3. If a pyosalpinx exists it should be removed surgically and radiation delayed for a week. The presence of sepsis both increases tissue anoxia and endangers the patient's life. The very small mortality associated with radiotherapy is due to sepsis.

4. Renal function should be assessed, and intravenous pyelography performed to exclude any involvement of the ureter.

5. X-ray examination of the bony pelvis and lumbar vertebrae should be carried out to exclude skeletal metastases, although these are rare.

Psychological

'Cancer' is still a fearful word; but the patient receiving radiotherapy is very likely to learn that cancer is her disease, and she should be prepared for this revelation.

The two routes of radiation should be described, and the patient told that she has a growth well within the curative power of modern radiotherapy. She should know what side-effects may occur during treatment, and how long she will be in hospital. Where the sexual function of the vagina is still important, she should be reassured that intercourse will still be feasible, although she will have no more periods.

EARLY COMPLICATIONS OF RADIOTHERAPY

Difficulties During Insertion of Radium

These arise from the variations in size and shape of the fornices and the extent of the tumour. Sometimes the cervical canal cannot be found, or the fornices are so distorted by fibrosis or invasive tissue that the colpostat cannot be properly applied. Technique has to be adapted to the needs of the individual patient, by using different sizes of applicator and by adjusting the dosage and increasing the proportion of external radiation.

Sometimes a fungating tumour will regress after one treatment sufficiently to allow the uterine tandem to be inserted. Dilatation of the canal must sometimes cause a cervical tear into the broad ligament if the growth is extensive; but if the tandem can be correctly placed, treatment should continue.

Pyrexia

Septic areas in a large tumour with a necrotic centre can never be completely eradicated before treatment and intracavitary radium often causes pyrexia. Antibiotic cover must be given, but if the temperature rises above 102° F, or symptoms and signs of peritonitis appear, the radium must be removed.

Sometimes the local infection becomes so purulent and offensive that it is no longer acceptable to the patient and nursing becomes difficult.

Reaction in the Urinary Tract

Some irritation of the bladder base is inevitable and frequency and dysuria may be complained of.

Reaction in the Alimentary Tract

Proctitis - diarrhoea, tenesmus, sometimes bleeding - is common and usually short-lived although it may take several months to disappear completely. Treatment is symptomatic, with chalk and opium mixture and steroid suppositories. The intestines are equally sensitive and their reaction is manifested by nausea and perhaps diarrhoea.

Reaction in the Vagina

A whitish membrane is seen to cover the vaginal epithelium after the first treatment, but this should disappear in about three weeks.

LATE COMPLICATIONS OF RADIOTHERAPY

Genital Tract

Ovarian function is destroyed and some patients may need the temporary support of oestrogens. The uterus ultimately becomes fibrotic, and pyometra sometimes develops. Some degree of vaginal atrophy is usual although often very slight, and subsequent sexual activity depends on the age of the patient and the amount of persistence displayed.

Urinary Tract

Fistula is the result of excessive destruction of blood vessels and inadequate collateral development. The incidence is now less than 1 percent, and fistula if it is going to appear usually does so within 2 years of treatment. Ureteric obstruction due to fibrosis is a very rare complication following intracavitary and external radiation unless there has been severe pelvic infection.

Alimentary Tract

Intestino-vaginal fistula may occur especially if a previous operation has produced adhesions between bowel and the pouch of Douglas. The radiotherapist must assess accurately the dose the bowel will receive, and because of the absence of skin damage with the modern apparatus used for external irradiation, late injury to the small intestine has become more common, although still amounting to less than one half percent. Rectal damage (ulceration, stenosis, fistula) amounts to about 2.4 percent in incidence, with fistula making up 1 percent.

Pelvic Skeleton

The risk of avascular necrosis and spontaneous fracture has become very small since the introduction of megavoltage apparatus. When such injuries were met with following treatment with 2-4KV machines the most common was fracture of the neck of the femur.

Skin Reactions

Surface erythema and ulceration were formerly limiting factors in X-ray dosage, but the high energy X-rays now used are much more penetrating, and skin reactions due to superficial ionisation are now negligible. Sometimes a degree of subcutaneous fibrosis may be observed a year or so after treatment.

RADIOSENSITIVITY AND RADIORESISTANCE

Various methods have been introduced for determining before or during treatment whether a tumour is sensitive or resistant, but none have been universally accepted. At present the only way to find out is to submit the tumour to irradiation and observe the result; and as radiation techniques improve, fewer and fewer tumours are being found resistant. At least two factors are involved.

1. Degree of vascularity. The more anoxic a tumour, the more it is resistant to irradiation.

2. Degree of malignancy i.e. the rapidity of metastasis. On the whole, the less differentiated tumours spread more quickly to lymph nodes. This is far from being an invariable rule, and the reasons for it are not known. Such tumours are reputed to respond quickly to irradiation and to recur quickly.

Some methods of forecasting radiosensitivity that have been used.

Classification of Broders.

Cells are divided according to their degree of 'de-differentiation'. Thus: Grade I, 0 to 25% de-differentiation; Grade II, 25 to 50%; Grade III, 50 to 75% Grade IV, 75 to 100%.

Spindle cells are regarded as the most de-differentiated; and in practice, grades II and III contain 70% of growths.

Serial Biopsy Method of Glucksman and Spear

This is based on differential counts of four types of cell: dividing (mitosis), degenerating, resting, and differentiating. Biopsies are taken before and after treatments, and a favourable response is shown by an increase in the proportion of degenerate and differentiating cells and a fall in dividing and resting cells.

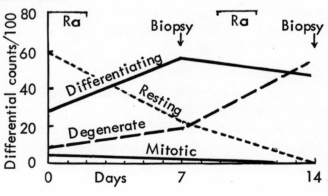

220

OPERATIONS FOR CERVICAL CARCINOMA

The best known consists of removal of the uterus and adnexa, most of the vagina and the fatty-fibrous tissue which 'pads' the pelvis and contains the lymph glands. This is known as the 'Wertheim hysterectomy' (although the original operation of Wertheim (1900) was less extensive).

The broad ligament is opened up and the ureter dissected off uterus and cervix. This is usually made difficult by the presence of inflammation.

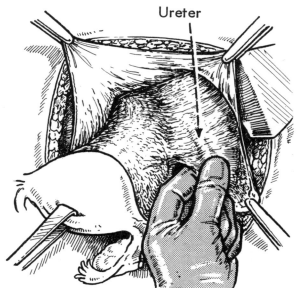

The ureter is being identified by palpation.

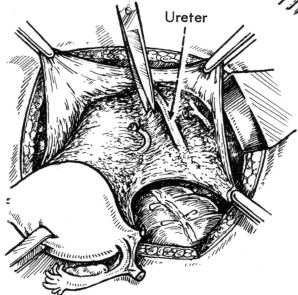

The ureter has been dissected clear down to the bladder and the uterine vessels divided.

The ureter can always be identified in the false pelvis and followed downwards, but dissection in the parametrium is difficult especially if the growth has infiltrated (stage II growth). The ureter has to be mobilised to protect it, but the more thorough the surgeon is, the greater the possibility of damage to the ureter's blood supply and development of fistula due to avascular necrosis.

RADICAL HYSTERECTOMY

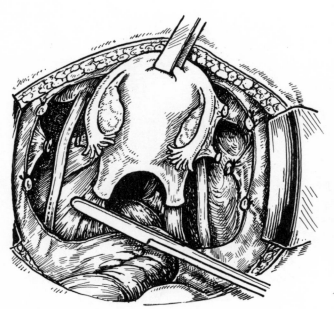

The separation of rectum is made difficult by the presence of inflammation and the depth of the pelvis. The rectal wall may be torn.

There is considerable variation in the distribution of the vessels arising from the internal iliac artery and care must be taken not to interfere with the supply to the rectum.

Rectum is stripped from uterus and vagina and uterosacral ligaments divided.

Venous oozing always complicates the operation, and damage to large veins causes severe haemorrhage. Ligatures tend to tear the thin vessels and blind clamping may damage the ureter or other structure. Pressure with a swab for two or more minutes until coagulation has occurred may be the only method of control.

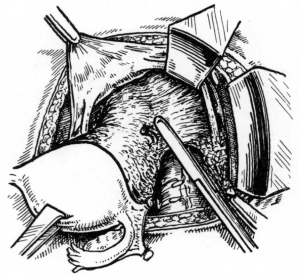

The transverse uterine ligaments are divided.

RADICAL HYSTERECTOMY

The vaginal stump is usually closed, but sometimes a drain is required because of oozing.

In this description the hysterectomy is shown first, to be followed by the lymphadenectomy; but many surgeons carry out a 'block dissection' removing pelvic nodes and fat and then the uterus and vagina all in one piece. The essential end-result is to clear the pelvis down to the muscle fascia, leaving only vessels, nerves and the rectum and bladder.

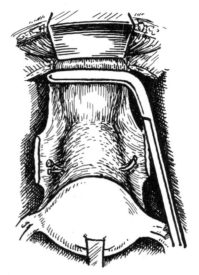

The vagina is severed below the special Wertheim clamp.

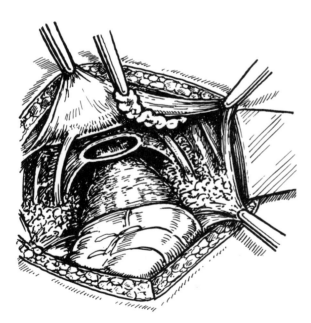

Dissecting out the fatty tissue and glands from the obturator fossa.

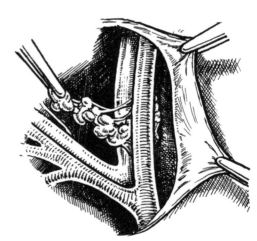

Dissecting out the external iliac glands.
(Other accessible groups of nodes are also removed.)

RADICAL VAGINAL HYSTERECTOMY

An extended vaginal hysterectomy can also be done. It is known as Schauta's operation; and because of its technical difficulties and the impossibility of gland dissection by the vaginal route, it is little practised in this country. Those few surgeons who have experience of it report good results, although not better than abdominal surgery or radiotherapy.

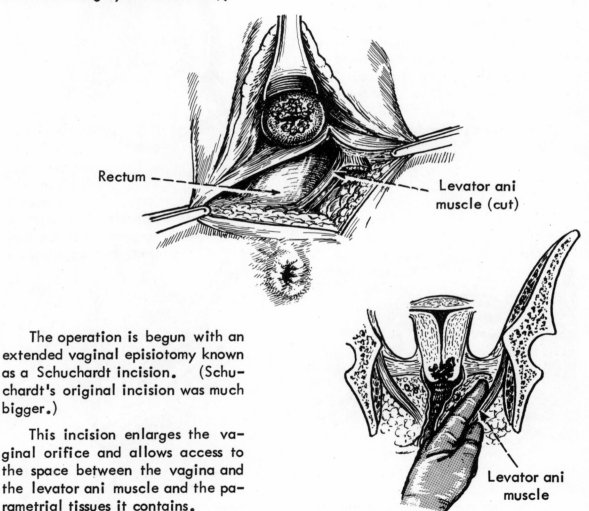

Rectum

Levator ani
muscle (cut)

Levator ani
muscle

The operation is begun with an extended vaginal episiotomy known as a Schuchardt incision. (Schuchardt's original incision was much bigger.)

This incision enlarges the vaginal orifice and allows access to the space between the vagina and the levator ani muscle and the parametrial tissues it contains.

RADICAL VAGINAL HYSTERECTOMY

SCHAUTA'S OPERATION

The object is to remove ovaries, tubes, uterus and vagina through the vulva.

The vagina is circumcised, i.e. a circular incision is made right round the vaginal wall.

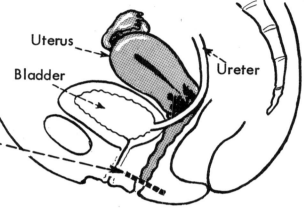

Uterus

Bladder

Ureter

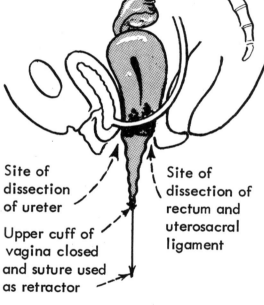

Site of dissection of ureter

Upper cuff of vagina closed and suture used as retractor

Site of dissection of rectum and uterosacral ligament

The upper part of the vagina is closed by sutures (closing off the cancerous cervix) and by traction downwards the areas of the ureteric canal, vesico-ureteric junction and posteriorly, the uterosacral ligaments become available for dissection. This is a difficult surgical exercise and may be accompanied by troublesome haemorrhage.

When the vagina with its contained cervix has been mobilised from bowel, bladder and ureter, the vesico-uterine pouch is opened and the uterine fundus pulled down to expose the adnexal ligaments for division. This allows removal of the whole genital tract other than the lower third of the vagina, and the operation area can now be closed.

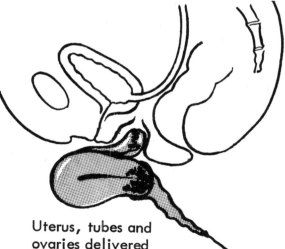

Uterus, tubes and ovaries delivered

PELVIC EXENTERATION

If the bladder or rectum or both are invaded by the growth, these organs can be removed along with the genital tract and pelvic lymph glands.

Anterior Exenteration
The bladder is more often invaded than the rectum. Cystectomy relieves the surgeon of the need for meticulous dissection of the ureters; but the urinary tract must be diverted.

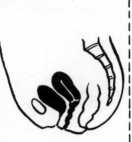

Organs removed

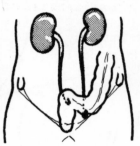

Uretero-colic implantation

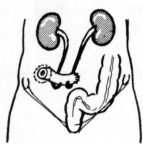

Ileal bladder

Posterior Exenteration
This is the most acceptable to the patient involving only a colostomy, but it is the least often indicated.

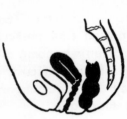

Organs removed

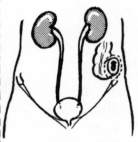

Colostomy

Total Exenteration
This leaves the patient with a colostomy and a urinary tract diversion and is a formidable operation.

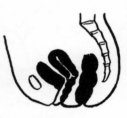

Organs removed

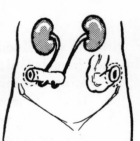

Ileal bladder and colostomy

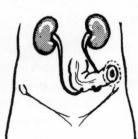

Wet colostomy (undesirable)

PELVIC EXENTERATION

These operations involve a long pelvic dissection, a urinary diversion (usually) and a perineal dissection. Such drastic surgery must be aimed at cure, and a 5 year cure rate of 20% can be achieved. Nevertheless the operation must also be considered for its short-term palliative effects.

The surgeon must be experienced, and the patient must be fit with good renal function, and should understand exactly what is proposed.

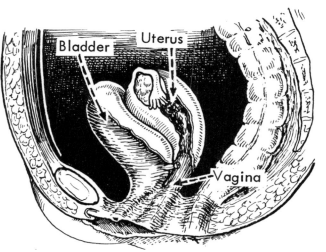

Anterior exenteration

Bladder, uterus and vagina are completely mobilised. The pelvis has been cleared, the urinary tract diverted and the abdomen closed.

The operative mortality is high perhaps in the region of 15%, but this figure will vary with the standard of selection observed by the surgeon.

Alternatives to these severe operations are:

a) In recurrent growths, a further dosage of irradiation may be possible.

b) Urinary and if necessary bowel diversion operations can be carried out and the pelvis treated by irradiation without the need to protect bladder or rectum.

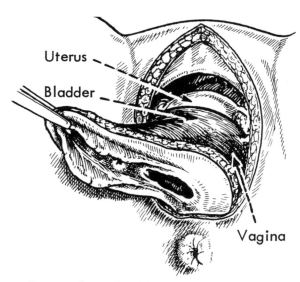

Removal of the bladder and genital tract from below, after the abdominal dissection.

COMBINED ABDOMINO-VAGINAL OPERATION

This operation has been developed by Howkins and may be compared to the abdomino-perineal excision of the rectum. If surgery is to be the treatment, the synchronous operation would be indicated where the vagina was invaded in its lower third by the tumour, or where the obesity of the patient was likely to make abdominal access alone more than usually difficult. Complete removal of the vagina is secured by this technique and the vaginal approach allows more protection for bladder, ureters and rectum in the depths of the pelvis. It is a more extensive operation than the standard Wertheim's hysterectomy and imposes a greater strain on the patient.

PREPARATION FOR RADICAL SURGERY

PHYSICAL

Cardio-respiratory and renal function must be investigated (this will include cystoscopy and intravenous pyelogram) and the existence of distant metastases as far as possible excluded. If urinary diversion is contemplated it is important that the patient has good renal function although some hydronephrosis is acceptable.

MENTAL

The patient and her husband or relatives should understand something of the magnitude of the operation, and if radiotherapy is a reasonable alternative they should be allowed to choose. If the patient is still sexually active she must be told that she will be made incapable of coitus; and if urinary or faecal diversion is required, there should be a full explanation with discussion of the various methods (as between rectal bladder with colostomy and ileal conduit with conservation of the rectum (see page 321).

COMPLICATIONS OF RADICAL SURGERY

OPERATIVE

1. Haemorrhage
There is continual oozing throughout a long dissection, and a large vein may suddenly tear. Pelvic blood vessels are often abnormally distributed.

2. Shock
This results from a long operation, with continual blood loss, fluctuating blood volume, and acidosis. A high standard of anaesthesia is required.

3. Damage to adjacent organs
The presence of malignant or inflamed tissue makes it easy to tear the bladder or rectum when separating them from the vagina. The ureter can be damaged at any point in the pelvis but is at greatest risk near the infundibulopelvic ligament and adjacent to the cervix and vagina. Dissection is extremely difficult if there has been lateral spread of the tumour.

4. Assessment of operability
Sometimes remote or peritoneal metastases are found as soon as the abdomen is opened. On occasion the surgeon will find as the operation progresses that a full clearance is impossible or too dangerous for the patient.

POST OPERATIVE

1. Ureteric fistula

2. Complications of urinary diversion

3. Urinary Retention
The bladder falls down into pelvis allowing stasis and infection to develop. Also bladder tone is inhibited at least for several days. Pyelograms done several months later very often show a still atonic bladder with narrowing of lower ureter from fibrosis and dilatation and hydronephrosis above.

4. Ileus is not uncommon.

5. Obstruction
This is encouraged by the displacement of viscera and the introduction of a colostomy.

6. Sepsis
This gives rise to thrombosis and anaemia.

7. Thrombosis and embolism
These risks are always present with pelvic surgery. Very rarely there may occur thrombosis of a large pelvic artery.

8. Lymphocyst formation
Cystic collections of lymphatic exudate occasionally form in the pelvis, sometimes reaching the size of a 20 week pregnancy and falsely suggesting recurrence. Such collections should be investigated and removed.

PAIN IN ADVANCED CANCER

Pelvic cancer spreads mostly by local invasion to the lateral walls of the pelvis, and up the lymphatic chains in the lumbosacral gutter.

Local invasion involves the sacral plexus and pelvic viscera; lumbar spread involves the lumbar plexus lying in the fibres of the psoas, and the lumbosacral trunk.

By the time the growth has extended to the nerve trunks there is usually lymphoedema and ureteric obstruction as well. Death from renal failure will be near and analgesic drugs the kindest treatment.

The occasion does arise however when some interference with pain fibres is necessary, and the help of a neurosurgeon is sought.

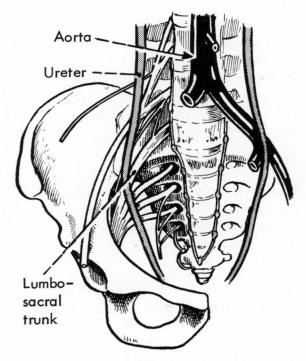

Aorta

Ureter

Lumbo-sacral trunk

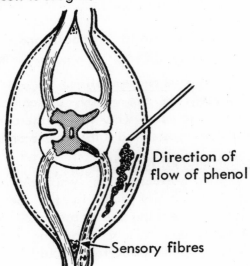

Direction of flow of phenol

Sensory fibres

Intrathecal Injection of Phenol

This is a technique requiring the special skill of the neurologist. The principle is to inject 1-2 ml of phenol in glycerine into the cerebrospinal space with the patient lying on her side in such a position that the phenol gravitates to the posterior roots through which the pain fibres enter the cord. About 3-6 months of relief is obtained. Phenol must be kept away from the sacral nerves supplying the sphincters; and this technique is not suitable for the relief of perineal pain.

PAIN IN ADVANCED CANCER

Antero-lateral Cordotomy

This is the treatment of choice if the pain to be abolished is unilateral.

Fibres entering the cord from the sensory roots cross over within 3 or 4 segments of entering, and dissociation into well-defined tracts occupies at least 5 segments in the thoracic region. Division of antero-lateral fibres at the level T2 will permanently interrupt pain and temperature fibres above the level of spinal integration.

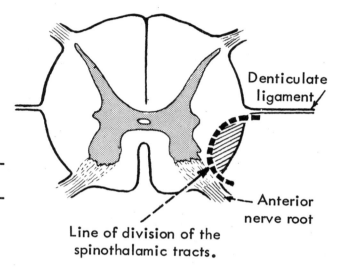

Denticulate ligament

Anterior nerve root

Line of division of the spinothalamic tracts.

There is usually some residual muscle weakness and the patient has a slight limp.   There is also constipation and temporary difficulty in starting micturition.   This operation does not affect the functioning of a colostomy but it is not suitable for patients in whom the ureters have been transplanted.

Bilateral Cordotomy

This is necessary for bilateral pain but carries much more disability. Permanent bladder and bowel dysfunction is the rule and the leg weakness is much more noticeable.

Posterior Rhizotomy (Section of a posterior root)

Three or four roots have to be severed because of overlap, and complete relief of pain is obtained at the expense of function. When proprioception and touch are lost the leg is useless. Paraesthesiae are troublesome and there is a tendency to ulceration, especially if the patient is bedridden.

COLPOSCOPY

Inspection of the genital tract under optical magnification.

The colposcope provides a x20 magnification and has been used principally as a means of detecting pre-invasive carcinoma of the cervix.

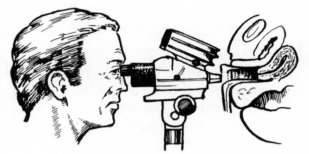

1. Much experience is needed for the interpretation of colposcopic appearances.

2. The number of 'suspicious cervices' amounts to about 1 in 10, most of which prove on biopsy to be benign.

3. The colposcope cannot be relied on to identify every pre-invasive carcinoma; and it cannot be used to inspect the cervical canal.

Colposcopy has been superseded by cervical smear examination as a means of screening large populations, and it is now seldom used in this country. It has been suggested that colposcopy and cervical cytology combined will increase the number of cancers detected.

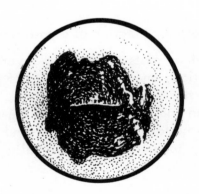

Normal cervix with ectropion

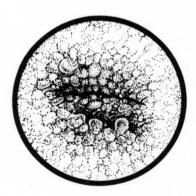

A 'suspicious' appearance

CHAPTER 10
DISEASES OF THE UTERUS

UTERINE POLYPS

ADENOMATOUS OR MUCOUS POLYP

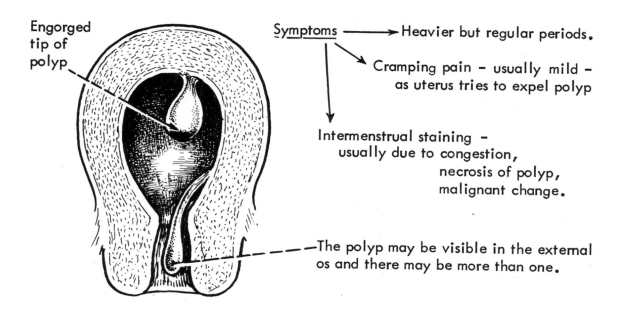

Engorged tip of polyp

Symptoms ——→ Heavier but regular periods.

Cramping pain – usually mild – as uterus tries to expel polyp

Intermenstrual staining – usually due to congestion, necrosis of polyp, malignant change.

—The polyp may be visible in the external os and there may be more than one.

PLACENTAL POLYP

This is due to survival of chorionic tissue on the uterine wall which has built up considerably with accretion of fibrin and debris.

The polyp may cause symptoms remote from the last pregnancy.

Symptoms are associated with increased size of uterine cavity, but intermenstrual bleeding may also occur.

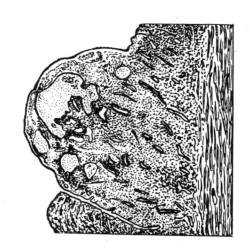

Treatment

All polyps must be removed – either by curettage or avulsion.

FIBROIDS

FIBROIDS (FIBROMYOMATA)

Fibroid is the gynaecological term for a leiomyoma of the uterus.

It is a circumscribed tumour of non-striped muscle with supporting fibrous tissue.

Though not encapsulated it can be shelled out from the uterine muscle.

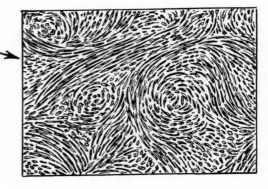

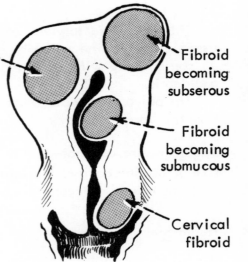

The cut surface is whorled, white and bulges.

Intramural fibroid

Fibroid becoming subserous

Fibroid becoming submucous

Cervical fibroid

Location of the fibroid describes the type.

They are sometimes conglomerate and multiple and vary in size from tiny (millet seed) to several centimetres in diameter.

Some fibroids develop a long pedicle and present as polyps.

FIBROIDS

The fibroid is the commonest tumour found in women (present in 15 to 20%) especially after 35 years of age.

They make the uterus bulky and irregular and enlarge the cavity so that there is a greater area of endometrium to be shed at menstruation. Congestion of the pelvis also increases the tendency to bleed, so periods may be heavy but the cycle is usually regular. The menopause is usually delayed. Fibroids are associated with infertility and nulliparity.

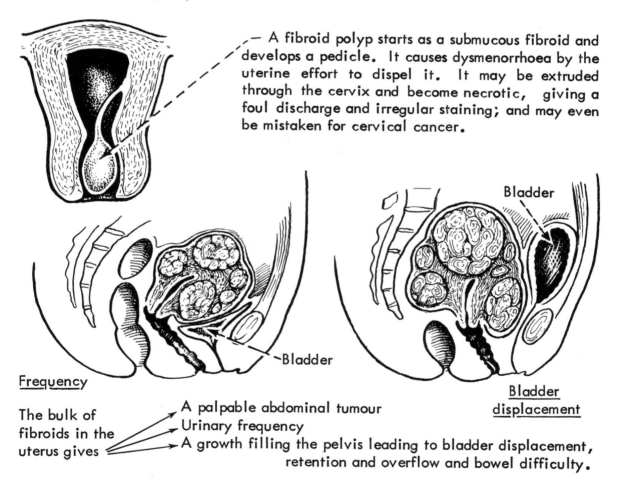

— A fibroid polyp starts as a submucous fibroid and develops a pedicle. It causes dysmenorrhoea by the uterine effort to dispel it. It may be extruded through the cervix and become necrotic, giving a foul discharge and irregular staining; and may even be mistaken for cervical cancer.

Bladder

~Bladder

Bladder
displacement

Frequency

The bulk of
fibroids in the
uterus gives

A palpable abdominal tumour
Urinary frequency
A growth filling the pelvis leading to bladder displacement, retention and overflow and bowel difficulty.

FIBROIDS

The diagnosis of fibroid is made by

1. History of menorrhagia
2. Palpable abdominal tumour
3. Vaginal examination - irregularly enlarged uterus and bulky ovaries (theca lutein cysts are common).

Curettage should be done as carcinoma of the body of the uterus and fibroids are said to be associated.

Fibroids tend to outgrow their blood supply and are subject to forms of degeneration. Necrobiosis (red degeneration) is found in pregnancy and usually only treatment of pain is required. Hyaline, mucoid and cystic degeneration occur and these may lead to calcification (womb stones). Sarcomatous degeneration is exceedingly rare.

Polypoid subserous fibroids may develop torsion of the pedicle and present with acute abdominal symptoms or, if the torsion is chronic, a parasitic tumour may be created (a tumour which has lost its own blood supply and developed a new one through adhesions).

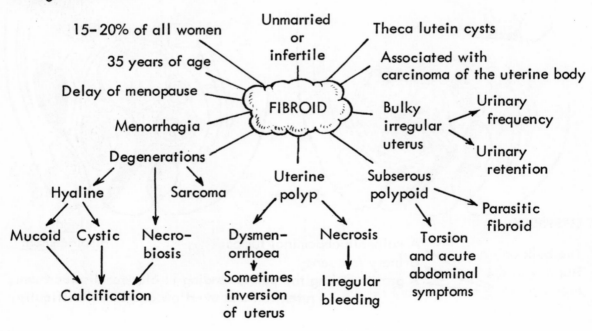

FIBROIDS

Treatment

Small fibroids found without symptoms should be ignored. Larger fibroids and those with symptoms can be dealth with in two ways :-
1. Remove the fibroids and leave the uterus (myomectomy). This is indicated when the patient wishes to keep her uterus.
2. Remove the uterus with the fibroids (hysterectomy).

MYOMECTOMY

The approach to the tumour is made through the anterior uterine wall if possible. The tumour is then shelled out by finger dissection or scalpel handle.

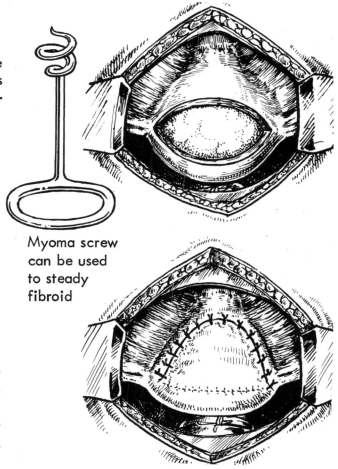

Myoma screw can be used to steady fibroid

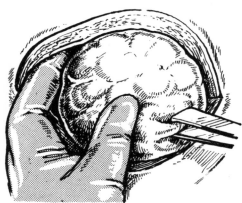

The resultant cavity is obliterated by buried sutures and the uterine wall flapped over to bring the suture line as low on the uterine wall as possible to obviate risk of adhesions.

ADENOMYOSIS

Ectopic endometrium in the uterine wall.

It may be localised resembling a fibroid, giving a firm irregular outline to the uterus; or diffused through a firm bulky uterus.

Blood drains into uterine cavity so "chocolate" cysts are absent but the patient complains of menorrhagia.

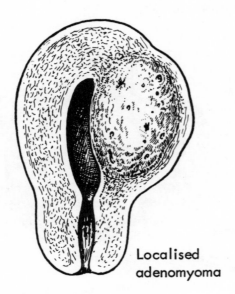

Localised
adenomyoma

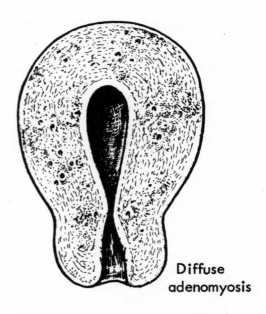

Diffuse
adenomyosis

Treatment

Hysterectomy (the tumour has no capsule).

ENDOMETRIOSIS

Endometrial deposits may appear externally on the uterus causing adhesions to other structures.

CHRONIC INVERSION of the uterus may give impression of tumour (p 259).

MYOHYPERPLASIA or CHRONIC SUBINVOLUTION are names given to a general-ised hypertrophy of the myometrium possibly a response to repeated pregnancies. This is a diagnosis usually made after hysterectomy.

CARCINOMA OF THE ENDOMETRIUM

CARCINOMA OF THE ENDOMETRIUM   (Carcinoma of the Uterine Body)

Malignant change begins in the glandular epithelium of the endometrium.

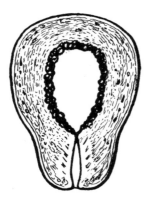

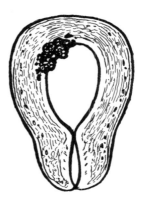

Diffuse Form
   The condition when diagnosed in-volves the whole endometrium.

Localised Form
   The growth begins in one area and tends to develop there both into the muscle and into the cavity, rather than involve the whole endometrium.

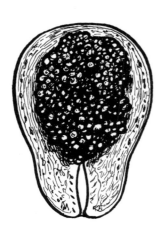

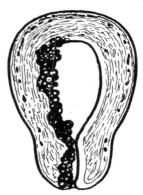

   An advanced growth will fill the whole cavity and may penetrate the muscle. There is a tendency to stop at the internal os, but cervical involvement can occur.

   If the growth invades the cervix, the condition is called carcinoma of body and cervix, and the treatment is as for cervical carcinoma (which is much more radical).

HISTOLOGY OF ENDOMETRIAL CARCINOMA

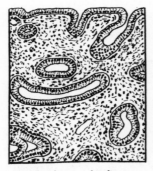

The histological pattern shows a wide variation between the highly differentiated and at the other extreme a tumour so undifferentiated as to resemble a sarcoma. In addition, there is between benign and malignant patterns the condition of 'atypical hyperplasia' – a marked increase of glandular tissue at the expense of stroma, which must be regarded with suspicion.

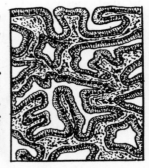

Normal epithelium

'Atypical hyperplasia'

Grade I Adenocarcinoma (Adenoma Malignum: Endometrial carcinoma in situ.)
This is very similar to atypical hyperplasia, but malignant cells are present. The muscle is not invaded.

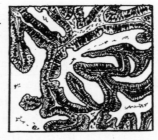

Grade II
Glands are smaller and closely packed, the muscle has been invaded and the appearances are obviously malignant.

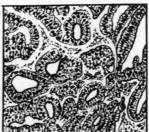

Grade III
Little glandular architecture is visible and the cells are undifferentiated. This is the most malignant type.

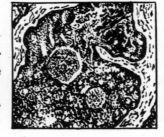

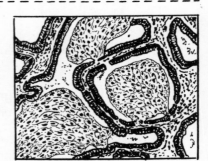

Squamous Metaplasia
(Adenoacanthoma: acantha, a thorn)
Areas of squamous metaplasia may be seen with any grade of malignancy and sometimes make it difficult to identify the origin of a very extensive tumour.

SPREAD OF ENDOMETRIAL CARCINOMA

Corpus cancer spreads less rapidly than cervical cancer probably because the myometrium is a fairly efficient barrier. This fact combined with the lower incidence of anaplastic growths accounts for the better results of treatment.

Local Spread

Slow invasion of the myometrium is the commonest spread. It may produce considerable uterine enlargement; or spread may involve the vaginal vault.

Venous Spread

This pathway might account for the occasional appearance of a low vaginal metastasis; but venous spread is not a common feature of uterine cancer.

Lymphatic Spread

The incidence of this (it is much debated) seems to be somewhere between 10 and 30%. All pelvic glands, including the internal iliacs, the parametrium, the ovaries, and the vagina may be involved, probably with equal frequency. Lymphatic spread is more likely to occur when the tumour is anaplastic and the uterine wall is deeply invaded.

Tubal Spread

Malignant cells can pass along the tube in the same way that peritoneal spill may occur during menstruation. This may account for isolated ovarian metastases.

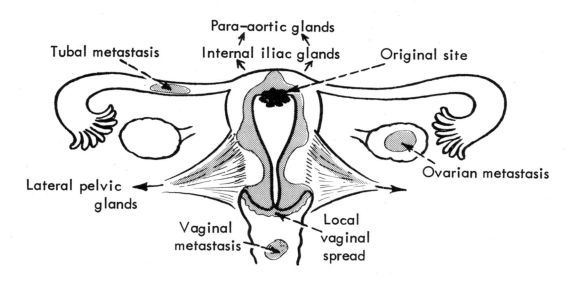

STAGING OF ENDOMETRIAL CARCINOMA

The classification given below is that of the Federation of Gynaecology and Obstetrics (F.I.G.O.) 1961.

Stage O The histological appearances are suggestive of cancer but not conclusive.

Stage I
The growth is confined to the corpus.

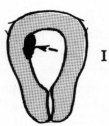

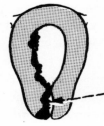

Stage II
The growth has extended to the cervix.

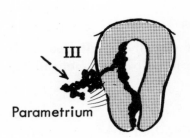

Stage III
The growth has extended beyond the uterus but not outside the pelvis and not into the bladder or rectum.

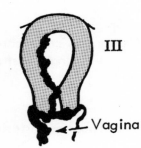

Parametrium

Vagina

Stage IV
The growth has invaded the rectum or bladder or structures beyond the pelvis.

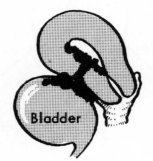

Bladder

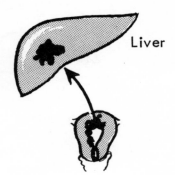

Liver

CLINICAL FEATURES OF ENDOMETRIAL CARCINOMA

AETIOLOGY

This is unknown. There is an association with obesity and diabetes and some abnormality of pituitary secretion is suspected. The disease usually appears after ovarian function has ceased, yet excessive oestrogenic stimulation may play some part since there are also associations with atypical endometrial hyperplasia, the late menopause, and oestrogen-producing tumours of the ovary.

CLINICAL FEATURES

Malignant change is less common in the endometrium than in the cervix; but as it is largely a disease of post-menopausal women (the average age is 55) the relative incidence of endometrial carcinoma is increasing with the ageing of the population.

The presenting symptoms will occasionally include pain or discharge from an ulcerated and purulent growth; but the only constant symptom is irregular bleeding at or after the menopause.

DIAGNOSIS is by examination of curettings. The cytology of the uterine cavity can be examined in the same way as the cervix, but the value of this technique has yet to be assessed.

Fractional Curettage

This is a technique designed to detect early cervical involvement. Its value is doubtful and it is not really feasible except in the earliest stages of the disease.

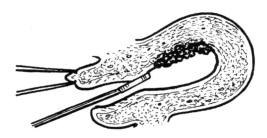

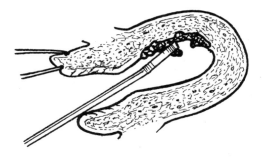

1. A cervical smear is taken, the canal is dilated a little, and curettings taken from the region of the internal os.

2. Dilatation is continued and a larger curette is used to obtain a biopsy from the cavity.

TREATMENT OF ENDOMETRIAL CARCINOMA

This is by a combination of surgery and radiotherapy, and it may be said that there are now two approaches:

Conservative Surgery

This is preceded by a course of intracavitary and intravaginal irradiation. About six weeks later a simple hysterectomy and salpingo-oophorectomy is carried out, with or without removal of a 2cm 'cuff' of vagina.

Radical Surgery

A modified course of intracavitary radiation is given, followed by a radical hysterectomy with removal of as much of the parametrial and vaginal tissue as possible, and also pelvic lymph nodes.

The arguments against radical surgery are:-

1. Even after a simple hysterectomy a 60% 5-year cure rate may be expected, which has compared well with the 40% cure rate for cervical cancer after the most arduous treatment.

2. The patients are on the average 15 years older than those with cervical cancer (the grandmother rather than the mother) and the mortality and morbidity of radical surgery is less acceptable.

3. The incidence of lymph node involvement (10-30%) is lower than in cervical cancer, and the internal iliac nodes which are the least accessible are often the first involved.

4. There is no incontrovertible evidence that radical surgery will improve the overall results.

The trend now is for a more flexible approach. If the growth has extended beyond the uterus, or is anaplastic, megavoltage irradiation is given as well as intracavitary; or surgery more extensive than simple hysterectomy is carried out. If the growth involves the cervix, the treatment is that of carcinoma of the cervix. If the patient is not suitable for surgery, or the growth is too extensive, radiotherapy only is given. By such methods, a 5 year survival rate of up to 75% is being claimed.

TREATMENT OF ENDOMETRIAL CARCINOMA

The following plan of treatment would be generally acceptable.

Intracavitary radium is given, perhaps 50mg for two periods of 24 hours a week apart. This gives the ionising radiations the benefit of a good blood supply which is necessary for the greatest effect.

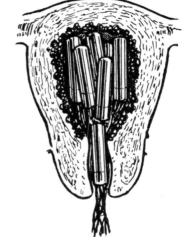

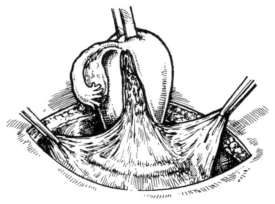

There are various ways of irradiating the vagina. The applicator shown is made of perspex and contains multiple sources, but a single source applicator may be used.

Six weeks later, total hysterectomy and salpingo-oophorectomy are carried out; and if the patient is not too obese a 'cuff' of vagina is removed with the uterus.

It is usual to close the cervix before beginning the operation, either with sutures or by plugging cervix and vagina with gauze soaked in mercuric chloride which kills any malignant cells that may be 'spilt' into the vagina.

Dissection must be carried down to dislodge the ureter from the vagina.

RECURRENCE OF ENDOMETRIAL CARCINOMA

The incidence of recurrence within 5 years is in the region of 30% and is accepted along with the 5 year survival rate as a measure of the effectiveness of the various systems of treatment.

Sites

Local recurrence is the commonest especially in the pelvic walls and vaginal vault; but endometrial carcinoma also recurs outside the pelvis in the para-aortic glands, the lungs, the skeleton, the lower vagina.

Prophylaxis

Pre-operative vaginal irradiation will very much reduce the chance of vaginal recurrence, and some radiotherapists advise pelvic megavoltage treatment as well. The basis of radical surgery is an attempt to clear the pelvis of lymphatic tissue which is not possible; and there is no agreement on whether lymphadenectomy if technically feasible is worth doing except on principle.

Treatment

Modern radiotherapy permits an attempt at cure, especially if the recurrence is restricted to the accessible vagina.

PROGESTERONE

This hormone is used for its anti-oestrogenic effect on the endometrium. Good results are most likely to be achieved in younger women and those with the most highly differentiated growths which are of course less malignant. Treatment must be maintained for about two months before any regression can be looked for and once seen to be effective, the drug must be continued. Histological changes observed are a return to a secretory type of cell, reduction in mitotic activity, and sometimes necrosis of the growth.

Two preparations are available.

Hydroxyprogesterone caproate (Primolut Depot) given intramuscularly, 250mg. twice or thrice a week.

Medroxyprogesterone acetate (Provera) given orally, 100mg. twice a day.

Progesterone in such large doses will produce some nausea and anorexia, but little fluid retention.

SARCOMA OF THE UTERUS

A malignant tumour arising from the connective tissue or muscle of the uterus. This is a rare disease in contrast to the common benign tumour of connective tissue and muscle, the fibromyoma or fibroid.

Clinical Features

The patient is usually over 50 and presents with a complaint of fairly heavy bleeding of recent origin, accompanied by pain. Pelvic examination reveals a large intra-uterine mass with friable tissue palpable through the os. The tumour may originate from the vagina in the younger woman and from the cervix in the child; but these are very rare conditions indeed.

Pathology

Tumour tissue may infiltrate the whole myometrium and fill the uterine cavity (diffuse, infiltrating) or arise from a pedicle (circumscribed type). This type often presents as a cervical or vaginal polyp. If the malignant change originates in a fibromyoma (which is very rare) the sarcomatous area has a yellowish fleshy appearance with areas of necrosis.

Differential Diagnosis

The growth is obviously malignant as a rule, but biopsy is required to distinguish sarcoma from the more common adenocarcinoma.

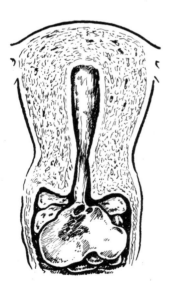

Pelvic examination in this case would suggest a cervical origin.

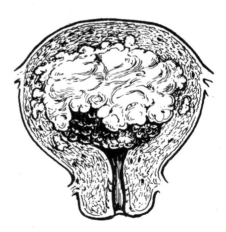

A diffuse infiltrating sarcoma.

SARCOMA OF THE UTERUS

Histological Appearances

The tissues of origin are the connective tissue and muscle of the myometrium or fibromyoma; or the endometrial stroma. These are composed of undifferentiated round- or spindle-celled masses. A special group of sarcomatous growths, the mixed mesodermal tumours, sometimes occur. In children striated muscle is often a feature and a characteristic polypoidal growth occurs – sarcoma botryoides. Later in life carcinoma, sarcoma and various mesodermal tissues such as cartilage may be found.

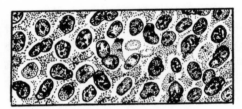

High power appearance of
round cell sarcoma.

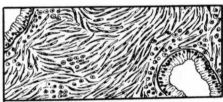

Low power view of spindle-cell sarcoma.

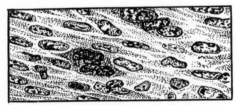

High power view of
smooth muscle sarcoma.

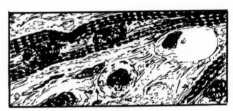

Striated muscle fibre in a mixed
mesodermal tumour.

Treatment

Sarcoma spreads by the blood stream and surgery should be limited to removal of the uterus and ovaries. If there are no remote metastases the patient should then be sent for external radiation.

Prognosis

This depends on the degree of spread and the histological differentiation and is generally poor. Circumscribed and pedunculated growths have a better prognosis than infiltrating ones, and the most hopeful outlook is in the case of a 'histological find' in a fibromyoma thought at operation to be benign.

CHAPTER 11
DISPLACEMENTS OF THE UTERUS

BACKWARD DISPLACEMENTS OF THE UTERUS

An alteration from the normal of the position of the uterus in the pelvis, often with an alteration in the curve of the uterine axis.

Normal Position

The uterus is approximately at right angles to the vagina and has a slight forward curve. This position has long been regarded as offering the best access to sperms at insemination; but it may well have some relation to man's assumption of the upright posture.

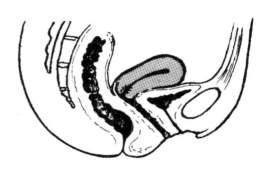

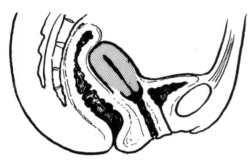

Retroversion

The long axis of the uterus is directed backwards.

Retroposition

The uterus is displaced backwards but the direction of its axis remains the same.

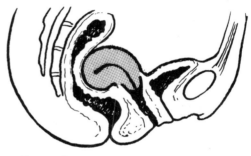

Retroflexion

The uterus is curved backwards. The cervix may remain in the normal position but is usually retroverted.

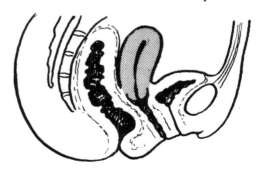

BACKWARD DISPLACEMENTS OF THE UTERUS

Causes of Displacement

'Complicated' displacement is due to the presence of some other condition such as a cyst or fibroid or endometriosis. 'Uncomplicated' displacement where there is no other abnormality, is of unknown aetiology; the uterus in some women appears to take up retro-displacement spontaneously.

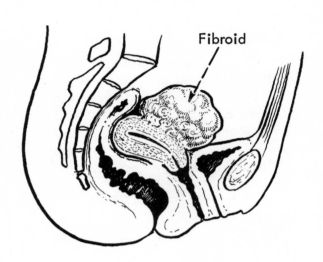

Fibroid

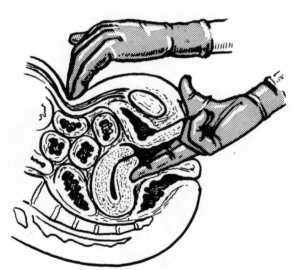

Diagnosis is by bimanual palpation. The vaginal hand palpates a mass in the pouch of Douglas, the abdominal hand detects the absence of a uterine corpus in the expected place. The possibility of tumours and inflammatory masses must be considered; and in fat women the diagnosis can only be made with confidence after an examination under anaesthesia and the careful passage of a sound to determine the direction in which the uterine cavity lies.

SYMPTOMS OF DISPLACEMENT

Consequences of Uncomplicated Displacement

1. Very often none at all. The manifestations of hysteria were classically attributed to movements of the womb round the abdomen; a retroverted uterus is an attractive focussing point for a variety of functional complaints. If a symptomless retroversion is discovered, it should not be mentioned to the patient.

2. If the uterus is not mobile, coitus may be unbearable if the husband's penis thrusts against the retroflexed uterus lying with prolapsed ovaries in the Pouch of Douglas. If such pain occurs it can easily be reproduced by pressing with the examining fingers. It is quite possible for the patient to present with a complaint of dyspareunia and to have a retroverted uterus which has nothing to do with her complaint.

3. Backache
   Dysmenorrhoea
   Menorrhagia

All these complaints are often difficult to explain and if a retroversion is found on examination, it is tempting to claim it as the cause. Very often the three complaints co-exist with a 'flabby' slightly enlarged parous retroverted uterus, a sequel to many pregnancies perhaps with some pelvic infection. In such a situation a 'pessary test' (vide infra) should be tried.

4. Infertility

The retroverted cervix, pointing away from the posterior fornix is said to be at a disadvantage during insemination, but experience with mechanical and barrier methods of contraception suggests that the spermatozoa in a normal ejaculate are capable of overcoming such an obstacle. Many women with retroverted uteri fall pregnant.

TREATMENT OF DISPLACEMENT

This should only be offered if the patient has symptoms.

1. Basculation

This means manual correction of the displacement (Fr. bascule, a cradle). The technique can only be acquired by experience and often an anaesthetic is required.

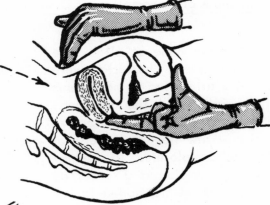

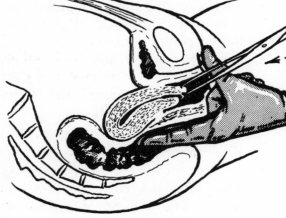

Correction with Forceps

This method may work where basculation fails. The cervix is pulled down by the forceps and the uterus thus dislodged is pushed forward by a finger in the rectum.

Correction with a Dilator

If the uterus is dislodged satisfactorily but cannot be pushed forward by the finger anteversion can sometimes be achieved by inserting a Hegar's dilator and rotating it at the same time as pressure is being applied from the finger.

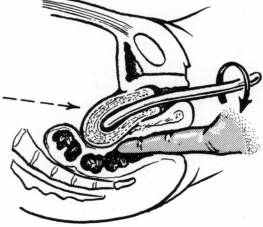

TREATMENT OF DISPLACEMENT

2. Insertion of Hodge Pessary

This is a rigid pessary of bakelite or perspex, oblong in shape and having an 'S' curve. It helps to maintain the anteverted position by pressing on the utero sacral ligaments.

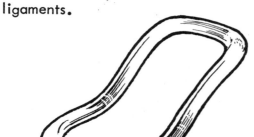

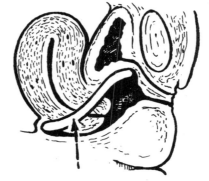

The pessary is kept in for a few weeks and if properly fitted should not interfere with coitus. When it is removed the uterus usually becomes retroverted again but the patient should not be told. If the symptoms have been relieved and only return when the pessary is removed, this constitutes a positive 'pessary test'.

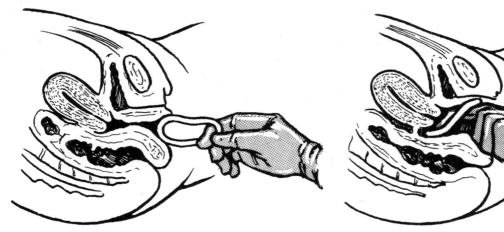

Inserting a Hodge Pessary.

SLING OPERATION ON UTERUS

This is seldom required and indicated only after at least one positive pessary test. Two operations are described both of them making use of the round ligaments to hold the uterus forward. These ligaments have a considerable capacity for stretching and a permanent correction can never be guaranteed.

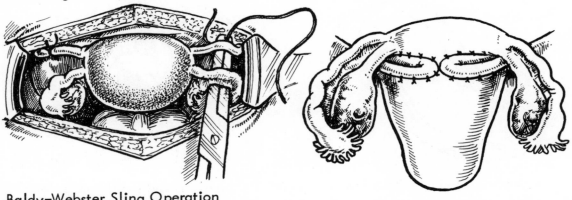

Baldy-Webster Sling Operation

Silk sutures are attached to the round ligaments and pulled back under the fallopian tubes so that the ligaments may be attached to the back of the uterus.

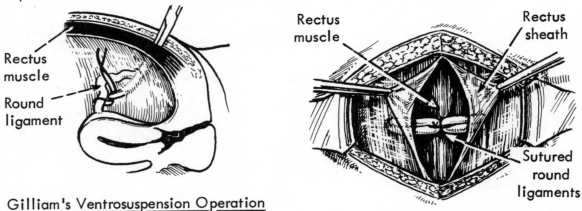

Gilliam's Ventrosuspension Operation

The sutures are attached as before and the loops of round ligament are pulled up through peritoneum and rectus muscle fibres, to be sutured to each other across the recti.

CHRONIC INVERSION OF THE UTERUS

The uterus is turned inside out through the cervix.

Causes of Chronic Inversion

(Acute inversion causing severe shock is an obstetrical problem.)

1. Unnoticed partial inversion after labour progresses to chronic inversion. This is caused by too much fundal pressure and cord traction in an effort to expel the placenta.

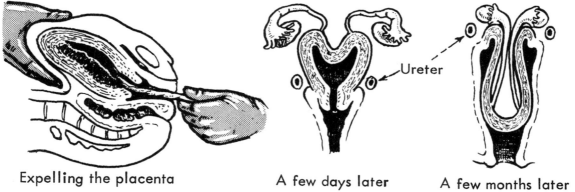

Expelling the placenta   A few days later   A few months later

2. Attempts of the uterus to expel an intracavitary tumour. The tumour is usually a fibromyoma and if the pedicle will not stretch, or if there is no pedicle, inversion develops.

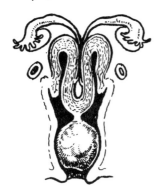

Note the short thick pedicle

If the cervix is also inverted, the vagina will follow, bringing the bladder with it. Note the position of the ureters.

CHRONIC INVERSION

Clinical Features

The patient complains of irregular bleeding and a sensation of 'something coming down'. Examination reveals an infected mass distending the genital canal.

Differential Diagnosis

Inversion should always be thought of. To attempt 'avulsion' of a uterus mistaken for a polyp would kill the patient.

1. The cervix should be palpated above the mass and a sound passed between it and the 'pedicle'. A very short cavity is suspicious.

2. Biopsy specimens should be taken.

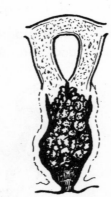

Carcinoma of the cervix

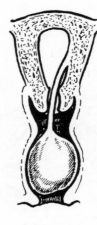

Uterine polyp with a long pedicle

3. Bimanual palpation (recto-abdominal if the vaginal mass is large) will reveal in a thin woman a hard ring where the uterine body should be. There may be a large tumour with no pedicle, masking a degree of inversion, and examination under anaesthesia is always necessary.

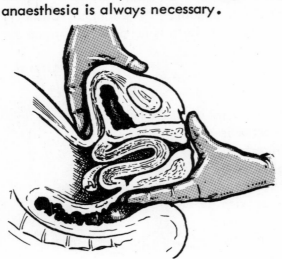

In this patient, the inversion behind the fibromyoma was not diagnosed with certainty until laparotomy.

Ureter

260

CHRONIC INVERSION

<u>Treatment</u>

Surgical correction of the inversion is best done by the abdominal route (Haultain's operation).

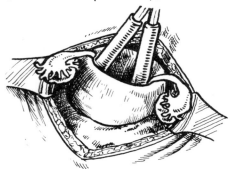

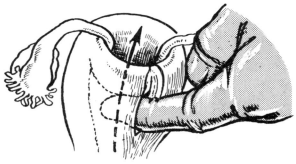

The constricting cervical ring is stretched.

The ring is divided and a finger passed into the vagina hooks up the inverted uterus.

Sometimes this correction may be prevented by the presence of a large tumour, unyielding or adherent tissues. In such cases subtotal hysterectomy should be done. The position of the ureters may be disturbed and they should if possible be identified. The 'upside down' anatomy makes the operating field unfamiliar.

<u>Pessary Treatment</u>

If the patient is unfit for surgery Aveling's repositor may be used. The plastic cup is applied to the inverted fundus and the rubber bands exert continuous upward pressure.

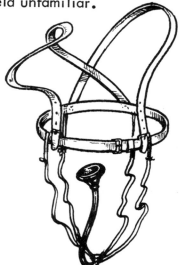

1. Fibrosis and infection should be treated with a week's course of oestrogen and antiseptic creams.
2. The repositor is painful in action and analgesics are required. Two attempts may be necessary.
3. The repositor must be removed before correction is complete lest it be trapped inside the uterus.

UTEROVAGINAL PROLAPSE

Herniation of the genital tract through the pelvic diaphragm.

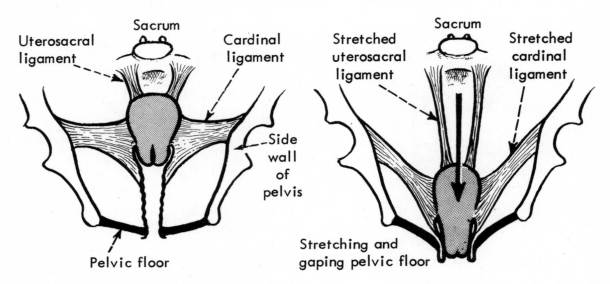

The uterus and vagina are held in the pelvis by the cardinal and utero-sacral ligaments and by the pelvic floor musculature, mainly the levatores ani.

When these ligaments and muscles become ineffective, the uterus and vagina descend (prolapse) through the gap between the muscles.

The Causes of Prolapse are:

1. The stretching of muscle and fibrous tissue which occurs with repeated child-birth.

2. Increased intra-abdominal pressure (as in fat women with chronic coughs) and in women who undertake heavy industrial work.

3. A constitutional predisposition to stretching of the ligaments as a response pre-sumably to years in the erect position. (Thus nulliparous women can develop prolapse: cf. the constitutional factor in the development of varicose veins.)

UTEROVAGINAL PROLAPSE

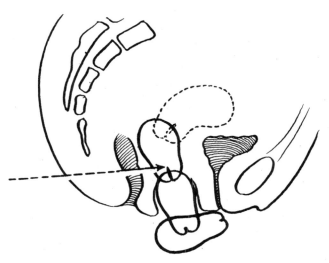

The uterus gradually descends in the axis of the vagina taking the vaginal wall with it. It may present clinically at any level, but is usually classified as one of three degrees.

<u>First degree</u>: cervix still inside vagina.

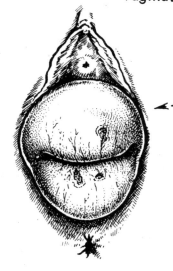

<u>Second degree</u>: the cervix appears outside the vulva. The cervical lips become congested and ulcerated.

<u>Third degree</u>: complete prolapse. In the picture the uterus is retroflexed, and the outline of bladder can be seen. There may be a rectal prolapse as well. This is sometimes called complete procidentia. (Procidentia means 'the parts of the body falling out of place'.)

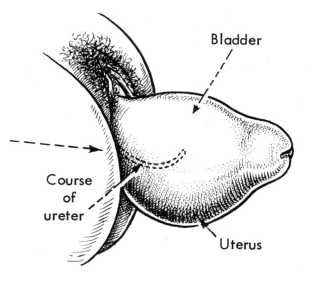

Bladder

Course of ureter

Uterus

CERVICOVAGINAL PROLAPSE

The prolapse is confined to the vaginal walls and related viscera. The cervix often prolapses because of elongation of the supravaginal cervix, but the uterus stays in the pelvis.

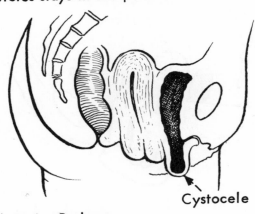

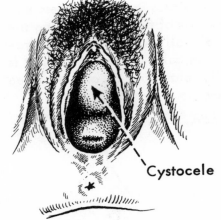

Cystocele

Cystocele

Anterior Prolapse

When the upper part of the anterior wall prolapses, there is an underlying failure of the investing fascia, and the bladder base also descends. This is called a cystocele.

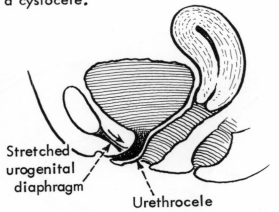

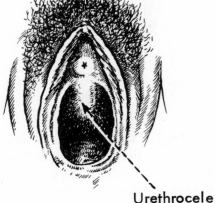

Stretched urogenital diaphragm

Urethrocele

Urethrocele

Sometimes the lower part of the vaginal wall prolapses and the urethra also descends. This is called a urethrocele and indicates stretching of the urogenital diaphragm which holds the urethra to the pubic bone.

PROLAPSE OF THE POSTERIOR WALL

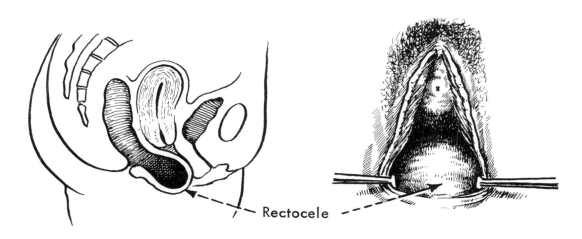

— Rectocele —

If the prolapse is at the level of the middle third of the vagina, the recto-vaginal septum is often involved and rectum prolapses with vaginal wall. This is called a rectocele. If the lowest part of the vagina prolapses, the perineal body is involved rather than the rectum.

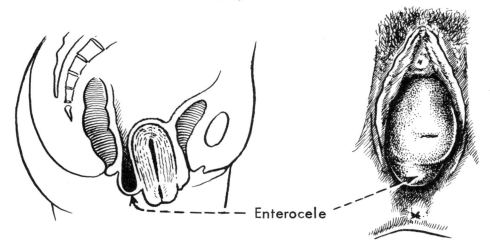

— Enterocele —

If the upper part of the posterior vaginal wall prolapses, the Pouch of Douglas is elongated and small bowel or omentum may descend. This is called an enterocele. Enterocele is usually associated with uterine prolapse, as in the picture, and is sometimes called 'vault prolapse' or 'hernia of the Pouch of Douglas'.

CERVICAL PROLAPSE

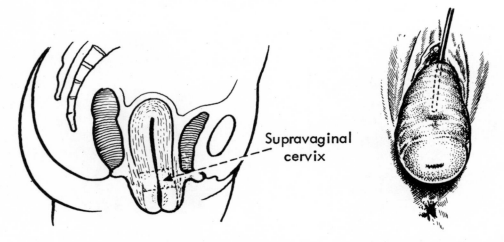

Supravaginal cervix

Most vaginal prolapse is associated with some degree of cervical descent, even though there is no uterine prolapse. This is due to elongation of the supravaginal cervix and may be so marked as to suggest uterine prolapse: but the uterus stays in the pelvis.

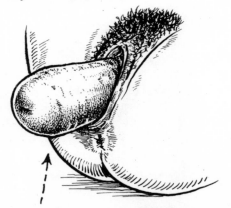

NULLIPAROUS UTERINE PROLAPSE is due to failure of the cardinal ligaments. The vaginal wall prolapses as well but there is no cystocele or rectocele. This prolapse is sometimes called 'vault' prolapse, confusing it with enterocele.

Diagnosis of Prolapse

This is most accurately made when the patient is anaesthetised. Prolapse of any kind is often not apparent until the woman has been walking about for some time, and the surgeon confirms the diagnosis only when he can apply traction with a volsellum. An enterocele sometimes cannot be identified until after the start of the operation.

CHANGES FOLLOWING PROLAPSE

In chronic prolapse the vaginal rugae are smoothed out and the epithelium becomes thickened and keratinised. Ulceration appears, partly from friction of clothes etc. and partly from congestion (cf. varicose ulcers). Reduction of the prolapse may require a period of rest in bed with glycerine dressings to reduce oedema. But true incarceration is very rare.

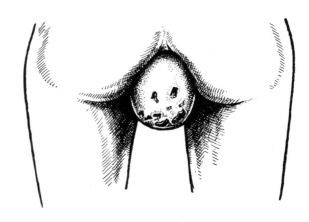

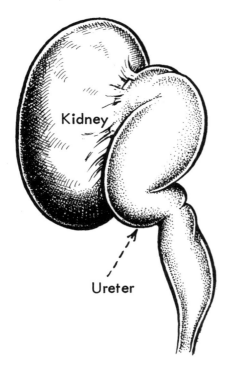

Changes in Urinary Tract

When cystocele is present, bladder emptying tends to be incomplete, causing hypertrophy. The intramural ureters may also be distorted, leading to reflux and ultimately hydronephrosis and dilatation of ureters. Infection is inevitable, and the renal infection is responsible for the hypertension and raised blood urea levels which are common in women with prolapse.

CLINICAL FEATURES OF PROLAPSE

The common complaints are:

1. 'Something coming down' when the patient is on her feet. The sensation is not there when she lies down.

2. A 'bearing down' sensation, analogous to the parturient woman's desire to push. This is probably caused by pelvic venous congestion, and pressure from the abdominal contents on an inadequate pelvic floor.

3. Backache. This is often due simply to the patient being overweight.

4. Increased frequency of micturition. This is at first due to incomplete emptying, but sooner or later is aggravated by cystitis.

5. Stress Incontinence.
This is by no means always present. Sometimes it is found that reduction of the prolapse causes stress incontinence.

6. Difficulty in voiding urine and defaecating. The patient may find that it is impossible to initiate micturition except by pushing up the cystocele with her finger. In the same way the rectocele must be pushed back to allow emptying of the rectum.

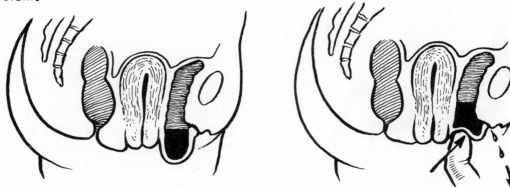

The onset may be gradual or quite sudden and is commoner after the menopause when the genital tract tissues begin to atrophy. Women tend to put off complaints of prolapse until they find their movements really inhibited, and their domestic duties have lightened sufficiently to allow them to spend some time in hospital.

DIFFERENTIAL DIAGNOSIS OF PROLAPSE

Prolapse may be complained of without being present, and not too much reliance may be placed on the history. The discomfort of senile vaginitis may suggest prolapse to the patient; or she is simply too fat and is feeling her weight at the most dependent part. The following conditions resemble prolapse on superficial examination.

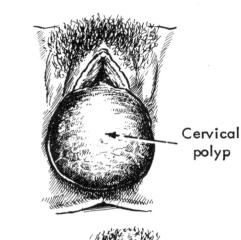

Cervical polyp

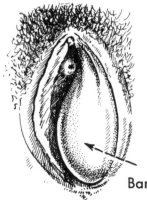

Cyst of Bartholin's gland

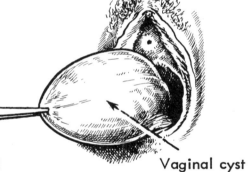

Vaginal cyst

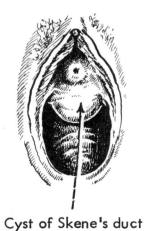

Cyst of Skene's duct

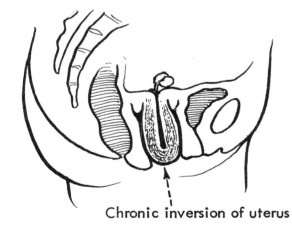

Chronic inversion of uterus

PESSARY TREATMENT

A ring pessary, usually of semi-rigid plastic is inserted into the vagina and so distends the vaginal walls that they cannot prolapse through the introitus.

The pessary is compressed into a long ovoid shape, lubricated and gently pushed into the vagina, where it resumes its circular shape and takes up a position in the coronal plane. It must not be too tight; and correct fitting is learnt by experience.

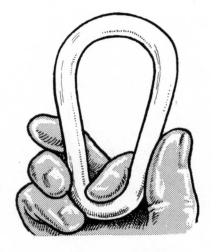

INDICATIONS for Pessary Treatment

1. The patient prefers a pessary. Pelvic surgery with its unavoidable risks should only be applied to a willing patient.

2. The prolapse is amenable to pessary support. If the perineal muscles are very deficient they will not hold a pessary. If too big a ring is required, the vaginal wall or cervix will prolapse through it.

3. The patient is not fit for surgery.

4. The patient wishes to delay operation temporarily (for example another pregnancy is anticipated).

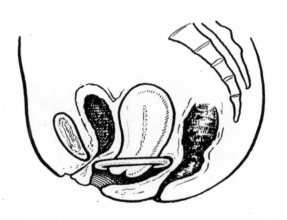

The pessary has acquired a bad reputation as a 'dirty thing' because of the profuse purulent discharge caused by rubber rings. This does not occur with plastic pessaries. The chief disadvantage is the need to change the ring every 4 or 6 months. An ill-fitting pessary can cause discomfort, constipation, dyspareunia and dysuria. If too tight or left in too long, vaginal ulceration will occur, and malignant change has been reported. If the pessary is properly fitted the patient should be unconscious of its presence and it should not interfere with intercourse.

PESSARY TREATMENT

TYPES OF PESSARY

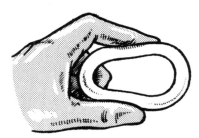 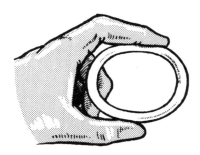 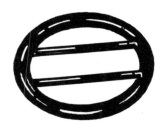

The semi-soft vinyl ring, useful when there is senile shrinkage of the introitus, making insertion of a big enough ring difficult. Vinyl rings also come out easily.

The semi-rigid poly-thene ring. This is the best pessary and goes in easily but may be difficult to extract.

The rigid bakelite pessary with bars is used to prevent a large pro-lapse from herniating through the ring; but the pelvic floor is usu-ally too stretched to re-tain it.

The stem pessary

This is used when the vaginal introitus is too slack to contain a ring pessary and the patient is too frail to stand operation. Such a pessary restricts move-ment and must be cleaned every day; but it may help to keep an old woman ambulant.

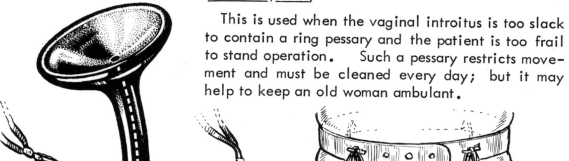

ANTERIOR COLPORRHAPHY
(AND REPAIR OF CYSTOCELE)

Surgical restoration of the normal anatomy is the best treatment. Reconstitution of the fibrous 'scaffolding' of the pelvic organs allows the musculature to function efficiently, provided it is not itself too fibrotic from prolonged stretching.

Cystocele, rectocele and vaginal wall prolapse are dealt with by anterior and posterior colporrhaphy. Uterine prolapse calls for shortening of the cardinal and uterosacral ligaments. Each 'repair' must be adapted to the extent of the prolapse, and perineal repair is often required as well.

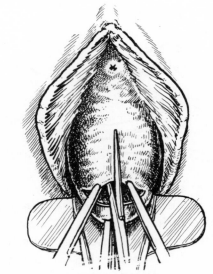

ANTERIOR REPAIR 1. Opening up the anterior vaginal wall.

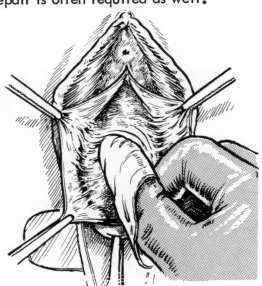

2. Mobilising cystocele from vaginal walls.

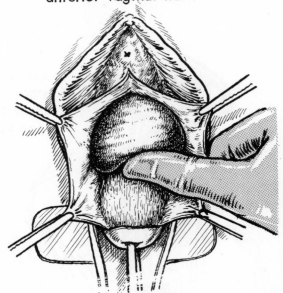

3. Mobilising cystocele from cervix.

ANTERIOR COLPORRHAPHY
(AND REPAIR OF CYSTOCELE)

The next step is obliteration of the cystocele protrusion by tightening the fascial layer between it and the vaginal wall, a layer which is often very difficult to identify. It has various names - pubovesical fascia, pubocervical ligaments (equating them with an anterior continuation of the transverse cervical ligaments) even fascia of Denonvillier. In practice, the bladder has a fascial envelope which can be used for the purpose.

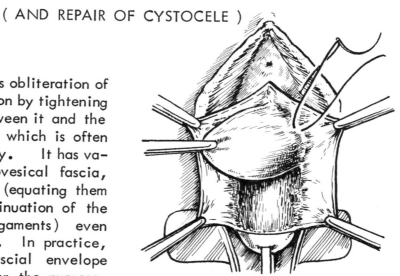

4. Placing the tightening suture as far laterally as possible.

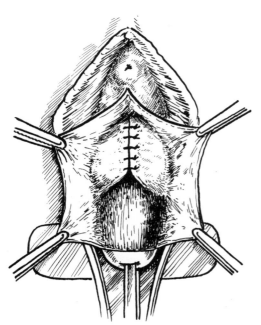

5. Obliteration of the cystocele completed.

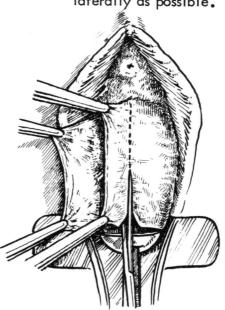

6. Removing redundant vaginal wall. This is followed by closure with a continuous catgut suture.

REPAIR OF UTERINE PROLAPSE

This involves at the least some shortening of the transverse cervical ligaments and usually amputation of the elongated supravaginal cervix. It is often done in conjunction with anterior and posterior repairs – the so-called Manchester or Donald–Fothergill operation – but only the operation for uterine prolapse would be required in, for example, nulliparous prolapse.

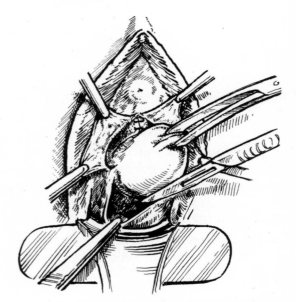

1. The cystocele has been repaired. The cervix is being stripped of vaginal wall.

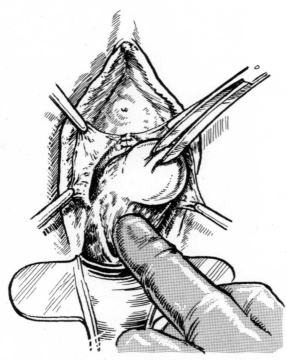

2. Posterior vaginal wall being stripped back.

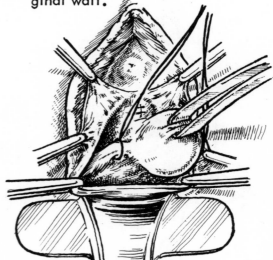

3. Elongated transverse cervical and uterosacral ligaments are sutured and divided.

REPAIR OF UTERINE PROLAPSE

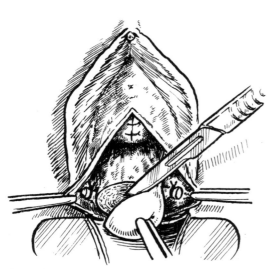

4. Amputation of cervical stump.

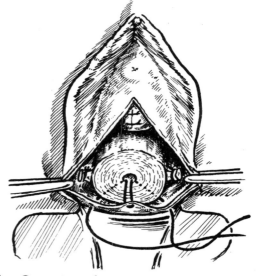

5. Covering the posterior stump with vaginal wall.

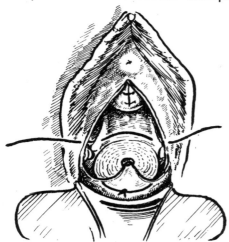

6. Tying the transverse cervical ligaments in front of the cervix and so shortening them and raising the uterus. (This is the so-called Fothergill suture: sometimes two are put in).

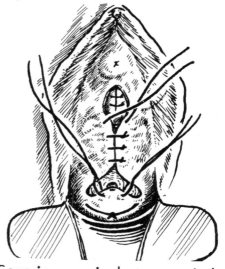

7. Covering cervical stump and closing the vaginal wall. On release of the cervical stump the uterus returns to the pelvis.

POSTERIOR COLPOPERINEORRHAPHY

(INCLUDING REPAIR OF RECTOCELE)

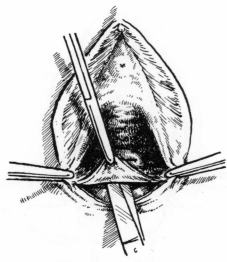

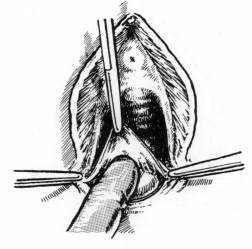

1. Mobilisation of the posterior vaginal wall.

2. Separating rectocele from posterior vaginal wall.

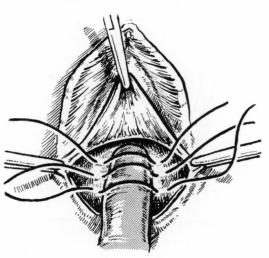

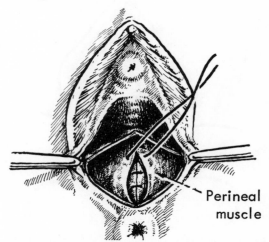

Perineal muscle

3. Obliterating the rectocele by tightening the fascial layer (cf. obliterating the cystocele.)

4. Excess vaginal skin is removed. The perineal muscles are sutured over the obliterated rectocele.
The skin and vagina are closed as in perineorrhaphy (p 155).

REPAIR OF ENTEROCELE

(Usually combined with repair of uterine prolapse
which is omitted here)

If the posterior vaginal fornix is seen to bulge downwards at
operation, an enterocele is suspected. The vaginal wall must be
stripped from the cervix and the
peritoneal sac shortened. If the
uterosacral ligaments are not too
attenuated, they should be sutured
together to act as a support, but
this is often not possible and support must be provided by a high
posterior colporrhaphy. Enterocele
is sometimes a sequel to a Manchester repair in which an early
vault prolapse has been overlooked.

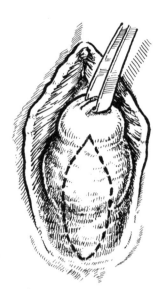

1. Dotted lines show the area of vaginal
wall which will be removed.

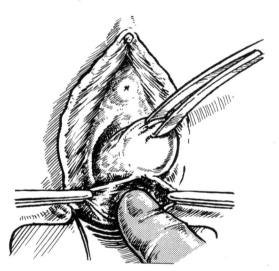

2. Vaginal wall is stripped from posterior cervix.

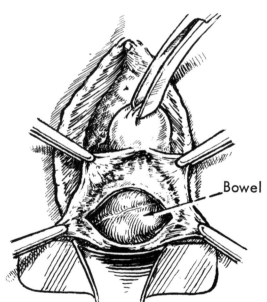

Bowel

3. The enterocele sac is identified
and opened.

REPAIR OF ENTEROCELE

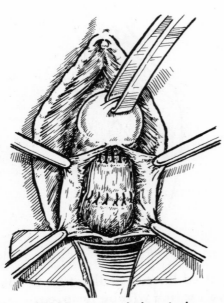

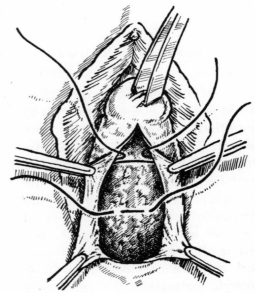

4. Once the sac is mobilised the neck is sutured as far up as possible and then sutured to the back of the cervix.

5. The posterior vaginal wall is now completely opened and the cervix pulled up. At this stage the utero-sacral ligaments can sometimes be apposed to form a support.

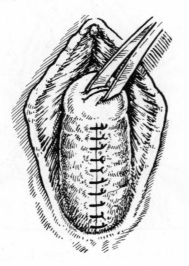

6. When the repair is completed and the vaginal wall closed, the suture line will run from the perineum up the vaginal wall and posterior fornix to the cervix.

REPAIR BY VAGINAL HYSTERECTOMY

Indications

1. When the prolapse is complete. In such cases the ligaments are very attenuated and a better result may be obtained by removal of the uterus.

2. When there is some non-malignant uterine condition – small fibroids, menorrhagia.

Some surgeons would rather remove the uterus than leave it when doing a repair. But the vaginal route no longer offers a greater safety margin than the abdominal; and except in cases of prolapse, vaginal hysterectomy is not much practised today.

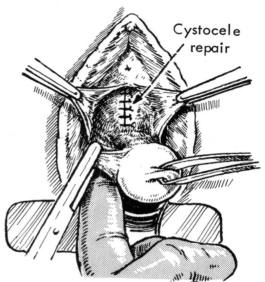

1. The bladder has been mobilised. The uterine ligaments are put on the stretch and divided.

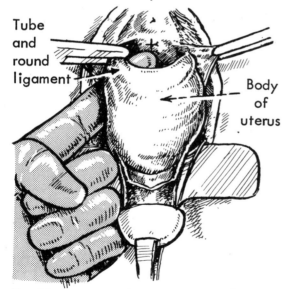

2. Utero-vesical pouch has been entered. Broad ligament structures put on the stretch and divided.

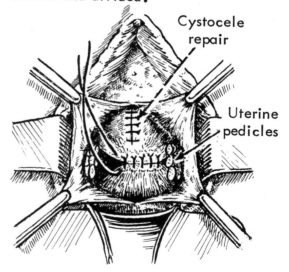

3. The uterus is removed and posterior peritoneal leaf is sutured to the peritoneum of the bladder.

REPAIR BY VAGINAL HYSTERECTOMY

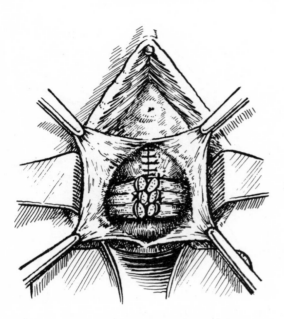

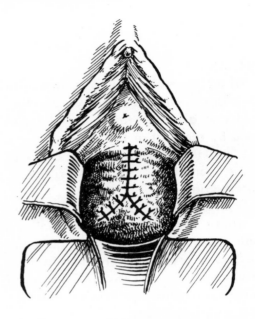

4. The lateral pedicles are sutured together to support the Pouch of Douglas.

5. The cystocele has been obliterated in the usual manner and the vaginal vault and anterior wall closed. Posterior colporrhaphy follows.

COMPLICATIONS

During Operation

1. Bleeding pedicles are more difficult to control than during abdominal surgery. The parametric structures should be clamped, divided and ligated in small rather than large bites.

2. With the uterus gone, there is a risk of distorting the ureters if the bladder fascia is tightened too much during repair of the cystocele.

After Operation

There is a tendency to vault haematoma which becomes infected and ultimately discharges per vaginam; but otherwise vaginal hysterectomy if done properly is not liable to any more complications than a repair operation.

LE FORT'S OPERATION FOR PROLAPSE

This is a short and simple procedure, designed for frail old women who would not be fit for a more extensive operation. It is not however, so reliable as a Manchester repair and has been made almost obsolete by modern advances in anaesthesia which allow so much more time to the surgeon.

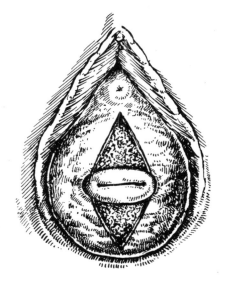

1. A triangular strip of tissue is removed from each vaginal wall.

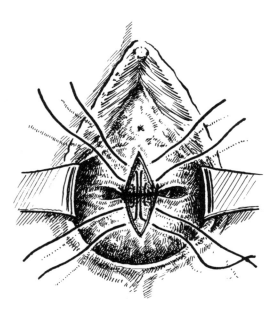

2. The edges are sutured together, anterior wall to posterior wall.

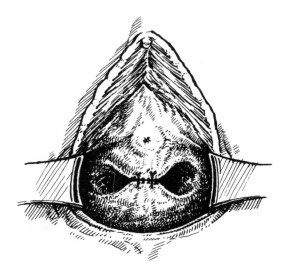

3. The vagina is now formed into two parallel 'pencil' vaginas.

SELECTION OF PATIENTS FOR OPERATION

1. The patient's symptoms must definitely be due to prolapse. This is probably the case if a pessary gives relief; but the effect of suggestion must not be discounted.

2. The patient must complain. If a woman with prolapse does not find it uncomfortable or inconvenient, no treatment should be offered.

3. The patient must be fit for operation. Neither youth nor age are themselves contraindications, but the anaesthetist must help to decide about the patient's fitness for operation, and the gynaecologist must consider whether the patient is likely to benefit from the increased freedom after a successful repair.

4. All pelvic operations carry a risk of embolism. A history of thrombosis would be a contraindication to surgery.

PRE-OPERATIVE PREPARATION

1. Cardiorespiratory system
In old patients, and when there is any history of chronic disease, X-ray and ECG examinations should be carried out, and a physician's opinion sought. Anaemia must be corrected.

2. Urinary Tract
The presence of hypertension, or a history of chronic infection call for some investigation - blood urea level, intravenous pyelogram, perhaps a renal function test. If urinary infection is present it must be treated before operation (but will probably recur post-operatively).

3. Ulceration of Prolapse
The patient should be given a week's nursing, with the prolapse replaced in the pelvis. This measure in itself, supported by application of dienoestrol cream will improve tissue vascularity and reduce local infection.

4. Menstruation and Recent Pregnancy
Surgery is accompanied by more bleeding during menstruation and for six months after pregnancy; and operation should be delayed in such circumstances.

POST-OPERATIVE COMPLICATIONS

Pain

The patient will need morphine 15mg when she recovers consciousness, and again in 4–6 hours.

Urinary complications

Urinary infection is very common, and dysuria is almost the rule even when no anterior repair has been done. Every effort should be made to get the patient to pass urine spontaneously, but if she cannot, a catheter must be passed as stasis is undesirable and distension very painful. Indwelling catheters and continuous drainage should not be resorted to until 48 hours of intermittent catheterisation have failed to bring about spontaneous voiding.

Catheters lead inevitably to infection, but this can at least be delayed by routine bladder irrigation with say 100ml of 2.5% noxytiolin twice daily. Specimens of urine should be sent regularly for culture and sensitivity reports. If incomplete emptying is suspected a catheter should be passed to check the amount of residual urine which should not be more than about 30ml.

Bleeding

This may occur soon after operation from a slipped ligature; or at about the 10th day when the catgut begins to disintegrate. The patient should be anaesthetised in theatre and the bleeding point picked up.

Recto-anal symptoms

Haemorrhoids are temporarily aggravated by colpoperineorrhaphy, but respond to Anusol creams and suppositories. If there is no bowel movement by the 5th day, an enema should be given.

Ambulation and Hygiene

Early ambulation should always be practised and the patient should be 'walking round her bed' in 24 hours. Thereafter she should take a bath or use a bidet at least once a day.

Thrombosis

Any signs of thrombophlebitis in the legs should be treated at once with anticoagulants and antibiotics, and the possibility of embolism borne in mind. If operation is undertaken in a patient with a history of thrombosis, prophylactic anticoagulant cover should be given either before or immediately after operation.

LATE COMPLICATIONS

1. Recurrence of Prolapse

i) Due to continuing extension of fibrous supports. This may be a congenital weakness or a result of excessive intra-abdominal pressure as from chronic bronchitis in a fat woman. (Cf. recurrence of inguinal hernia due to imperfect healing.)

ii) Faulty Technique.

Vaginal repair operations call for some experience. An unsuspected and unlooked for enterocele may appear.

iii) Faulty Indications for Operation

The patient's symptoms may have been due to vaginitis, or a neurotic response to stress, or even chronic constipation.

2. Stress Incontinence

Sometimes this appears for the first time after a repair operation, or it is not specifically complained of and ignored during operation.

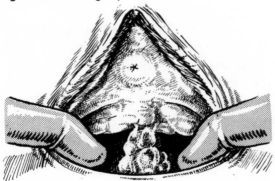

Vaginal wall adhesions

3. Dyspareunia

The surgeon must enquire before the operation about the patient's sexual activity and must be careful to leave a functional vagina where this is required (even although this may make support of the prolapse more difficult).

Causes are:

i) Too early resumption of intercourse before healing is complete and vaginal epithelium normal.

ii) Too small a vaginal orifice. Usually stretching will occur, but if necessary a perineoplasty can be done (page 157).

iii) Too narrow or too short a vagina. A narrow vagina can sometimes be widened at the expense of length by the equivalent of a perineoplasty. Nothing can be done if the vagina is too short beyond prescribing an oestrogen cream and counselling perseverance.

iv) Adhesions between vaginal walls. To prevent this the vagina is packed for 24 hours post-operatively. They are caused by sepsis, and are occasionally so tough that they have to be divided under anaesthesia. Adhesions are not common and are most likely to occur in older women who are not sexually active.

CHAPTER 12
STRESS INCONTINENCE

PHYSIOLOGY OF MICTURITION

There are many causes of urinary incontinence, only some of which can be treated by surgery. Accurate diagnosis of the cause calls for some consideration of the problems of bladder physiology.

Intravesical Pressure

The bladder displays the phenomenon of adaptation to increased urinary volume so that urine is normally stored at low pressure. The bladder wall relaxes its tone as urine is secreted from the ureters, and pressure rises very little until over 400ml. of urine are contained.

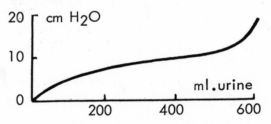

It will be seen that the pressure does not exceed 20cm of water until the bladder is full.

Intra-urethral Pressure

The urethra can normally resist pressures between 20 and 50cm (much higher than the bladder exerts except when full). This pressure is maintained by the tone of the urethral wall assisted by the external sphincter.

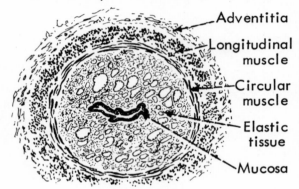

Cross section of urethra

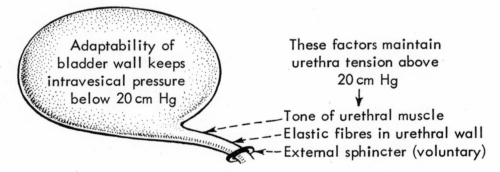

Adaptability of bladder wall keeps intravesical pressure below 20 cm Hg

These factors maintain urethra tension above 20 cm Hg
↓
Tone of urethral muscle
Elastic fibres in urethral wall
External sphincter (voluntary)

Urine is contained in the bladder as long as the intra-urethral pressure is greater than the intravesical pressure.

PHYSIOLOGY OF MICTURITION

Nervous Control of Micturition

The exact mechanism is not yet understood, but micturition may be described as an autonomic reflex which can be consciously inhibited or facilitated in the trained individual.

Distension stimulates the stretch receptors in the bladder wall and a desire to void reaches consciousness when about 300ml. of urine are in the bladder. This stimulus passes via the parasympathetic, and reflex detrusor contractions can be inhibited until about 700ml. are secreted, by which time the external sphincter is strongly contracted.

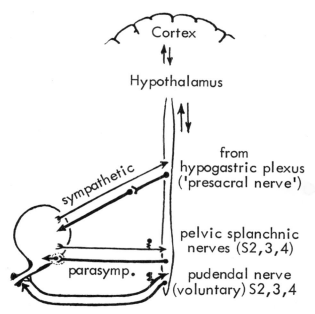

from hypogastric plexus ('presacral nerve')

pelvic splanchnic nerves (S2,3,4)

pudendal nerve (voluntary) S2,3,4

Relaxation of this sphincter is usually a conscious act at the onset of micturition, and is sometimes psychologically inhibited, as in a patient unused to a bedpan or urinal.

Function of the External Sphincter

This striated muscle is innervated by the pudendal nerve.

1. It contracts voluntarily to maintain urethral pressure when the individual wishes to resist the desire to void urine. As everyone knows, this contraction cannot be maintained indefinitely.

2. It contracts reflexly if the posterior urethra should momentarily open under stress of coughing, laughing etc.

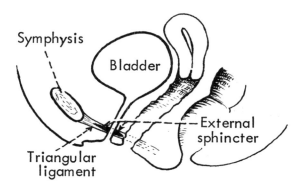

3. At the end of micturition it contracts and forces the last drops of urine back into the bladder. (The urethra is normally empty.)

PHYSIOLOGY OF MICTURITION

Changes During Micturition

The 'detrusor muscle' is the three muscular coats of bladder <u>and urethra</u>. As the distal end of the urethra is fixed, the effect of detrusor contraction is to open the internal urethral meatus.

<u>Coronal plane</u>

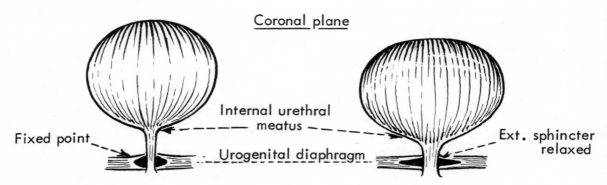

Fixed point

Internal urethral meatus

Urogenital diaphragm

Ext. sphincter relaxed

<u>Resting Bladder</u>. The muscle is not contracting, but maintaining tone. The urethra is long, closed, and empty.

<u>Micturition</u>. Detrusor contraction opens the internal urethra. Urine enters and reflexly stimulates further detrusor contraction.

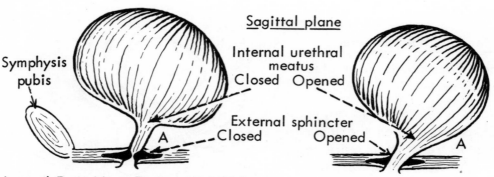

Sagittal plane

Symphysis pubis

Internal urethral meatus
Closed   Opened

External sphincter
Closed   Opened

A

A

Lateral Erect View During Micturition

The internal urethral meatus undergoes dilatation (funnelling). The urethra shortens, and moves a little backwards and downwards. The point A marks the urethrovesical (UV) angle which can be seen on X-ray urethrocystography to be obliterated during micturition.

CAUSES OF STRESS INCONTINENCE

STRESS INCONTINENCE

This is a response to a sudden increase in intra-abdominal – and hence intra-vesical pressure.

Any increase in intra-abdominal pressure, as from coughing, is distributed equally to bladder and urethra, so that no leakage should occur.   (Yet about 50% of parous women occasionally experience stress incontinence.)

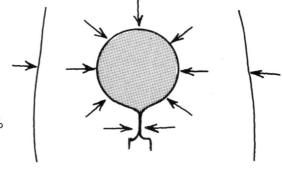

Causes of Stress Incontinence

1. <u>Displacement or damage to urethral supports</u>.

This is usually a consequence of parturition followed by the physiological atrophy of pelvic tissues associated with the menopause. Vaginal prolapse is often present.   Sometimes the damage is the result of surgical operations in the periurethral area.   (Repair of prolapse or fistula.)

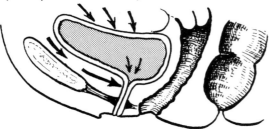

Coughing stress applied equally to bladder and urethra. No incontinence.

2. <u>Congenital weakness of the urethral sphincteric mechanism</u>.

This is at present our only explanation for the rare appearance of true stress incontinence in a nulliparous woman with no history of trauma. (Cf. the constitutional disposition of some women to the development of varicose veins.)

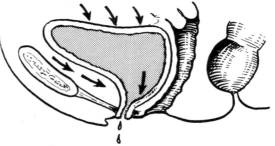

Same stress in presence of a prolapsed and scarred urethrovesical junction.

It is postulated that when the urethrovesical junction is poorly supported and more or less permanently in the micturition position, an increase in intra-abdominal tension acts on the urethra as an opening rather than as a closing force.

DISTURBED BLADDER FUNCTION

Urgency Incontinence.

The patient is unable to inhibit detrusor contraction and must void urine forth-with. The commonest cause is irritability due to cystitis, but all forms of bladder pathology must be considered, including tuberculosis, calculus and carcinoma. Urethritis and even vaginal discharge from cervicitis are also causes; and urgency and stress incontinence may occur simultaneously.

Fistula Incontinence is described on page 324 et seq.

Overflow Incontinence

Sudden retention is rare in women except after pelvic floor operations. Spasmodic destrusor contractions force a little urine into the urethra, and the stretched muscle takes several days to regain its tone.

When obstruction to outflow occurs gradually, as from pressure by a pelvic tumour or an incarcerated gravid uterus, the detrusor has time to hypertrophy and for a time forces urine out; but eventually the bladder becomes atonic and painless and urine dribbles out only when the intra-abdominal pressure is raised.

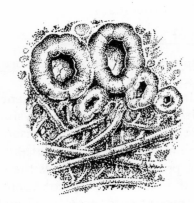

Atonic, distended, trabeculated bladder due to tumour.

Neurological disease

Failure of detrusor inhibition is the commonest symptom and is the cause of senile incontinence. It is also a symptom, although not usually the presenting one, of multiple sclerosis. Full sensation is present, but the incontinence is of the urgency type and cannot be resisted.

Failure of bladder sensation is a result of diseases which interrupt the posterior columns of the cord: such as tabes, syringomyelia, occasionally multiple sclerosis. Chronic overdistension leads to an atonic bladder and overflow incontinence, and infection is a common complication.

FREQUENCY

FREQUENCY (Excessive frequency of micturition) is due to abnormal bladder irritability. It differs from urgency in that the stimulus to micturate can for a short time be resisted (i.e. voluntary inhibition of detrusor action is retained).

Frequency is usually diurnal – occurring only during waking hours – although it may prevent the onset of sleep.

Nocturnal frequency indicates a more severe degree of bladder irritation; although it may be difficult to decide whether the irritation has wakened the patient or whether the desire to micturate is felt simply because the patient is awake.

Frequency results from any source of irritation to bladder or urethra – cystitis, urethritis, tumour, calculus, cystocele (stretching of the bladder base, and incomplete emptying). It is one of the earliest symptoms of pregnancy. If no organic cause can be found, the frequency is attributed to habit or neurosis (the 'psychogenic bladder').

PAIN in the urinary tract is usually lateral and is referred to the loins. In chronic cases when the ureters are involved, it is more difficult to distinguish from pelvic pain.

Pain on micturition ('like passing red-hot needles') is called dysuria, and indicates a cystitis or a urethritis possibly gonococcal. Sometimes the dysuria is in fact due to a vaginitis when the inflamed epithelium is irritated by the dribbling of urine. Such pain is most acute at the end of micturition.

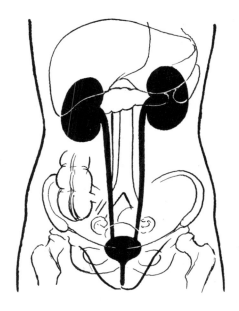

HAEMATURIA may be due to organic disease, infection, or calculus: but it is a complaint sometimes incorrectly made, when the blood is really coming from the genital tract.

INVESTIGATION OF INCONTINENCE

The object is to identify stress incontinence which can be lessened by gynaecological treatment: and to exclude other causes which are associated with disturbed bladder function. The history is often inconclusive, but the following points are suggestive:

STRESS INCONTINENCE

Gradual onset after one or more pregnancies.

Urine appears <u>only</u> after effort (stress) such as coughing, laughing, running for a bus.

Only small quantities of urine are passed, whether the bladder is full or not.

DISTURBED BLADDER FUNCTION

History of a 'weak bladder' even before pregnancies: or childhood enuresis.

Incontinence preceded by a strong desire to micturate, but not by stress. The patient 'has to run'.

Occurs usually with a full bladder, and larger amounts are passed.

Stress incontinence combined with urgency incontinence due to bladder infection or cystocoele is quite common. Continuous incontinence suggests fistula (page 324).

The degree of severity is indicated by extent to which the patient feels socially restricted.

EXAMINATION

Signs of infection (urethritis) and scarring from previous surgery are looked for, and the usual bimanual and speculum examinations are made (pp 75–77).

Demonstration of Stress Incontinence

The labia are separated and the patient asked to cough and strain. If no urine appears, the test should be repeated with the patient standing up.

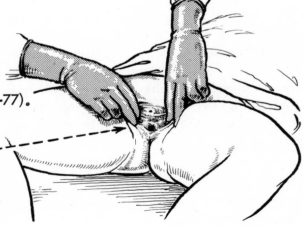

INVESTIGATION OF INCONTINENCE

The diagnosis is often not clear, and some of the following procedures may be necessary.

Culture of Urine

This is a routine procedure in all cases of incontinence, but several mid-stream specimens may be required before the urine can definitely be passed as sterile. Culture of urine obtained by suprapubic aspiration may be necessary.

Renal Function

This is affected by chronic infection, and estimation of the blood urea should always be done. Clearance tests may be indicated, and renal pyelography is an easily performed examination although it is seldom of help in diagnosing the cause of incontinence.

Cystometry

This means the determination of bladder tone and its response to gradual distension with normal saline at body heat. This will provide a measurement of capacity (the normal bladder can hold about 700ml.) and of any residual urine after voiding (as with cystocoele). About 50ml. are instilled at a time and the bladder wall given time to accommodate. The manometer indicates detrusor contractions, and if these are frequent, and occur early on, an 'irritable bladder' is diagnosed. Cystometry cannot determine the cause.

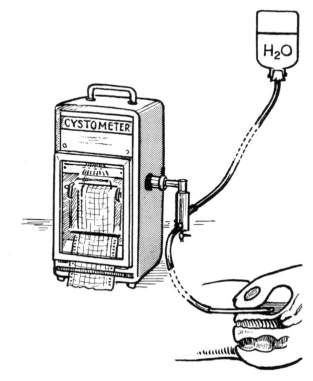

INVESTIGATION OF INCONTINENCE

URETHROCYSTOGRAPHY

The bladder is filled with a contrast medium, and lateral X-ray pictures are taken at rest, straining, and micturating.

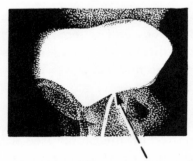

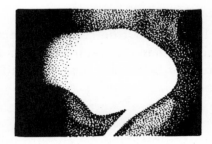

Normal resting X-ray.   Note the well formed posterior UV angle.

Normal micturating X-ray.   Note urethral dilatation, downward displacement of UV junction, flattening of UV angle.

If the appearances on straining are those of micturition, stress incontinence is diagnosed.   This is a difficult and specialised technique, uncomfortable for the patient, and not infallible; but it is the best way of demonstrating urethral mobility in cases where there is no obvious prolapse, or much peri-urethral scarring.

In practice, patients who complain of lack of bladder control can be allocated to one of three groups:

1. Those with obvious stress incontinence.
2. Those with obvious disturbed bladder function but no stress incontinence.
3. Those in whom the diagnosis is not clear and whose complaint may involve more than one condition.

It is in this last group that cystometry and urethro-cystography may be of value. Surgery cannot guarantee a cure of stress incontinence and may exacerbate the patient's condition if wrongly applied; so it is important to be as precise as possible in the selection of patients for operation.

The treatment of functional as opposed to stress incontinence is best left to the urologist.

SURGICAL TREATMENT

The object is to restore the urethrovesical junction to its correct position below the symphysis, and to narrow the dilated urethra.

The 'cure' of stress incontinence is a somewhat subjective concept depending on the persistence of the surgeon's enquiry and on the stoicism of the patient. A woman who has endured the discomfort of one operation may decide that the degree of incontinence which remains is not sufficient to justify a second ordeal. Many operations produce a temporary improvement which would be found not to be sustained if the patient were followed up for two years. The condition will not invariably be relieved until we have a better understanding of the exact mechanism of bladder control and stress incontinence. It is the common experience that about three quarters of one's patients will be improved, and a successful outcome is variously attributed to:

1. Elevation of the urethrovesical junction.
2. Restoration of the radiological posterior urethrovesical angle.
3. Lengthening of the urethra.
4. Personal eccentricities of technique.

Plan of Treatment. It is usual to begin with physiotherapy and follow with one or more surgical procedures if no success is achieved.

First: Physiotherapy (if prolapse is absent or slight).

Second: A vaginal buttressing operation, especially if prolapse is present.

Third: A repetition of the vaginal buttressing; or one of the urethral sling operations.

Fourth: For the twenty percent who continue to suffer from stress incontinence, the electrical stimulation of the pelvic muscles (page 296) may offer some hope. Otherwise there is no alternative to a urinary diversion operation.

Success in this field depends very much on the careful exclusion of other causes of incontinence, and on the technical skill of the surgeon.

PHYSIOTHERAPY

This takes the form of stimulating the pelvic floor with electrical current (faradism), and exercises for the pelvic muscles. The object is to 're-educate' the muscles and obtain a permanent improvement in muscle tone.

Faradism

This is applied through two electrodes, an indifferent one over the sacrum and an active electrode applied to the vagina. Current is applied in 2 second 'surges' with a 2-3 second interval, and treatment gradually extended to 40 minutes.

A dozen treatments may be needed, but there should be early signs of improvement.

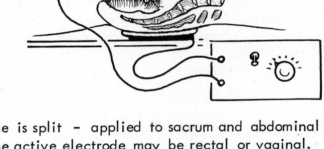

Sometimes the indifferent electrode is split - applied to sacrum and abdominal wall to reduce discomfort - and the active electrode may be rectal or vaginal. Another technique is to apply several maximal stimuli under anaesthesia on one occasion only. In some cases this will completely restore muscle tone.

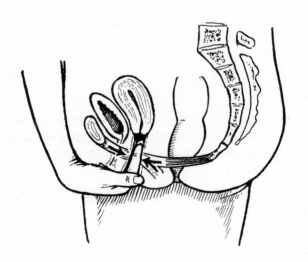

Exercises

These include repeated pressing together of the buttocks and thighs, and stopping the urine stream during micturition. The patient should also be instructed to insert two fingers into the vagina just above the plane of the levator muscles, and contract these to grip the fingers as tightly as possible. This is the best exercise and provides the patient with a direct measure of her progress.

VAGINAL URETHROPLASTY

This is the commonest operation and usually the first choice. It is sometimes called a 'buttressing' operation or Kelly's operation, and it is an attempt to prevent urethral dilatation on straining by tightening the paraurethral tissues; and to raise and support the urethra by suturing the fascia beneath it.

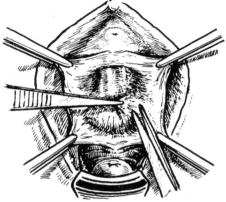

1. Anterior vaginal wall is carefully dissected from the urethrovesical area.

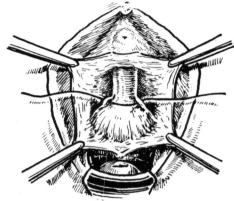

2. At the level of the urethrovesical junction, a silk suture picks up the periurethral fascia on either side of the urethra. This suture is repeated above and below.

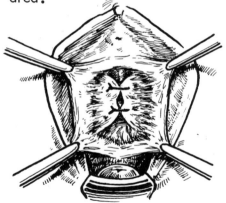

3. After tying the silk sutures, the bladder fascia (sometimes called pubo-cervical fascia) is pulled together with catgut to give added support.

The repair of cystocoele if present is proceeded with in the usual manner. Dysuria is inevitable for the next few days and catheterisation will be required, but indwelling catheters are to be avoided.

ALDRIDGE'S OPERATION

Fascial strips are cut from the aponeurosis of the external oblique, passed through the rectus muscles and joined under the urethra. This operation is done in conjunction with a vaginal urethroplasty.

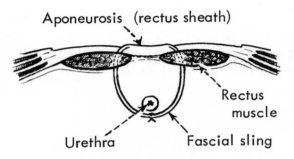

Aponeurosis (rectus sheath)

Rectus muscle

Urethra

Fascial sling

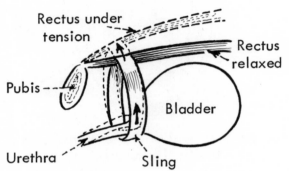

Rectus under tension

Rectus relaxed

Pubis

Bladder

Urethra

Sling

Rationale of the Operation

When the recti contract and move anteriorly under stimulus of coughing, sneezing etc. the sling supports the urethrovesical junction and prevents it from being forced down into the micturition position.

Points in Technique

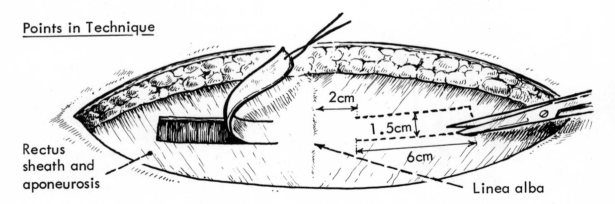

2cm

1.5cm

6cm

Rectus sheath and aponeurosis

Linea alba

(After completion of the vaginal urethroplasty)

A wide suprapubic incision is required to expose the external oblique aponeurosis. This is elevated with scissors and two strips are cut, 6cm long and 1.5cm wide.

ALDRIDGE'S OPERATION

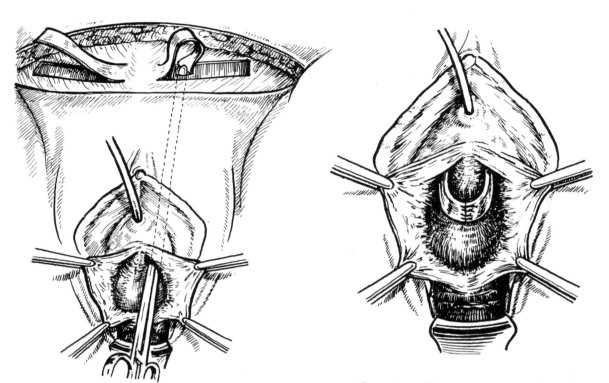

By blunt dissection the bladder and urethra are displaced sideways, and forceps are passed up and pushed between the fibres of the rectus muscle.

The fascial strips are pulled down and sutured under the urethrovesical junction. This sling must not be too tight and there should be room to pass a finger tip between sling and urethra.

As in other sling operations, catheterisation for a week is necessary. If the sling is too tight it will cause chronic retention and infection; if too loose it will be ineffective.

MOIR'S OPERATION

This operation makes use of a strip of mersilene gauze instead of fascial strips which may be difficult to obtain and require a wide incision in the abdominal wall.

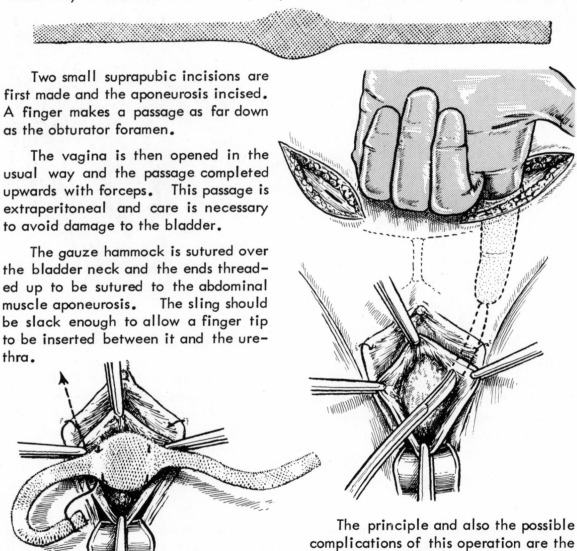

Two small suprapubic incisions are first made and the aponeurosis incised. A finger makes a passage as far down as the obturator foramen.

The vagina is then opened in the usual way and the passage completed upwards with forceps. This passage is extraperitoneal and care is necessary to avoid damage to the bladder.

The gauze hammock is sutured over the bladder neck and the ends threaded up to be sutured to the abdominal muscle aponeurosis. The sling should be slack enough to allow a finger tip to be inserted between it and the urethra.

The principle and also the possible complications of this operation are the same as for Aldridge's operation.

MILLIN'S OPERATION

This is the provision of a fascial sling for the urethra, done entirely through an abdominal incision.

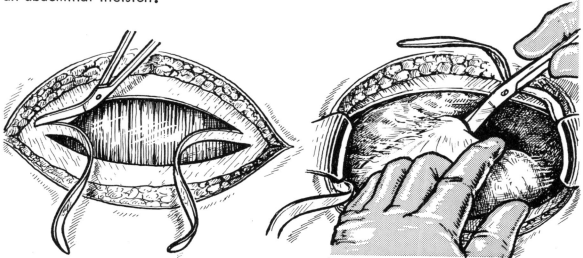

1. Cutting fascial strips. (These are attached laterally).

2. The urethra is freed from the vaginal wall.

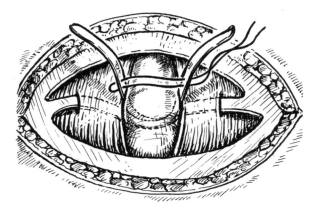

3. The slings are led through the recti and under the urethra, and sutured in front of the urethra.

This operation is little practised today.

1. Dissection of the urethra from a fibrotic vaginal wall is difficult from below and even more so from above.

2. There is often difficulty in obtaining sufficiently long fascial strips.

3. It is difficult to assess the correct tension for the fascial slings. If they are too tight, a urethrovesical fistula may develop.

MARSHALL-MARCHETTI-KRANZ OPERATION

The urethrovesical junction is made to adhere firmly to the anterior vaginal wall by suturing the vaginal tissue to the back of the symphysis pubis.

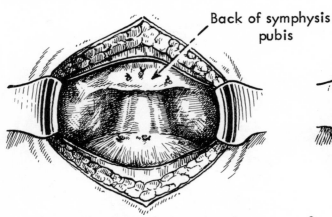

Back of symphysis pubis

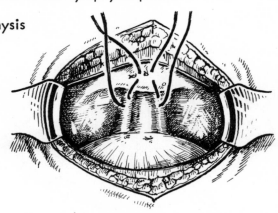

1. The urethrovesical junction is exposed in the space of Retzius. Adhesions are divided and all bleeding points picked up. The urethra must be dissected to within 1cm of the external meatus.

2. A Foley's catheter in the bladder helps to identify the urethrovesical junction. Silk sutures pick up <u>vaginal</u> tissue on either side and suture it to the pubic periosteum.

Closure is with a suprapubic drain for 48 hours in case of urinary leakage or haematoma formation. Haematuria is common and continuous catheterisation is required for 7 days.

The object of this operation is to provide elevation and support for the UV junction and proximal urethra.

Periosteitis is sometimes a late complication and the operation is difficult in the presence of excessive obesity. If too acute an angle is produced, the patient may have difficulty in emptying her bladder.

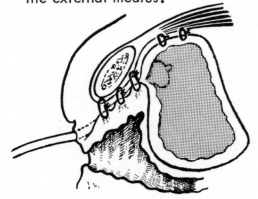

3. Additional sutures are added between bladder muscle and rectus muscles. (This step is sometimes unnecessary.)

OTHER URETHROPEXY TECHNIQUES

LAPIDES' OPERATION

This is a modification of the Marshall-Marchetti-Kranz operation. The urethra is itself sutured to the symphysis and periosteum, the sutures passing through the urethral lumen. The object of this technique is to correct the 'concertina' shortening of the urethra on straining, which is thought to be a factor in the causation of stress incontinence. It is more traumatic to the urethra.

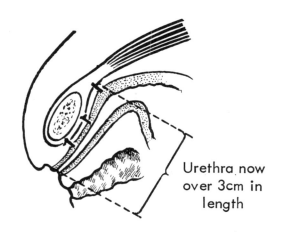

Urethra now over 3cm in length

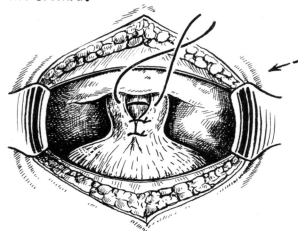

BALL'S OPERATION

This operation consists of an anterior plication of the urethrovesical junction in conjunction with the posterior urethroplasty, so as to create good anterior and posterior urethrovesical angles. To do this, the urethra must be well mobilised and all bleeding controlled.

The theoretical basis of Ball's operation rests on the ability of the intact urethra to contract by itself if free to do so; and on the equal distribution to urethra and bladder of raised intra-abdominal pressure.

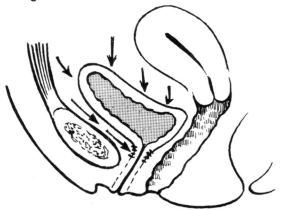

INTERPOSITION OPERATIONS

The body of the uterus is pulled forward to lie between the bladder and the vagina. This is an obsolete operation for prolapse which has been re-examined in recent years with a view to providing support for the urethrovesical junctions in patients with intractable stress incontinence.

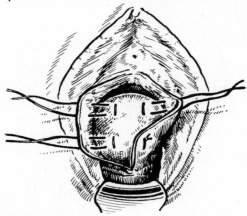

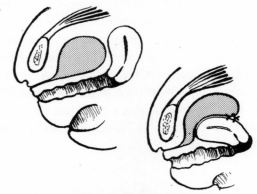

Vaginal approach.
The vaginal wall is opened, bladder mobilised and vesico-uterine peritoneum opened. The body of the uterus is pulled through and sutured to the vaginal wall.

Abdominal approach (Louros' operation)
Through an abdominal incision the vesico-uterine pouch is divided. The uterus is first sutured in an acutely anteverted position by a Gilliam ventrosuspension operation. The vesico-uterine peritoneum is opened and the vesical edge sutured to the lower part of the back of the uterine body.

Interposition operations are objectionable for the following reasons:

1. A subsequent pregnancy would obviously have disastrous effects on the bladder and urethra.
2. In a woman still sexually active, the acutely anteverted uterus may cause dyspareunia.
3. If malignant or other disease subsequently develops in the uterus, treatment would be much more difficult.

If the operation were to be indicated as a last resort, sterilisation would have to be done at the same time.

ELECTRICAL CONTROL OF STRESS INCONTINENCE

This is in essence a sort of permanent physiotherapy and is still an experimental technique. The results are poor if the pelvic muscles are poor, but electrical control is indicated if surgery fails or is contra-indicated.

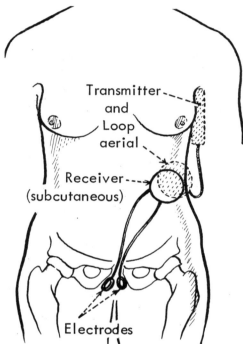

Platinum-iridium electrodes are sutured to the periosteum of the pubic rami, and the leads are led subcutaneously to a small radio receiver implanted in the abdominal wall. This receives signals from a battery-powered transmitter strapped under the patient's armpit, and passes these signals as electrical impulses to the pudendal nerves. The current is switched off to allow micturition.

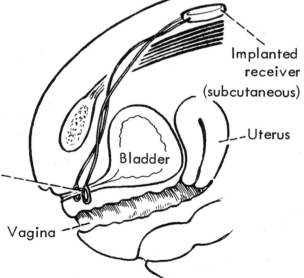

Another method is to enter the space of Retzius and dissect down to the surface of the levator ani muscles. The electrodes are then sutured direct to the muscles. This is technically more difficult but avoids any complications caused by ulceration of electrodes through the skin which may occur when perineal implantation is used.

ELECTRICAL CONTROL OF STRESS INCONTINENCE

Electrodes may also be attached to vaginal pessaries or perspex anal plugs which do not require surgical implantation and may be as effective.

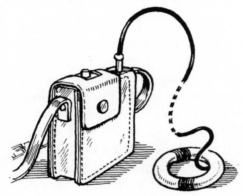

A vinyl pessary with electrodes attached in such a way that flexing the pessary does not fracture the wire.

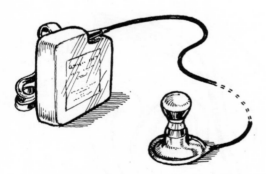

An anal plug. Insertion and removal are easier for the patient but may be less acceptable to her than the vaginal pessary.

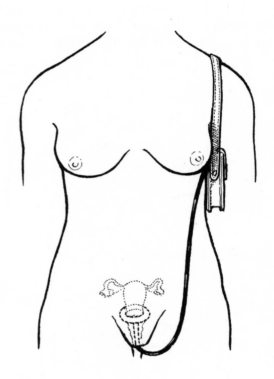

The electronic apparatus designed for incontinence control is now extremely reliable, and such methods are worth a trial.

About a 50% success rate may be expected; and patients who have failed to achieve control by any other treatment are extremely grateful.

CHAPTER 13
THE URETER

ANATOMY

The ureter enters the pelvis retroperitoneally by crossing over or near the bifurcation of the common iliac artery.

It is itself crossed by the ovarian vessels and is near the fold of peritoneum which forms the infundibulopelvic ligament.

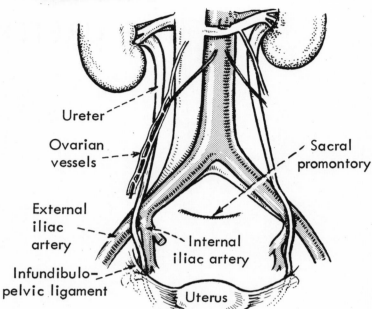

It passes down and medially behind the ovarian fossa and is in close relation to the internal iliac artery. In the healthy subject its shape can be made out beneath the peritoneum and its movements observed (vermiculation).

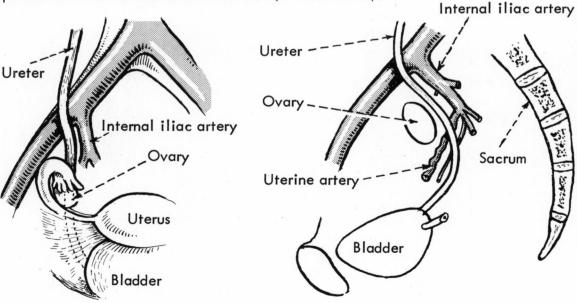

ANATOMY

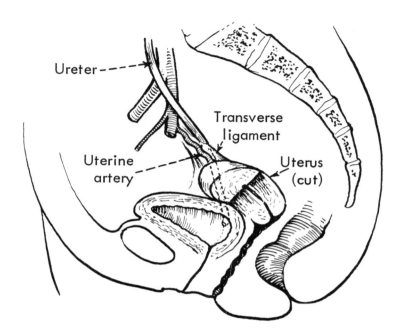

The ureter then passes beneath the base of the broad ligament, through the transverse uterine ligament and into the bladder. In this parametrial part of its course it lies alongside the vaginal fornix and passes under the uterine artery.

Ureter

Transverse ligament

Uterine artery

Uterus (cut)

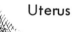

Uterus

Cervix

Vagina

Ureter

Trigone of bladder (cut)

This picture shows the parametrial part of the ureter with the connective tissue removed. Note that the assymmetry of the uterus and vagina makes the left ureter have a much closer relationship with the vaginal fornix than the right.

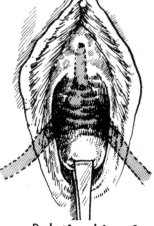

Relationship of bladder base to vagina.

BLOOD SUPPLY

The ureter is supplied by branches from the main arteries with which it is in relation, principally the renal and ovarian arteries. The pelvic vessels are variable; and because the blood enters mostly at the upper and lower ends the peri-ureteric anastomoses are important.

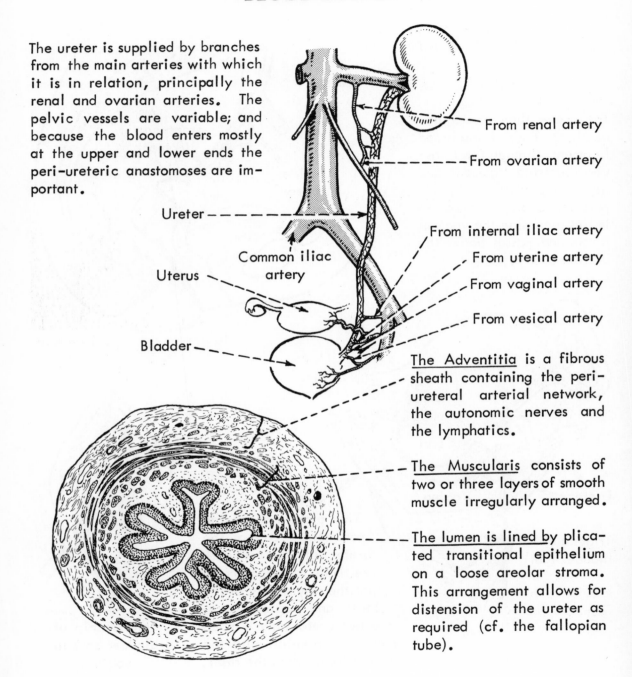

From renal artery

From ovarian artery

Ureter

Common iliac artery

From internal iliac artery

From uterine artery

From vaginal artery

From vesical artery

Uterus

Bladder

The Adventitia is a fibrous sheath containing the peri-ureteral arterial network, the autonomic nerves and the lymphatics.

The Muscularis consists of two or three layers of smooth muscle irregularly arranged.

The lumen is lined by plicated transitional epithelium on a loose areolar stroma. This arrangement allows for distension of the ureter as required (cf. the fallopian tube).

INJURY TO THE URETER

The ureter will occasionally be damaged no matter how much skill and care are exercised.

1. The ureter is not easily demonstrated or dissected where it is in closest relationship to the genital tract; and not always easily palpated.

2. The ureter's course is to some extent variable, and under pressure it will gradually change its position in the pelvis. A large tumour filling the pelvis will displace it laterally; a tumour in the broad ligament may displace the ureter outwards and upwards; and double ureters are occasionally met with.

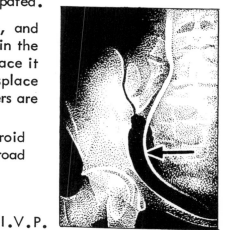

I.V.P.
showing lateral displacement

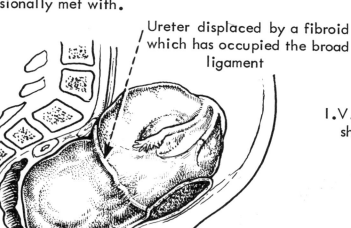

Ureter displaced by a fibroid which has occupied the broad ligament

3. The ureter may be embedded in malignant or inflammatory tissue, making dissection almost impossible.

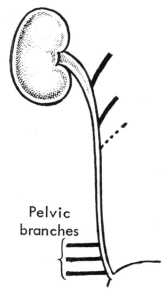

Pelvic branches

4. Radical surgery may destroy so much of the pelvic blood supply that the pelvic ureter becomes ischaemic, leading to fibrotic narrowing or fistula.

INJURY TO THE URETER

The ureter is most commonly injured :-

1. Entering the Pelvis.

The ureter descends medial to the infundibulopelvic ligament, and if displaced by inflammation or tumour, may be so close as to be caught in a clamp applied to the ligament.

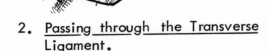

Ureter

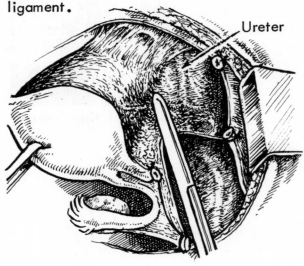

Ureter

2. Passing through the Transverse Ligament.

If the clamp is applied too far out from the uterus the ureter will be included. The uterosacral ligament also must be clamped close to the cervix.

3. In the vesico-uterine ligament

as the ureter turns round the vagina into the bladder. This ligament must be displaced laterally before excision of the uterus if the ureter is to be safe. Unfortunately the more the lateral displacement the greater the disturbance of the venous plexus and the greater the bleeding.

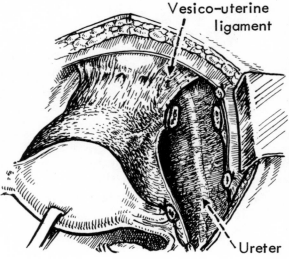

Vesico-uterine ligament

Ureter

PREVENTION OF INJURY

In simple hysterectomy where ureter is not exposed it should be palpated if possible where it lies alongside the vaginal fornix. It conveys a rubbery incompressible sensation to the fingers; but some engorged veins feel the same; and much fat or inflamed tissue make the palpation difficult.

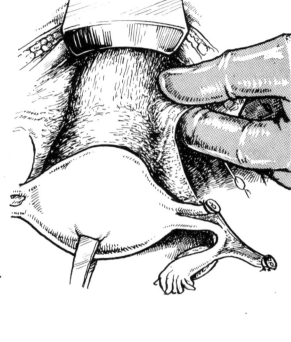

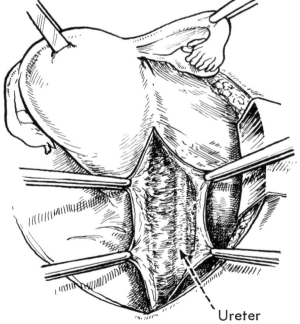

Ureter

The course of the ureter should be examined before starting the dissection. Vermiculation can usually be observed through the peritoneum, but if there is any doubt the peritoneum should be incised and reflected medially so that the ureter may be traced down to where it enters the transverse ligament.

PREVENTION OF INJURY

In radical hysterectomy the ureter must be dissected clear of the uterine artery before the artery is divided.

Never pass pedicle ligatures deeper than necessary.

Do not apply haemostatic forceps blindly when there is sudden haemorrhage. Apply swab pressure and try to identify the bleeding point.

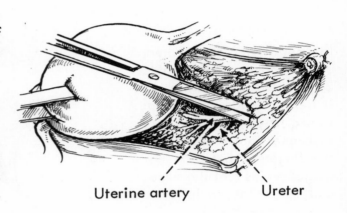

Uterine artery   Ureter

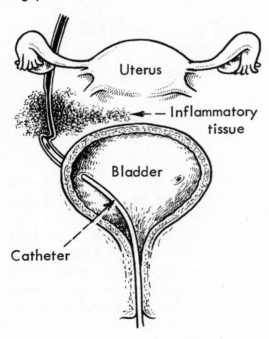

Kinking of ureter obstructs the catheter. Force would cause perforation.

Pre-operative Passage of Ureteric Catheters.

This is an old method of protection and can be extremely useful in the presence of dense fibrosis, endometriosis etc. It makes palpation of the ureters very easy and the catheters tend to displace the ureters outwards, away from the uterus.

But:

1. A catheterised ureter can still be clamped or ligated.

2. Catheters aggravate the complications of urinary infection.

3. Catheters may be obstructed or the ureters may be damaged, if there has been much fixation of tissues by inflammatory or malignant invasion.

URETER IN VAGINAL OPERATIONS

When there is prolapse and when the cervix is drawn down, the position of the adjacent ureters is also altered. The prolapsed uterus pulls down its arteries which in turn displace the ureters, and the bladder base is also involved in the prolapse.

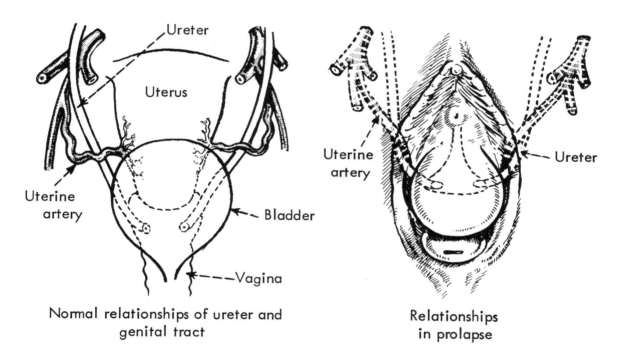

Normal relationships of ureter and genital tract

Relationships in prolapse

During vaginal hysterectomy or in 'complete procidentia' (page 263) the ureter can sometimes be palpated laterally, and when the cystocele is being obliterated, sutures placed too deeply or too far laterally will catch the ureter. The removal of the uterus removes the 'splint' and support of the trigone; and too much infolding of the bladder may distort and obstruct the ureters in their passage through the bladder wall.

315

REPAIR OF DAMAGED URETER

Damage Observed at Operation
(It is frequently *not* observed).

If the damage amounts to bruising by clamp or ligature, a ureteric catheter should be passed in case fistula develops. This is most easily done through an incision in the bladder. (The ureter tends to expel its catheter.) 'Urine will find a way out'; and it is advisable also to drain the operation area through the abdomen.

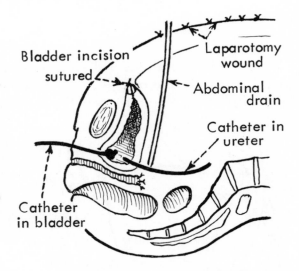

Bladder incision sutured

Laparotomy wound

Abdominal drain

Catheter in ureter

Catheter in bladder

If the ureter is lacerated or divided, the ends should be trimmed and anastomosed over a catheter. The same drainage is required and this technique carries a risk of subsequent stenosis with ultimately the loss of the kidney. An alternative is the vesico-ureteric anastomosis which is best done through the opened bladder. This method carries no risk of stenosis, but reflux is more likely. It is important that the implanted area should not be under tension.

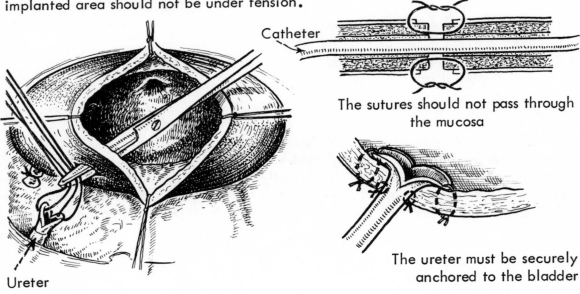

Catheter

The sutures should not pass through the mucosa

Ureter

The ureter must be securely anchored to the bladder

316

REPAIR OF DAMAGED URETER

If neither ureter anastomosis nor implantation are possible, the gynaecologist
should ask for the immediate assistance of
a urologist. If such help is not available,
some temporary procedure should be carried out which will preserve the function
of the kidney.

Cutaneous Ureterostomy

This is a simple procedure provided
enough ureter can be mobilised to avoid
tension. There is no absorption problem
and the difficulty in collecting the urine
does not arise in the short term as a catheter is passed up to the renal pelvis.

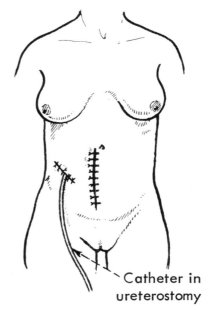

Catheter in
ureterostomy

Other methods are uretero-colic anastomosis and nephrostomy or pyelotomy. This
calls for a flank incision and the kidney may have to be partly delivered through it
to allow insertion of the catheter. A nephrostomy does not always drain well, and
it is a procedure best left to the urologist.

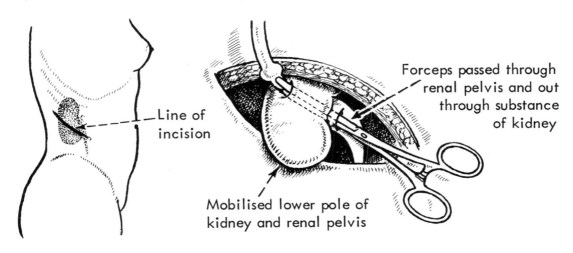

Line of
incision

Forceps passed through
renal pelvis and out
through substance
of kidney

Mobilised lower pole of
kidney and renal pelvis

REPAIR OF DAMAGED URETER

The urologist if he contemplates an immediate permanent repair, has two methods of 'lengthening' a ureter which is too short.

1. Fashioning a tube from the bladder wall.

2. Replacement by an isolated length of ileum.

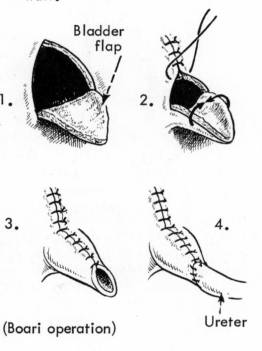

(Boari operation)

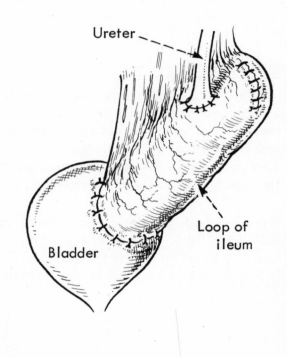

Both these methods may be followed by pyelonephritis with eventual loss of renal function; and if the other kidney were healthy the best treatment for the patient might be nephrectomy.

There may on occasion be an indication for simple ligation of the cut ureter. When this happens the kidney if healthy often undergoes symptomless atrophy and if the ureter is repaired within a month or so, renal function may be restored. Alternatively hydronephrosis slowly increases and the kidney substance is destroyed by the pressure.

TREATMENT OF DAMAGED URETER

TREATMENT OF DAMAGED URETERS ____ [Injury NOT Observed at Operation
(the more usual situation)]

Clinical features. These are variable.

a) If only one ureter is occluded there may be no disturbance, and the kidney silently atrophies.

b) If both ureters are occluded there will be anuria, or fistula will develop either vaginal or abdominal.

c) More often the patient is acutely ill for no obvious reason, and at this stage the gynaecologist should be suspicious of ureter involvement. There is pyrexia, a persistently high pulse, loin pain if hydronephrosis is developing, and ileus if there is internal fistula.

Urine may track retroperitoneally and escape through the abdominal wound, but usually there are symptoms of pelvic abscess and obstruction which demand laparotomy and drainage. Urine is soon observed in the drain; and at this stage if not sooner a urologist should be consulted.

Diagnosis. Two questions must be answered.
a) Is the fistula in bladder or ureter?
b) If ureteric, which side?

If urine is passing per vaginam, ureteric and vesical fistulae may be distinguished by methylene blue test (p327).

Cystoscopy and retrograde pyelography will help to identify the damaged side, and an attempt is made to pass catheters up to the renal pelvis. If this is not possible it suggests ligation of the ureters.

Time of appearance of fistula.

An early fistula (in the first week) suggests division or partial occlusion.

Appearance about the 10th day suggests ligation and subsequent sloughing.

Appearance after 3 weeks or later suggests ischaemic necrosis.

TREATMENT   All urinary fistulae have a tendency to spontaneous closure provided the urinary stream can be diverted. This is done by an abdominal drain, ureteric and bladder catheters or by nephrostomy, and if the patient can be kept fairly comfortable for three or four weeks in this manner there is a chance of spontaneous closure. If this does not occur or if the drainage is unsatisfactory (as is often the case with a temporary nephrostomy) then the abdomen must be opened, all ligature material removed that can be found and one or other of the repair operations described above is carried out.   The best is a uretero-vesical implantation without interposition of flaps or ileum;   and sometimes the urologist may find it necessary to effect a permanent diversion of the urine or remove an infected and functionless kidney.

URINARY DIVERSION OPERATIONS

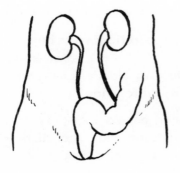

Uretero-colic Anastomosis

The ureters are implanted into the sigmoid and urine is passed per rectum. It is an easy operation and psychologically acceptable to the female. No collecting bag is needed and the rectum can with practice hold urine for up to four hours.

Disadvantages

1. If the ureter is passed obliquely through bowel wall to provide some valve formation against reflux, there is a high incidence of stenosis leading to hydronephrosis and ultimately pyelonephritis.

2. If a wide stoma is made to prevent stenosis, there is inevitably reflux infection.

3. The bowel selectively absorbs acid radicals, mainly chloride causing severe acidosis. The patient has to watch her diet and take alkali mixtures.

4. If used with a colostomy – a 'wet colostomy'– the result is too unpleasant to be acceptable.

Coffey Method

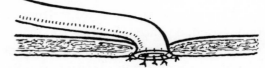

An oblique tunnel led to stenosis (1910)

Nesbit Method

A wide stoma led to reflux (1949)

Leadbetter Method

Combined wide stoma with oblique tunnel (1951)

Indications
1. The older patient (say over 60 years).
2. The frail patient who might not stand a more complicated operation.
3. The patient psychologically incapable of dealing with a urinary stoma.

URINARY DIVERSION OPERATIONS

RECTAL BLADDER

The ureters are implanted into the rectum and faeces are diverted by a colostomy. This method reduces (although it does not abolish) the risk of ascending renal infection and chloride absorption; and might be an acceptable alternative to the patient who 'prefers' a colostomy to a ureteroileostomy. The anal sphincter must be competent and the patient requires to void urine at least every four hours.

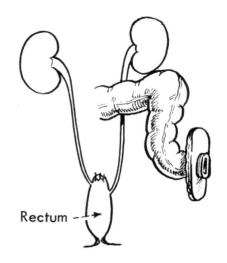

Rectum

- -

COMPLICATIONS OF DIVERSION PROCEDURES

HYPERCHLORAEMIC ACIDOSIS

The transitional epithelium of the urinary tract absorbs nothing, while one of the bowel's main functions is to absorb water and electrolytes. The acid urine which is diverted to the bowel is gradually alkalinised by the selective absorption of acid radicals mainly Cl^-, leading to hyperchloraemic acidosis in the patient. The condition is aggravated by the impaired excretion of acid by the infected and hydronephrotic kidney.

Nearly all patients will show the biochemical changes - base deficit, raised chloride and urea levels - and about a quarter experience symptoms of nausea and weakness. In acute cases there is vomiting, dehydration and coma.

Treatment

1. Encourage frequent voiding of urine to reduce absorption. A rectal catheter may be needed for a while, especially at night.
2. Increase the fluid intake.
3. Prescribe Sod. Bicarbonate up to 2g (30gr.) thrice daily. In acute phases, intravenous treatment with bicarbonate is needed.

ASCENDING INFECTION

This is the commonest complication and may be regarded in some degree as inevitable. However the modern approach to pyelonephritis with prolonged courses of a variety of antibiotics has improved the prognosis for this condition.

THE ILEAL CONDUIT

THE ILEAL CONDUIT

The ureters are anastomosed to an isolated loop of ileum which is implanted in the skin as an ileostomy.

This not inconsiderable surgical procedure helps to avoid the pyelonephritis and chloride absorption which follow bowel implantation, and the many complications of permanent cutaneous ureterostomy which include stenosis, pyelonephritis, abscess formation and difficulties in collecting urine.

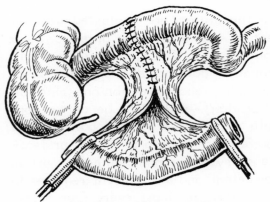

Isolating loop of ileum

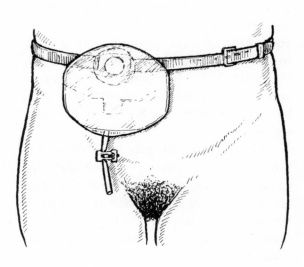

Ureters implanted
in loop of ileum

The ileal conduit is fashioned with wide stomata (both skin and ureteric) and in theory merely acts as pipe carrying a free flow of urine, so that there is no stenosis and no stasis, no absorption and no acidaemia, no reflux and no ascending infection.

The collecting apparatus consists of a rubber or plastic flange held to the skin by a watertight adhesive, and supported by a belt. The urine passes into a bag which can be drained without being taken off.

CHAPTER 14
FISTULA

URINARY FISTULA

(L. fistula: a pipe).   A pathological connection between the urinary tract and an adjacent structure through which urine escapes.   A fistula between the bladder base and the vagina is the condition most often seen.

AETIOLOGY

1. The exposed bladder wall is torn or penetrated during a vaginal operation, or during total abdominal hysterectomy. This is the commonest cause in this country.

A tear develops during mobilization of the bladder

Prolonged pressure of vertex on the vagina during obstructed labour. In a few days slough forms.

2. The vaginal wall and bladder are torn during an obstetric operation: or pressure necrosis develops during a prolonged and difficult labour.

3. The ureter is damaged or made ischaemic during a pelvic operation, especially radical hysterectomy.   This produces a uretero-vaginal fistula.

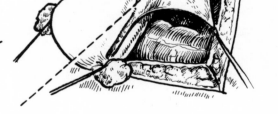

Exposing ureter in radical hysterectomy.

CAUSES OF FISTULA

4. Radiation burns following treatment for carcinoma of the cervix. This fistula may appear several years after treatment.

5. Untreated or recurrent cancer of bladder or genital tract. (This may also be complicated by radiation effects.)

6. Chronic tuberculosis or syphilis. Fistula may complicate surgical treatment of pelvic tuberculosis.

7. Congenital fistula. An accessory ectopic ureter may open into the vagina. This condition should be recognised in childhood.

SITES OF URINARY FISTULA

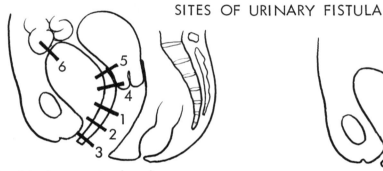

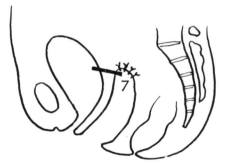

1. Vesico-vaginal: the commonest.

2. Urethro-vesico-vaginal: closure usually followed by stress incontinence.

3. Urethro-vaginal: the only fistula not causing incontinence.

4. Vesico-cervico-vaginal: due to a cervical tear during delivery.

5. Utero-vesico-vaginal: due to a tear of the lower segment and bladder.

6. Vesico-intestinal: may arise from sepsis following major surgery, or from tuberculosis.

7. Vault fistula following hysterectomy.

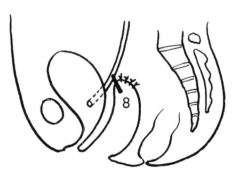

8. Uretero-vaginal: follows ureteric damage at hysterectomy.

PATHOLOGY OF URINARY FISTULA

If the cause is a tear, urine escapes at once but the wound may not immediately become infected, and primary union can occur in a week or two provided the urinary stream is diverted.

If the cause is pressure necrosis, the affected area will form a slough which eventually drops out leaving a fistula.

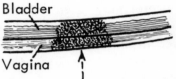

Bladder

Vagina

Area of necrosis which sloughs.

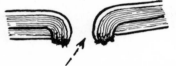

Bladder wall tends to prolapse through fistula.

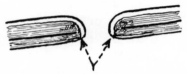

Scar tissue forms and the fistula becomes lined with transitional epithelium.

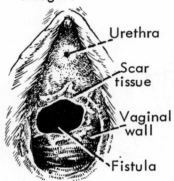

Urethra

Scar tissue

Vaginal wall

Fistula

Large fistula of bladder base with much scarring.

If the fistula is large (over 2cm diameter) spontaneous healing is unlikely and scar tissue gradually forms a dense white ring round the edge of the fistula, even fixing it to a pubic ramus.

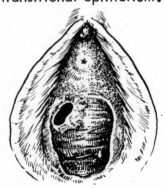

Fistula fixed to the pubic ramus by scar tissue.

Urinary fistulae have a natural tendency to close by granulation, fibrosis and contraction.   Factors interfering with this are:

1. The continual flow of urine.   2. Sepsis.
3. Persistence of a causative factor such as malignancy or radiation necrosis.

If the urinary stream is diverted by a catheter and good bladder drainage maintained, and if the sepsis is dealt with, the natural decrease in size will occur, and many fistulae of 1cm diameter or less, may be expected to close in 2 or 3 months.

SYMPTOMS OF FISTULA

Incontinence may immediately follow the injury, but usually the patient has several days of dysuria and haematuria with symptoms of urinary infection. A discharge appears followed by sloughing, and the patient finds her vulva and perineum are constantly wet. This is soon followed by excoriation of the skin accompanied by a strong ammoniacal smell and incrustation of vulva and vagina with urinary salts. The whole area becomes extremely tender.

DIAGNOSIS

This is usually easy, but if the patient says she also passes urine normally, two conditions must be considered.

1. <u>A very small fistula</u>. Most of the urine is retained in the bladder and passed per urethram. Sometimes quite large quantities of urine may be held temporarily in the vagina while the patient is resting, and she will say that she seems to be dry at night. Small 'pin-hole' fistulae may persist for years and be mistaken for stress incontinence.

A nylon thread passed through a pinhole fistula.

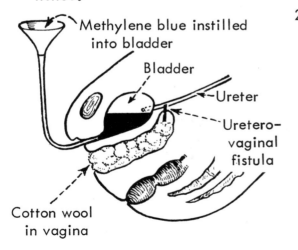

Methylene blue instilled into bladder

Bladder

Ureter

Uretero-vaginal fistula

Cotton wool in vagina

2. <u>A uretero-vaginal fistula</u> produces a constant trickle of urine, but the bladder is still intact and will continue to function. The usual test is to instil methylene blue solution into the bladder. Cottonwool in the vagina will not be stained if the fistula is ureteric. During cystoscopy the dye is injected intravenously to identify the ureteric openings, and cottonwool in the vaginal vault will then be stained. An intravenous pyelogram will show contrast medium leaking into the vagina.

EXAMINATION OF FISTULA

EXAMINATION   In all but the most straightforward cases, this should be made with the patient anaesthetised.

Position of the Patient

If the fistula is low down on the vaginal wall, the lithotomy position is best, but sometimes access is awkward unless some modification of the 'knee elbow' position is used.   One of the main difficulties in repairing a fistula is to obtain good access.

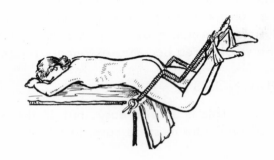

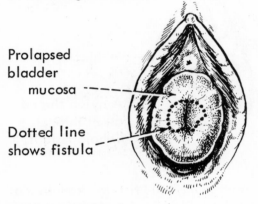

Prolapsed bladder mucosa - - - - - - -

Dotted line shows fistula

Ureteric Orifices

These may be at the edge of a large bladder base fistula, and their situation must be known, lest they be involved in the suturing. Cystoscopy is required during which the fistula must be plugged somehow with a finger or a fingerstall filled with water and distending the vagina.

Another way is to plug the hole with a Foley's catheter passed through the fistula.

Examination of the Fistula

The second difficulty in operative repair is the obtaining of a suture line not under tension from scar tissue. It is essential to know the exact size and situation of the fistula, and the extent of cicatrization and fixity. Prolapsing bladder mucosa may have to be pushed back to determine the margins of the opening; there may be more than one fistula.

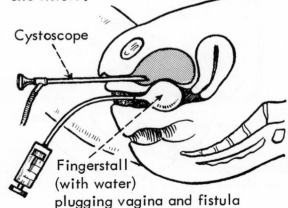

Cystoscope

Fingerstall (with water) plugging vagina and fistula

TREATMENT OF FISTULA

A period of bladder drainage is usual. Fistulae do have a tendency to 'grow smaller' and local infection must be dealt with. The object is to obtain a small fistula surrounded by reasonably healthy, supple, vascular vaginal wall which will allow suturing without tension. If the fistula is small it may even heal spontaneously.

It is sometimes difficult to devise a method of drainage which will leave the patient dry and comfortable; and the longer catheterisation is maintained, the greater the chance of renal infection.

Small Fistula

Suction drainage through a urethral catheter will usually suffice, while the patient lies on her side or in the semi-prone position.

It is seldom worthwhile continuing this treatment for more than three weeks.

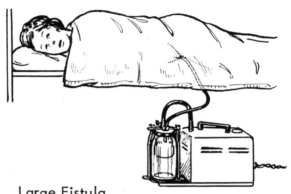

Large Fistula

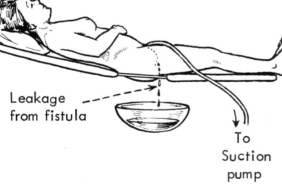

Leakage from fistula

To Suction pump

When damage is extensive, and especially when the urethra is involved, it will usually be impossible to keep the patient dry. Suction is applied through a suprapubic catheter and the patient is nursed in some form of orthopaedic bed which allows free drainage of urine through the fistula. This treatment may be worth maintaining for up to three months.

During this period, antibiotics must be given and local applications include bland vaginal creams such as acriflavine emulsion, and the application of a barrier cream such as benzalkonium chloride (drapoline) to excoriated skin.

OPERATIVE TREATMENT

Two problems must be overcome:
1. Access to the fistula.   2. Avoidance of wound tension.

<u>Access.</u>   The patient must be in a position which provides the surgeon with the most comfortable approach.   The urologist might prefer to work through the bladder from above, but most gynaecologists will be more at ease when operating per vaginam. The patient may have to be in the modified knee-elbow position described on p328.

Sometimes an extended episiotomy may be necessary if the fistula is at the vault, but this must be done with caution. Entry into the ischio-rectal fossa produces free bleeding, and there is a risk of cutting the pudendal and haemorrhoidal nerves.

Meatus

Extended episiotomy

Sucker

Traction sutures

The operating field must be kept clear of urine and blood by continuous suction.   The fistulous area must usually be brought within reach by traction with sutures or Allis's forceps.

Suitably delicate instruments must be provided

Paring scissors

No 11 Swann–Morton blade

Mosquito forceps

Toothed dissecting forceps

OPERATIVE TREATMENT

Classical Technique with Saucerisation

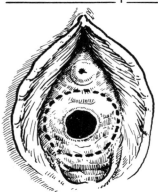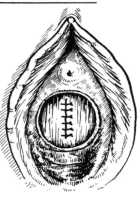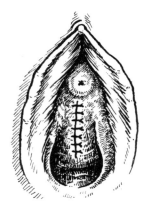

Vaginal skin is dissected as shown. This leaves a rather large wound ('saucerisation') but it is necessary to achieve healthy vascular skin edges and to avoid tension in the sutures over the fistula. The bladder mucosa should not be cut but it is probably good practice to close the bladder wound with fine catgut sutures. The vaginal wall is then closed with interrupted silk sutures.

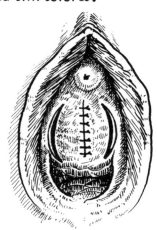

If cicatrization is excessive, and the wound does not seem completely free from tension, relaxation incisions cutting through fibrous bands will allow the wound to close easily ('par glissement'). These incisions may require a vaginal pack to control bleeding but they heal in a few days.

After Treatment

Catheter drainage is continued for a week and antibiotic cover is given. The catheter is then clamped for gradually increasing periods and withdrawn on the ninth day. The sutures are removed on the tenth day, usually with the patient anaesthetised. If there is any doubt about healing, the catheter is replaced for another week.

THE FLAP-SPLITTING TECHNIQUE

This method is used when the fistula is fixed, and mobility difficult to achieve; this is particularly so in the region of the proximal urethra. The 'flaps' consist of vaginal and bladder wall and they are separated sufficiently to allow closure in two layers without tension.

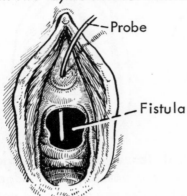

1. A large fistula involving proximal urethra and urethrovesical junction.

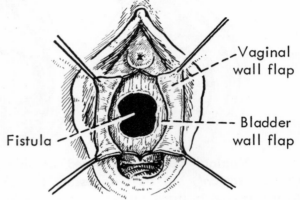

2. Dissection of vaginal wall from bladder.

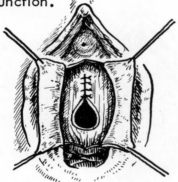

3. Closure of bladder wall with fine catgut. The vaginal wall is then closed in the usual manner, with silk.

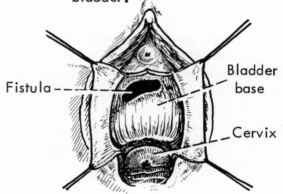

4. Sometimes the whole bladder base must be mobilised from vagina and cervix to provide enough mobile bladder tissue.

A fistula in this area even when successfully repaired, will affect bladder control, and treatment for stress incontinence is usually required some months later.

VAGINAL VAULT FISTULA

This may occur after hysterectomy, and emphasises the problems of inaccessibility and fixity of tissues by scar formation. It might be most easily reached through the abdominal approach, but if sexual function is not important, closure by colpocleisis (lit. closing of vagina) is a good method. The technique is called Latzko's operation, and to permit access an extended episiotomy is made and retractors and traction sutures are required.

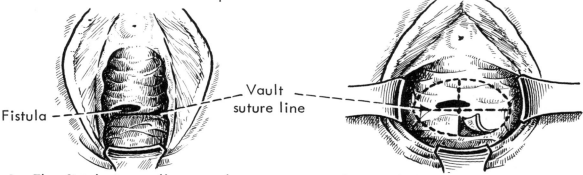

1. The fistula is usually very close to the vault suture line and may also be close to the ureteric orifices.

2. Vaginal vault tissue is removed in quadrants as shown. (Piecemeal dissection is easier.)

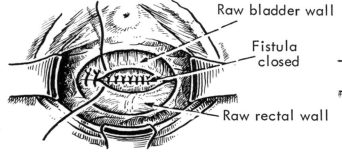

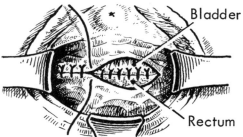

3. The fistula is closed and a second row of sutures apposes raw bladder to raw rectal wall.

4. The vaginal wall is closed transversely with silk sutures.

This technique is applicable only to vault fistulae. If it were applied to a fistula further down the vagina, the vesico-rectal suture line would be under tension. Any colpocleisis must shorten the vagina to some extent.

URETHRAL FISTULA

Operation is difficult because of the thinness of the urethral wall and its adhesion to the vaginal wall. If the fistula is small and scar tissue minimal, the edges should be pared and the fistula closed with silk sutures. Catheter drainage must be maintained for 10 days.

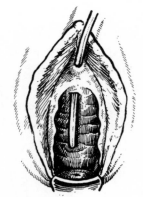

Complete or Partial Destruction of Urethra

Various reconstruction operations have been devised, and Martius' technique is shown here, as illustrating the principle. A new tube must be formed, and then supported by some means so that stress incontinence is prevented or minimised.

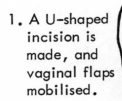

1. A U-shaped incision is made, and vaginal flaps mobilised.

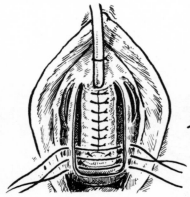

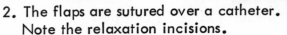

2. The flaps are sutured over a catheter. Note the relaxation incisions.

The new urethra will become lined with epithelium. Before the vaginal wall is closed, a buttressing operation(p297)is done if the tissues are sufficiently mobile. If not a Marshall-Marchettie-Kranz procedure may be possible, which would avoid the fistula field; or one of the operations for interposing fresh tissue with its own blood supply, to provide a supporting shelf beneath the urethra.   Reconstruction operations run the risk of sloughing of ischaemic tissues.

INTERPOSITION OPERATIONS

An adjacent tissue or structure is placed between bladder and vagina to provide support with a fresh blood supply. This may be required where there has been much trauma and especially when fistula is due to radiation necrosis.

<u>Uterine interposition</u> (p 304) is the oldest procedure, but the uterus of course is liable to its own diseases and will probably have been irradiated.

<u>Interposition of Bulbospongiosus Muscle</u> (Martius' Operation). A pedicle of this muscle and attached fatty tissue is interposed.

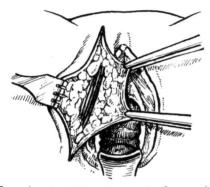

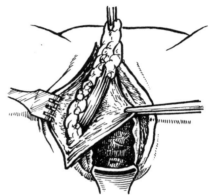

1. An incision is made lateral to the labium majus.

2. A pedicle of musculo-fatty tissue is prepared. Haemorrhage is troublesome.

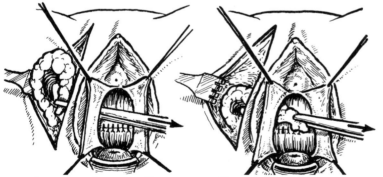

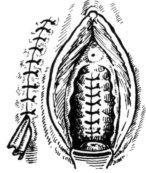

3. The pedicle is pulled medially under the labium minus and sutured over the closed fistula and bladder neck.

4. The incisions are closed. Note the drain in the labial wound.

INTERPOSITION OF THE GRACILIS MUSCLE

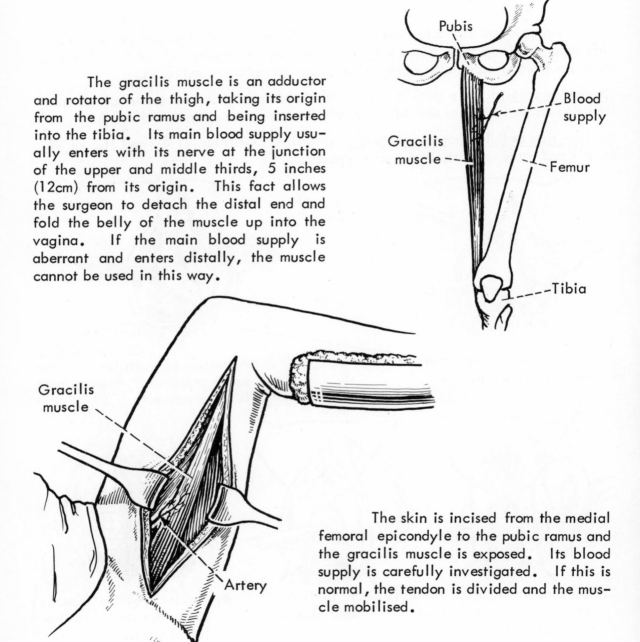

The gracilis muscle is an adductor and rotator of the thigh, taking its origin from the pubic ramus and being inserted into the tibia. Its main blood supply usually enters with its nerve at the junction of the upper and middle thirds, 5 inches (12cm) from its origin. This fact allows the surgeon to detach the distal end and fold the belly of the muscle up into the vagina. If the main blood supply is aberrant and enters distally, the muscle cannot be used in this way.

Pubis

Blood supply

Gracilis muscle

Femur

Tibia

Gracilis muscle

Artery

The skin is incised from the medial femoral epicondyle to the pubic ramus and the gracilis muscle is exposed. Its blood supply is carefully investigated. If this is normal, the tendon is divided and the muscle mobilised.

INTERPOSITION OF THE GRACILIS MUSCLE

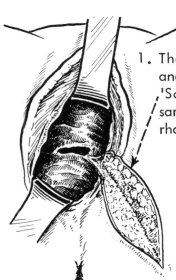

1. The fistula must first be closed and a large episiotomy (the 'Schuchardt incision') is necessary to allow access. Haemorrhage must be dealt with.

2. A fairly large area of sclerotic vaginal wall is removed and the fistula closed with two layers of catgut sutures.

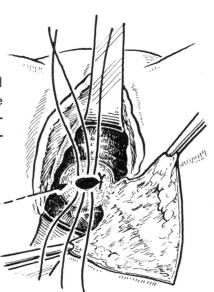

3. A tunnel is dissected under the fascia lata, so that the gracilis may be pulled through into the vagina, in front of the pubic ramus.

4. The muscle is sutured across the fistulous area and the vaginal wall closed over it.

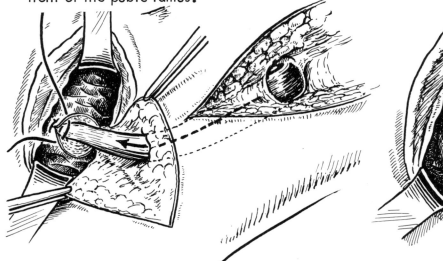

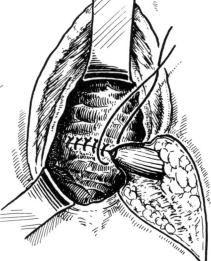

INTERPOSITION OF THE RECTUS MUSCLE

If there has been no abdominal irradiation, this muscle has advantages over the gracilis.

1. The blood supply is multiple and point of entry of the arteries is not critical.

2. It is more accessible.

A disadvantage is the likelihood of ventral hernia.

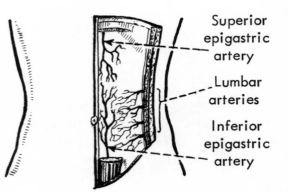

Superior epigastric artery

Lumbar arteries

Inferior epigastric artery

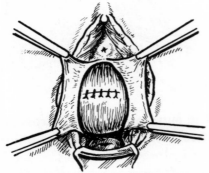

1. The fistula is mobilised and re-paired.

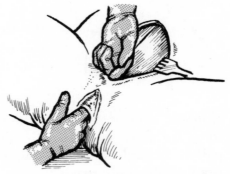

2. Using abdominal and vaginal approach a tunnel is dissected from the space of Retzius to the vagina.

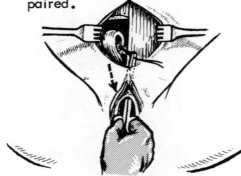

3. The rectus sheath is opened and the lower half of one muscle is mobilised and pulled into the vagina.

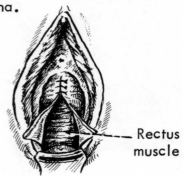

Rectus muscle

4. The muscle is sutured across the fistula and the vagina closed.

INTERPOSITION OF OMENTAL FAT (METHOD OF BASTIAANSE)

This technique was developed to deal with large fistulae following combined radium and surgical treatment of cervical carcinoma. The principle is to introduce into the vagina tissues not damaged by radiation: the bladder fundus, the wall of the sigmoid, the omentum.

A transverse colostomy is made 3 weeks before operation, so that the vaginal area may be cleared of faeces.

1. By vaginal dissection, the peritoneal cavity is entered between bladder and rectal mucosa.

2. By abdominal dissection, the bladder fundus and recto-sigmoid are mobilised and an omental pedicle fashioned.

3. The fistulae are closed and the omental fat sutured between them.

(This kind of surgery calls for very careful dissection in a very difficult field of operation; and would only be undertaken by an expert.)

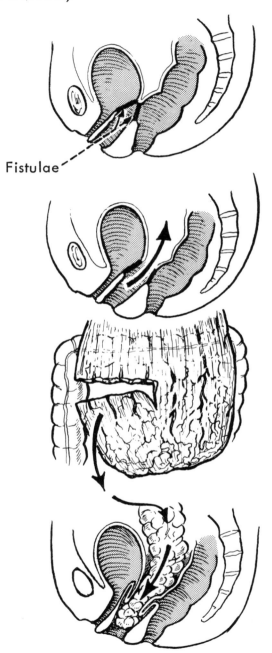

Fistulae

TRANSVESICAL REPAIR

Nearly all fistulae can be repaired by the vaginal route, but it is occasionally necessary to open the bladder to gain access. Repair by this route is more difficult than it looks, and it is an operation best left to the urologist.

The space of Retzius (supra-pubic space) is opened and the bladder incised by a transverse incision.

Polythene catheters are inserted into the ureters. The vagina should be packed beforehand to push the bladder base upwards.

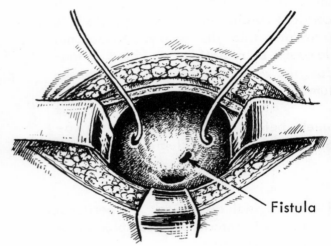

Fistula

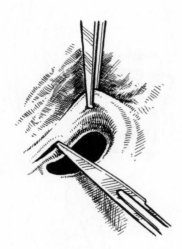

Bladder wall is mobilised from vagina.

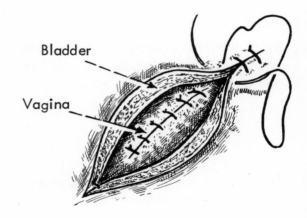

Bladder

Vagina

The vagina is closed with catgut and then the bladder wall.

CHAPTER 15
DISEASES OF THE BROAD LIGAMENT AND FALLOPIAN TUBE

BROAD LIGAMENT CYSTS

BROAD LIGAMENT CYSTS (Parovarian cysts)

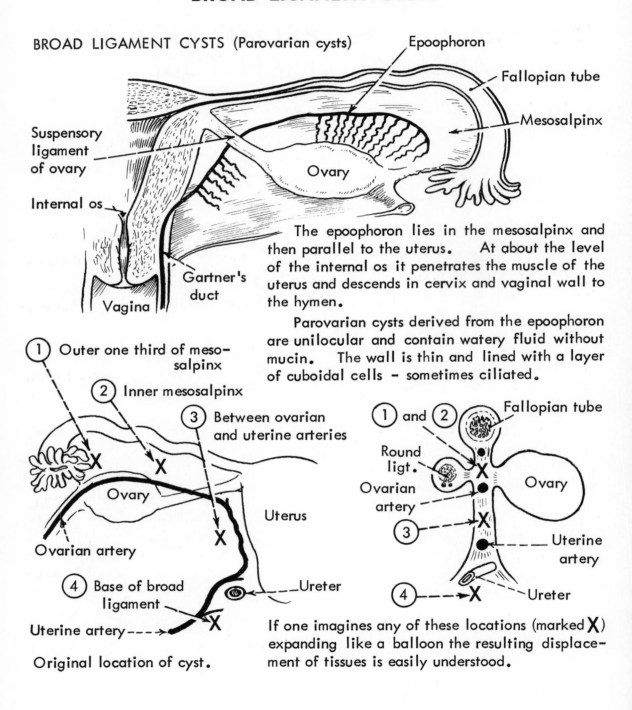

The epoophoron lies in the mesosalpinx and then parallel to the uterus. At about the level of the internal os it penetrates the muscle of the uterus and descends in cervix and vaginal wall to the hymen.

Parovarian cysts derived from the epoophoron are unilocular and contain watery fluid without mucin. The wall is thin and lined with a layer of cuboidal cells – sometimes ciliated.

① Outer one third of meso-salpinx

② Inner mesosalpinx

③ Between ovarian and uterine arteries

④ Base of broad ligament

Original location of cyst.

① and ② Fallopian tube

Round ligt.

Ovarian artery

③

④

If one imagines any of these locations (marked **X**) expanding like a balloon the resulting displacement of tissues is easily understood.

BROAD LIGAMENT CYSTS

Diagnosis

On palpation the cyst, which is not mobile, may displace the uterus and is closely related to it. An ovarian cyst with adhesions may feel very similar and it is seldom possible to distinguish between the two before laparotomy.

Operation

Great care must be taken in identifying tissues as the location of the original site of cyst determines displacement and characteristics.

In the outer third of the broad ligament the cyst tends to develop a pedicle.

In the middle of the broad ligament the tumour is sessile but relatively fixed.

The ovarian vessels are displaced and may be stretched leading to interference with ovarian blood supply.

It is possible for the ureter and uterine artery to be displaced outwards, but usually they are below and medial to the cyst.

The tumour may increase in size and strip the peritoneum off the pelvic walls and spread laterally and posteriorly obliterating the pouch of Douglas.

The broad ligament is incised anteriorly where the blood vessels are few and the cyst is enucleated digitally. The oozing area is now exposed and should be obliterated. Care is necessary to avoid damage to blood vessels, ureter and bladder. Redundant broad ligament may require to be excised.

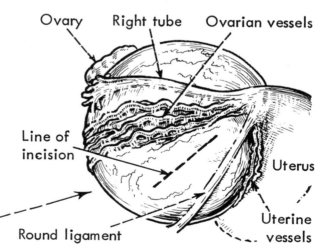

Broad ligament cyst of right side displacing uterus to left.

Ovary   Right tube   Ovarian vessels

Line of incision

Uterus

Round ligament

Uterine vessels

CARCINOMA OF FALLOPIAN TUBES

The fallopian tubes are peculiar among the genital organs for the ease with which they succumb to infection, and their almost total resistance to malignant change. The average gynaecologist may expect to see perhaps one case in a professional lifetime of primary carcinoma of the tube.

Pathology

The growth is usually a papillary adenocarcinoma of the tubal epithelium, which grows inwards rather than invade the tubal musculature, and secretes a copious serosanguinous fluid. The tube wall is much distended and eventually ruptures. Both tubes are liable to be affected simultaneously. Primary sarcoma and chorioncarcinoma have been reported.

Clinical Features

The patient is usually postmenopausal and her complaints are of pelvic pain and sometimes of watery yellowish discharge. This last is said to be pathognomonic, but only appears if the proximal tube is not closed by infection. There may be irregular post-menopausal bleeding and carcinoma of the corpus uteri is suspected.

Treatment

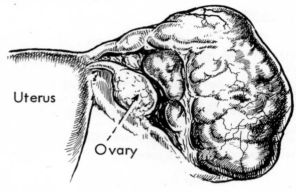

Carcinoma of the right tube. It would be impossible to distinguish this from ovarian tumour except at laparotomy.

Differential Diagnosis

1. Carcinoma of the corpus.
   This is excluded by curettage.
2. Salpingitis. This may well coexist, and in a postmenopausal woman is by itself an indication for laparotomy.
3. Ovarian tumour.

At laparotomy the growth may be so necrotic as to suggest pyosalpinx, but the possibility of cancer must be borne in mind.

Surgical removal of tubes, ovaries and uterus, followed by external irradiation. The prognosis depends on the extent of spread, but is not good.

STERILISATION

This in practice means permanent interruption of the fallopian tubes.

The only certain method of surgical sterilisation is to remove the ovaries. Any operation on the tubes can end in failure, proved by a pregnancy in an aggrieved and possibly litigious patient. But such incidents are very infrequent and large numbers of women undergo sterilisation.

The <u>Principle of Operation</u> is to interrupt continuity of the tubal cavity and seal the ends. There is a natural resistance to this (cf. recanalisation of veins) so interruption of the muscular wall is also necessary. Even then a fistula may develop and allow passage of an ovum.

TECHNIQUES

1. <u>Simple ligation</u>
Silk can be sloughed off and catgut is absorbed. The likelihood of recanalisation is obvious and this operation is not adequate.

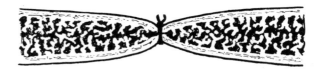

2. <u>Ligation of a loop</u>

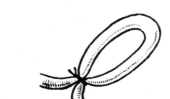  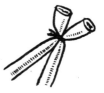

One suture can be used : . . . . or two : . . . . or the end can be cut off

Several months later the end result is the same, a thin short band of fibrous tissue connecting two blind ends.

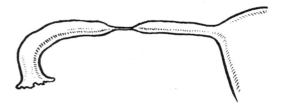

3. Partial Salpingectomy

This has the advantage of allowing the blind ends to be further
apart, but a fistulous ostium is still
a possibility.   Total salpingectomy
is more rational.

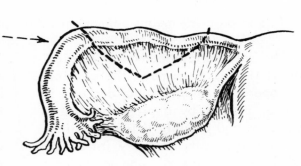

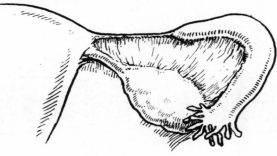

4. Diathermy Coagulation

This can be done under laparoscopic control (p 79).   One electrode is
a plate attached to the patient's leg,
the other is the forceps holding the
tube.   About an inch of tube, usually
the proximal end is coagulated.   The
appearance a few months later is much
the same as partial salpingectomy.

Risks of Sterilisation

1. Sepsis
Salpingitis is an occasional sequel
and total salpingectomy has the merit
of avoiding this.

2. Thromboembolism

3. Tubal Pregnancy
This is extremely rare, but can follow any sort of damage to the fallopian
tube.

The best method is ligation of a loop which can be carried out through a small
suprapubic incision.   Bilateral salpingectomy is a rather more extensive procedure
than is justified by the probability of recanalisation. Whatever method is used, the
chance of restoring continuity is slight, and the patient should be told that the
operation is irreversible.

RESTORING TUBAL PATENCY

These operations are feasible if the blockage is due to a previous sterilisation, or to post-inflammatory adhesions and fibrosis in only part of a tube. But even in the most favourable case - the young woman seeking reversal of tubal ligation - the chance of success is unpredictable.

Salpingostomy

If the block is at the distal end, the tube can be re-opened and a cuff of tubal wall turned back. Reclosure is common and a solid polythene rod should be threaded to be removed per vaginam 6 weeks later. Unfortunately the isthmal and interstitial parts are often too narrow to take such a splint.

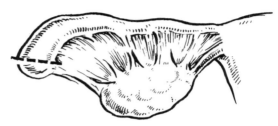

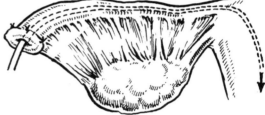

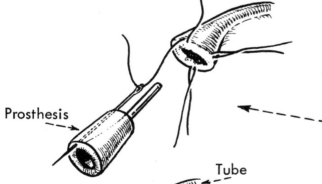

Tube

Prosthesis

Tube

Prosthesis in place

Mulligan's Operation

A plastic fimbrial prosthesis is sutured over the blocked fimbrial end after it has been opened. This technique offers a better chance of obtaining a new ostium that will remain open. The disadvantage is the second laparotomy which is required 3 months later to remove the prosthesis.

RESTORING TUBAL PATENCY

Tubal Anastomosis

The blocked part is excised and an end-to-end anastomosis is carried out. Again it may be impossible to pass the polythene rod into the uterus.

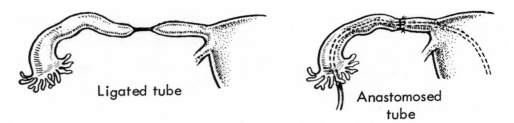

Ligated tube

Anastomosed tube

Uterotubal Implantation

This is done when the block is shown by hysterosalpingography to be at the uterine end of the tube. The blocked length is excised, a new hole is made in the uterine cornu with a reamer (like an apple corer) and the tube threaded through.

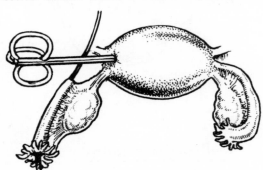

The reamer is boring a hole. Note the polythene rod in the remaining part of the tube.

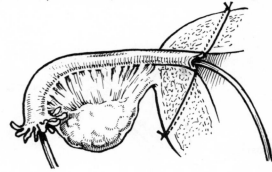

The tube is guided into the new hole and sutured into place.

Such operations are not difficult provided fine instruments are used. The uterus tends to expel the polythene rods and they must be sutured to the peritoneum with their free ends reaching to the cervix or vagina whence they are removed after 6 weeks. These rods cause a good deal of discomfort and uterine bleeding. All operations on the tubes are associated with an increased incidence of ectopic pregnancy if conception should occur.

ECTOPIC PREGNANCY

Implantation of the fertilised ovum outside the uterine cavity. By far the commonest site is the fallopian tube.

Aetiology

Ectopic pregnancy must be regarded as fortuitous, but there are some recognised predisposing factors such as salpingitis which tend to delay the passage of the ovum.

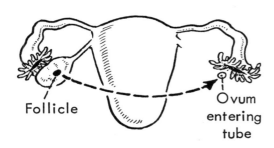

Follicle

Ovum entering tube

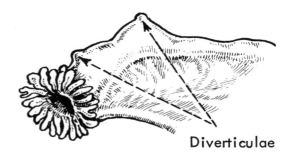

Diverticulae

Migration of the ovum across the pelvic cavity suggests that it may be a day or so older before it enters the tube.

Congenital abnormality of the tube such as hypoplasia or diverticulum formation. This picture shows two diverticulae.

Implantation

There is no proper decidual membrane in the tube and the ovum, once the trophoblastic villi begin to develop, burrows rapidly through the mucosa and embeds in the muscular wall of the tube, opening up maternal blood vessels, and causing necrosis of muscle and connective tissue cells.

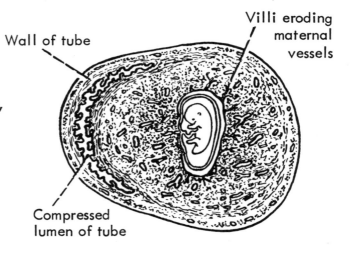

Wall of tube

Villi eroding maternal vessels

Compressed lumen of tube

SITES OF IMPLANTATION

Sites of Implantation

The ampulla is the commonest followed by the isthmus, but the developing ovum can implant anywhere in or out of the uterus.

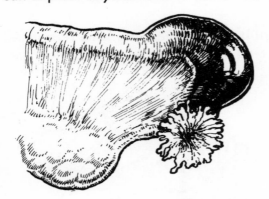

Ampullary implantation. Note the thinning of the tube wall.

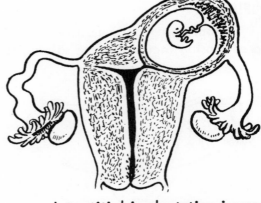

Interstitial implantation is very rare but very dangerous because rupture is accompanied by bleeding from uterine arteries.

Effect on the Uterus

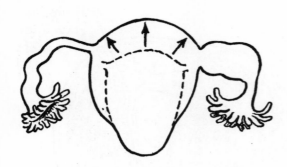

In the first 3 months the uterus enlarges almost as if the implantation were normal. This is a source of confusion in diagnosis.

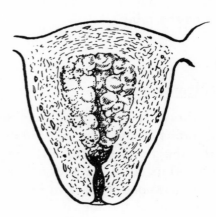

Decidua grows abundantly, and degenerates and bleeds when the ovum dies. Rarely it is expelled entire as a decidual cast.

RUPTURE OF THE TUBE

The muscle wall of the tube has not the capacity of uterine muscle for hypertrophy and distension, and tubal pregnancy nearly always ends in rupture and the death of the ovum.

RUPTURE INTO LUMEN OF TUBE (TUBAL ABORTION)

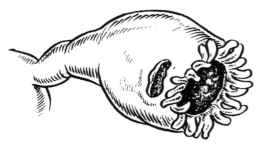

This is usual in ampullary pregnancy at about 8 weeks. The conceptus is extruded, complete or incomplete, towards the fimbriated end of the tube, probably by the pressure of accumulated blood. There is a trickle of bleeding into the peritoneal cavity, and this may collect as a clot in the pouch of Douglas. It is then called a pelvic haematocele.

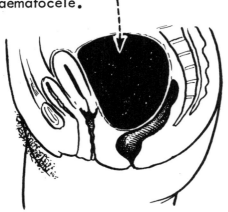

RUPTURE INTO THE PERITONEAL CAVITY

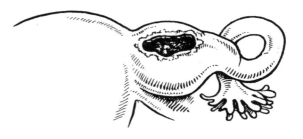

This may occur spontaneously, or from pressure (such as straining at stool, coitus or pelvic examination) and occurs mainly from the narrow isthmus before 8 weeks, or from the interstitial portion at 12 weeks. Haemorrhage is likely to be severe.

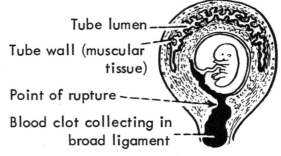

Tube lumen

Tube wall (muscular tissue)

Point of rupture

Blood clot collecting in broad ligament

Sometimes rupture is retroperitoneal between the leaves of the broad ligament — broad ligament haematoma. Haemorrhage in this site is more likely to be controlled.

DIAGNOSIS OF TUBAL PREGNANCY

Tubal pregnancy can present in many ways and misdiagnosis is common.

PAIN in the lower abdomen is always present and may be either stabbing or cramp-like – 'uterine colic'. It may be referred to the shoulder if blood tracks to the diaphragm and stimulates the phrenic nerve, and it may be so severe as to cause fainting. The pain is caused by distension of the gravid tube, by its efforts to contract and expel the ovum, and by irritation of the peritoneum by leakage of blood.

VAGINAL BLEEDING occurs usually after the death of the ovum and is an effect of oestrogen withdrawal. It is dark brown and scanty ('vaginal spotting') and its irregularity may lead the patient to confuse it with the menstrual flow. In about 25% of cases tubal pregnancy presents without any vaginal bleeding.

INTERNAL BLOOD LOSS will, if gradual, lead to anaemia. If haemorrhage is severe and rapid (as when a large vessel is eroded) the usual signs of collapse and shock will appear. Acute internal bleeding is the most dramatic and dangerous consequence of tubal pregnancy but it is less common than the condition presented by a slow trickle of blood into the pelvic cavity.

PELVIC EXAMINATION in the conscious patient will demonstrate extreme tenderness over the gravid tube or in the pouch of Douglas if a haematocele has collected. If the pregnancy is sufficiently advanced and rupture has not occurred, a cystic (and very tender) mass may be felt in the fornix; but often tenderness is the only sign elicited.

PERITONEAL IRRITATION may produce muscle guarding, frequency of micturition, and later a degree of fever, all leading towards a misdiagnosis of appendicitis.

SIGNS AND SYMPTOMS OF EARLY PREGNANCY must be expected, all of which can confuse the clinical picture. When implantation occurs in the isthmus, tubal rupture may occur before the patient has missed a period, and pregnancy tests may be negative until the 40th day.

ABDOMINAL EXAMINATION will demonstrate tenderness in one or other fossa. If there has been much intra-peritoneal bleeding there will be general tenderness and resistance to palpation over the whole abdomen.

DIAGNOSIS OF TUBAL PREGNANCY

Differential Diagnosis

This includes salpingitis, abortion, torsion of the pedicle of a cyst or rupture of a cyst and perhaps appendicitis. The clinical problem is to decide whether or not laparotomy is required, and there are various procedures short of this which may be of help.

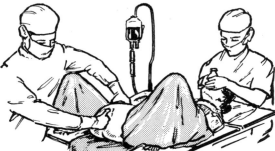

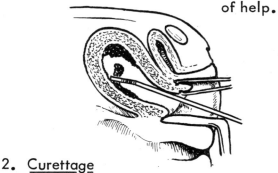

1. Examination under Anaesthesia
This is not likely to yield more information than in the conscious patient. It should always be done in theatre because of the risk of starting haemorrhage.

2. Curettage
If products of conception are obtained, a co-existing tubal pregnancy is very unlikely. Decidua alone means an ectopic but the histological report must be awaited.

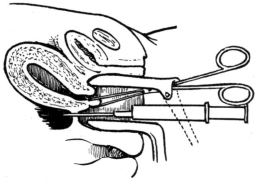

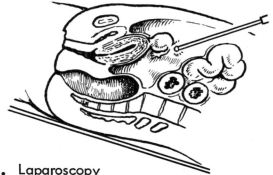

3. Culdocentesis
The passing of a wide-bore needle through the posterior fornix. Old blood is very suggestive, but the absence of blood does not exclude an ectopic pregnancy.

4. Laparoscopy
This is undeniably useful in borderline cases, but it is not always possible to distinguish through the laparoscope between a salpingitis and an intact tubal pregnancy especially if there are many adhesions.

TREATMENT OF TUBAL PREGNANCY

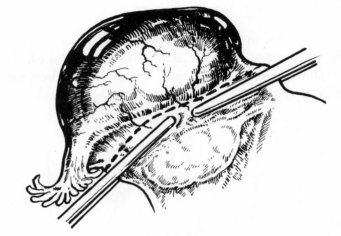

1. Haemorrhage and shock must be treated but if there is delay in obtaining blood the operation should be proceeded with. The patient's condition will improve as soon as internal bleeding is controlled.

2. If a tubal pregnancy is found the blood should be sucked and mopped out and salpingectomy performed. Conservation and repair of the tube even if possible is unwise because of the danger of recurrence, and should not be attempted unless there is a compelling reason such as previous loss of the other tube in a patient who very much wants a child.

Natural History of Ectopic Pregnancies

Rupture or abortion is almost inevitable in tubal pregnancy but absorption must very occasionally occur, and forty years ago it was common practice to encourage natural resolution by vaginal drainage of a pelvic haematocele.

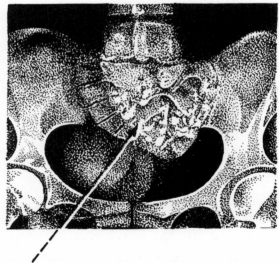

Abdominal pregnancies usually present as obstetrical problems, but in such cases the foetus may also be absorbed or passed per rectum or present as a bizarre gynaecological problem with lithopaedion formation.

Lithopaedion is the name given to calcification of the foetus. This X-ray picture shows one which took $4\frac{1}{2}$ years to develop.

CHAPTER 16
DISEASES OF THE OVARY

CLINICAL FEATURES OF OVARIAN TUMOURS

Ovarian tumours arise at any age but are most common between 30 and 60. The older the patient the more likely is the tumour to be malignant.

Because of the lack of any specific symptom, uncomplicated tumours are often large by the time the doctor is consulted. Menstrual function is seldom upset and any irregularity is attributed to the patient's 'time of life'. She may have noticed that her clothes were getting tight; and if the abdominal swelling has coincided with amenorrhoea, she perhaps believes herself pregnant.

PRESSURE SYMPTOMS

These are commonly an in-creased frequency of micturition and a dull pain in the lower abdomen. If the tumour becomes very big, there may be respiratory embarrassment and oedema or vari-cosities in the legs, and a charac-teristic 'ovarian cachexia' develops, due perhaps to interference with alimentary function.

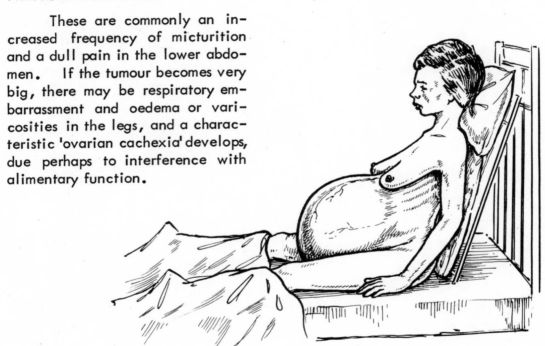

The clinical features are very different if the tumour is hormone secreting or is subject to some complication.

PHYSICAL SIGNS OF OVARIAN TUMOURS

Small tumours remain in the pelvis and will only be detected on bimanual examination.

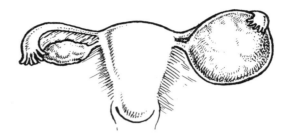

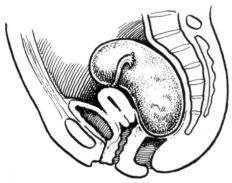

←———————— Larger tumours fill the pelvis and usually lie between the uterus and sacrum. If the patient is not too fat the uterus can be distinguished on palpation as separate from the tumour.

A tumour occupying the abdomen causes a midline swelling and is usually tense.

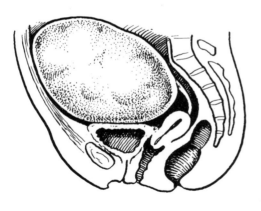

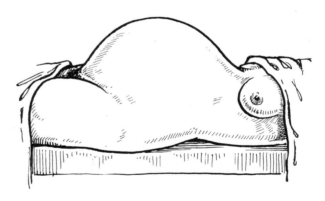

Little can be done at this stage to classify the tumour or exclude malignancy; but very large tumours are likely to be benign; a primarily malignant tumour would have killed the patient before reaching such a size.

PHYSICAL SIGNS OF OVARIAN TUMOURS

If the patient is very thin irregularities may be palpated, and sometimes two tumours may be suspected.

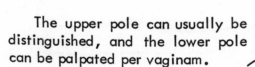

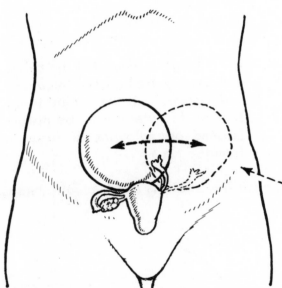

Some tumours of moderate size have a long pedicle composed of the attenuated broad ligament and fallopian tube, which allows the tumour to be displaced from side to side, or to occupy a high abdominal position.

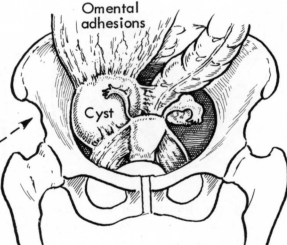

Omental adhesions

Cyst

The upper pole can usually be distinguished, and the lower pole can be palpated per vaginam.

Adhesions, inflammation, displacement of pelvic organs may all exist along with a tumour and confuse the examiner.

DIFFERENTIAL DIAGNOSIS

An experienced examiner will recognise an ovarian tumour, mainly because ovarian tumour is, in the circumstances, the most likely diagnosis; but all abdominal swellings should be subjected to X-ray or ultrasound examination.

Two very obvious mistakes must be avoided.

1. The midline swelling due to a full bladder.

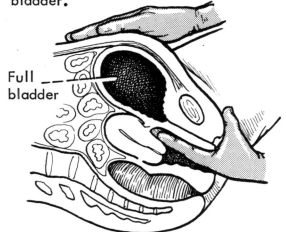

Full bladder

2. The 16 week pregnancy. The gravid uterus at this stage has a very soft isthmic region which can resemble the pedicle of a cyst.

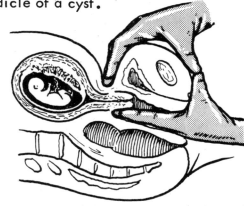

ASCITES. A fluid thrill may be elicited from an ovarian cyst, and ascites and tumour may coexist; but as a rule the distinction should be easily made.

<u>Ascites</u>

The bowel floats on the fluid. The percussion note is resonant over the top of the swelling and dull over the flanks.

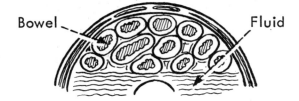

Bowel   Fluid

<u>Tumour</u>

Percussion note is dull over the top of the swelling and resonant in the flanks.

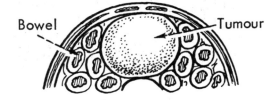

Bowel   Tumour

DIFFERENTIAL DIAGNOSIS

Uterine Fibroids

A large midline intramural fibroid (p 236) may be impossible to distinguish from a solid ovarian tumour until the abdomen is opened and an entirely different surgical problem encountered.

An ovarian tumour will displace the uterus forwards or downwards where it may sometimes be made out separately on vaginal examination.

An intramural fibroid will obscure the uterus. The cavity is often elongated.

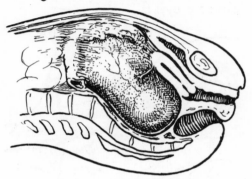

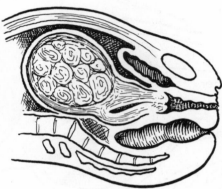

Ultrasound examination should be able to distinguish between fibroid and ovarian cyst; but many ovarian tumours are solid, and some fibroids undergo cystic degeneration.

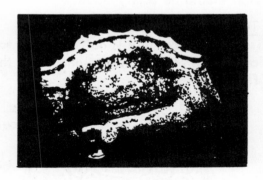

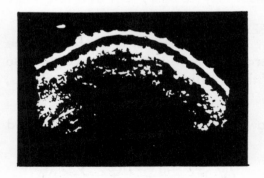

Sonogram of fibroid   Sonogram of cyst

DIFFERENTIAL DIAGNOSIS

Pelvic Inflammation

The swelling palpated per vaginam may be due to an adherent mass of uterus, tubes, 'chocolate' ovarian cysts, and bowel.

A tuberculous pyosalpinx may give the same sensation.

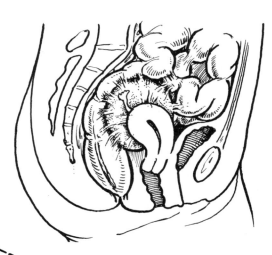

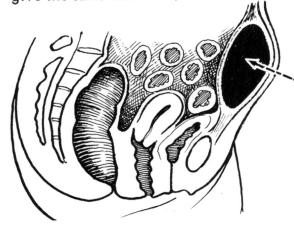

Rectus Sheath Haematoma

This rare condition presents as a fixed abdominal mass, accompanied by pain; and usually follows sudden exertion such as severe coughing. It should be thought of when the pelvis is found to be empty of any tumour.

The Fat Abdominal Wall

The fat patient may be convinced she has a tumour although she is only putting on weight ("phantom tumour"). Palpation is difficult; but the percussion note in the lower half of the abdomen will be resonant.

The Atonic Abdominal Wall

This is seen in old women who display a tense and distended abdomen. There is however resonance to percussion in every area.

Hydatid Cyst
Pancreatic Cyst
Large Hydronephrotic
   Kidney
} These are all rarities in this country, but must be considered if the physical signs are equivocal and especially if the swelling is not in the mid-line.

DIFFERENTIAL DIAGNOSIS

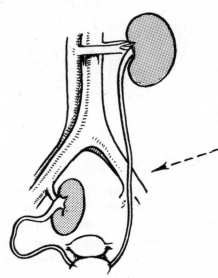

Broad Ligament Cysts

The distinction is not likely to be made before laparotomy, when the intact ovary is observed on the back of the swelling.

Ectopic Kidney or Spleen

These abnormalities are rare but as they are usually detected for the first time on bimanual examination they must be borne in mind. The ectopic kidney can lie anywhere in the pelvis and derives its blood supply from the iliac vessels. The ureter often runs a tortuous course.

Retroperitoneal Tumours

Retroperitoneal in the surgical sense means behind the peritoneum of the posterior abdominal wall. Such tumours are rare but may arise from any connective tissue, lipoma being the commonest. Examination reveals a fixed tumour; but the lipoma may be deceptively fluctuant. The tumour may displace the ureter and is in close relation to large vessels.

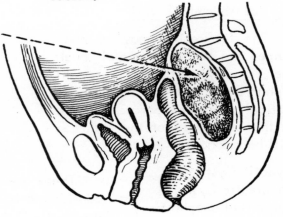

TORSION OF THE PEDICLE

COMPLICATIONS OF OVARIAN TUMOURS

TORSION OF THE PEDICLE
(Axial rotation)

This is the commonest complication and may occur with any tumour except those with adhesions. The thin-walled veins of the pedicle are obstructed first while the arterial supply continues. As a result there is haemorrhage into the tumour and into the peritoneum, and if not treated gangrene will occur. Very rarely the pedicle atrophies and the tumour obtains a new blood supply through its adhesions to surrounding viscera
(parasitic tumour).

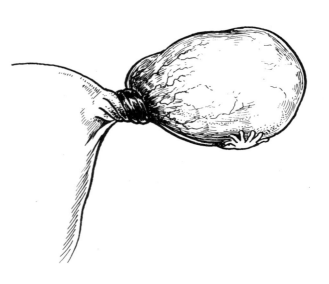

CLINICAL FEATURES

Subacute

The patient complains of recurrent abdominal pain which passes off as the pedicle untwists. There is a rise in pulse and temperature during the bleeding; and over a period anaemia develops.

Acute

The signs and symptoms are those of an acute abdominal condition. The problem becomes one of differential diagnosis to exclude those conditions in which laparotomy is not needed, and laparoscopy may be useful.

DIFFERENTIAL DIAGNOSIS

1. 'Surgical Conditions' (i.e. those conditions commonly seen and dealt with by a general surgeon.)

>   Acute appendicitis
>   Obstruction
>   Diverticulitis

2. Ruptured Cyst

This may occur alone or in conjunction with torsion. Rupture is not particularly upsetting to the patient unless the contents are irritant.

TORSION OF PEDICLE

DIFFERENTIAL DIAGNOSIS

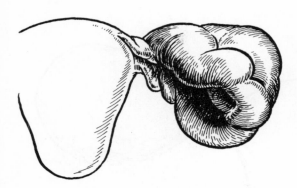

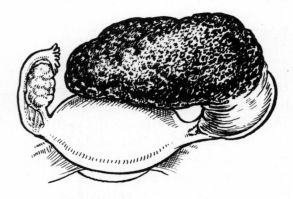

<u>Acute Pelvic Inflammation</u> with tubo-ovarian abscess.

Signs of infection are more marked. A cyst which has undergone rotation is usually larger than the diffuse swelling of pelvic inflammation.

<u>Ectopic Pregnancy</u>

The swelling is usually small although extremely tender and the history suggestive; but in a young woman this condition must always be considered.

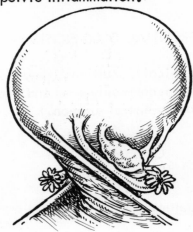

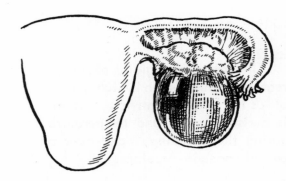

<u>Torsion of a Fibroid</u>

Normal organs very rarely if ever develop axial rotation, but a uterus enlarged by a fibroid may do so.

<u>Ovulation Bleeding</u>

If the ovulation bleeding is greater than usual the woman may show quite marked signs of peritonism. The corpus luteum may thereafter become exaggeratedly cystic and mislead the examiner.

RUPTURE OF OVARIAN CYST

Rupture may be either traumatic or spontaneous.

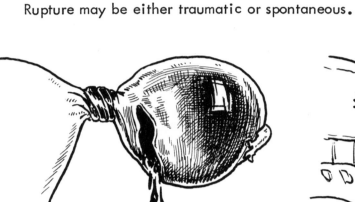

1. Following torsion of a pedicle.

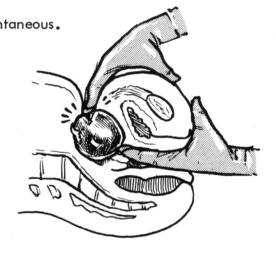

2. During bimanual examination.

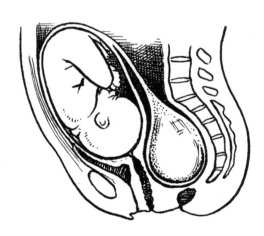

3. During labour when the cyst is impacted in the pelvis.

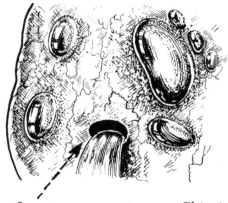

4. Spontaneous rupture. This is not uncommon, especially with malignant cysts, when the epithelial tissue outgrows the connective tissue.

RUPTURE OF OVARIAN CYST

PSEUDOMYXOMA PERITONEI

This rare condition occasionally but not inevitably follows the rupture of a pseudomucinous cystadenoma (p 371). The epithelial cells implant on the peritoneum and continue to secrete a gelatinous pseudomucin; this material is not absorbed, or secretion is faster than absorption; and the abdominal cavity is eventually filled with the jelly, while the secreting cells spread over the parietal and visceral peritoneum. A reactive peritonitis with adhesions is a sequel, and the patient must be operated on at intervals for removal of as much of the exudate as possible. The disease develops slowly over several years, but will eventually cause the patient's death from cachexia or obstruction. A similar condition is reported chiefly in males, from a ruptured mucocele of the appendix vermiformis.

ASCITES

Ascites (Gk.askos: a wine skin) means free fluid in the peritoneal cavity, and its presence in association with an ovarian tumour is strongly suggestive of malignancy. The cause is unknown; but any large tumour may be accompanied by ascites (cf. the small quantities of free fluid sometimes seen at caesarean section).

ASCITES and HYDROTHORAX

The fluid may track via the lymphatic system from the peritoneal to the pleural cavity. Hydrothorax may accompany ascites due to any cause, or may occur as an accompaniment of a lung tumour. The so-called Meigs' syndrome describes the specific condition of ascites and hydrothorax in conjunction with a benign ovarian fibroma.

FEATURES SUGGESTIVE OF MALIGNANCY

1. Age. If patient is over 50 the chance of malignancy is over 50%. Tumours in childhood are usually malignant.

2. Rapid growth.

3. Ascites (almost pathognomic).

4. Solid tumours especially when bilateral.

5. Multilocular cysts with solid areas. (At least 10% of cysts are malignant.)

6. Pain. Pressure pain can occur with any tumour; but referred pain suggests malignant involvement of nerve roots.

EXTRAPERITONEAL DEVELOPMENT

Some ovarian tumours develop to a considerable size between the layers of the broad ligament or retroperitoneally in the direction of the kidney. This is only discovered at operation and the condition must be appreciated and the right plane of cleavage found.

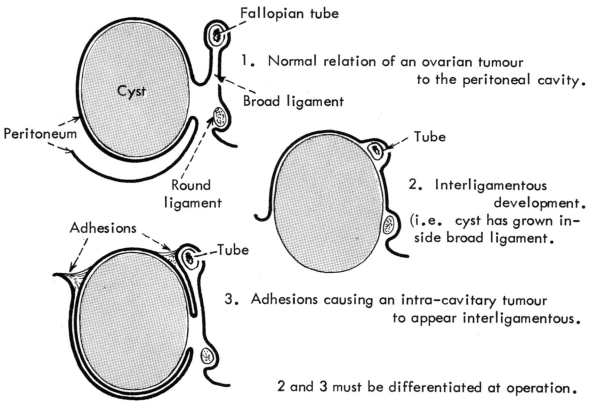

Fallopian tube

1. Normal relation of an ovarian tumour to the peritoneal cavity.

Broad ligament

Cyst

Peritoneum

Round ligament

Tube

2. Interligamentous development. (i.e. cyst has grown inside broad ligament.

Adhesions

Tube

3. Adhesions causing an intra-cavitary tumour to appear interligamentous.

2 and 3 must be differentiated at operation.

INFECTION

Ovarian tumours seldom become infected nowadays but sepsis can be a complication of any trauma to the tumour, including torsion of the pedicle, rupture, and injudicious aspiration of a cyst.

SURGICAL TREATMENT OF OVARIAN TUMOURS

Ovarian tumours must be removed; but this maxim will occasionally be modified by circumstances. Three degrees of excision are recognised :-

1. **Resection**: A portion of the ovarian cortex is removed. This procedure is restricted to some cases of polycystic ovary disease.

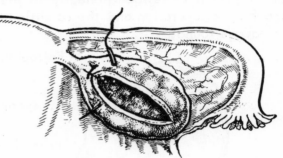

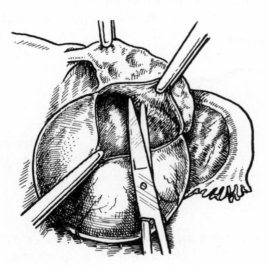

2. **Cystectomy**: Enucleation of the tumour from its capsule of ovarian tissue, thus preserving ovarian function.

Indications: A tumour apparently benign in a woman under 45.

This operation would not be feasible in the case of a very large tumour, or where there had been previous inflammation.

3. **Ovariotomy**: Removal of an ovary containing a tumour. (Removal of an ovary not containing a tumour is called oophorectomy.)

Indications: (a) Malignancy. (The uterus and other ovary are also removed.)

(b) The patient is over 45, or she wishes no more children and the other ovary is normal.

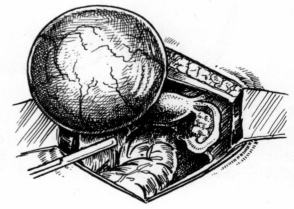

SURGICAL TREATMENT OF OVARIAN TUMOURS

The foregoing summary of the operating position ignores some points which are important in practice. The difference between benign and malignant is often ill-defined, and some women over 45 wish to retain ovarian function. Young women with 'suspicious' tumours provide the most difficult problem, and it is proper to treat them by conservative surgery until malignancy is certain, even although this means two operations.

Removal of the Uterus

Ovarian tumours commonly spread by the blood stream, but most surgeons will remove the uterus. Some prefer to leave it for subsequent use as a radium container, but it is accepted that intracavitary radium cannot reach the pelvic nodes. If the tumour is benign hysterectomy is sometimes done for prophylactic reasons in the older patient.

Tapping an Ovarian Cyst

This is a palliative measure when the cyst is causing dyspnoea and the patient is unfit for operation. At operation large cysts are better dealt with this way before excision, rather than making an incision from xiphisternum to pubis. The theoretical objection is the dissemination of malignant cells, but these very large cysts that need decompression are nearly always benign.

Tapping can be done satisfactorily by passing a suction cannula through a very small incision in the cyst.

Involvement of Other Organs

When the disease has spread beyond the genital tract, a laparotomy and biopsy is usually the only justifiable surgery. However if the omentum is invaded it should be removed with a view to reducing ascites and prolonging survival. Bowel resection (perhaps with a colostomy) is indicated if it will allow complete removal of secondary deposits.

DEALING WITH THE TUMOUR PEDICLE

The pedicle is made up of the fallopian tube, and broad and ovarian ligaments and the infundibulopelvic fold; and contains the anastomosing uterine and ovarian vessels which will be much distended if the tumour is large.

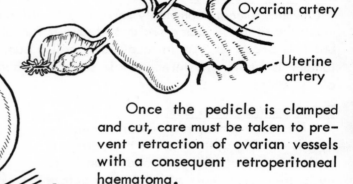

Ovarian artery

Uterine artery

Once the pedicle is clamped and cut, care must be taken to prevent retraction of ovarian vessels with a consequent retroperitoneal haematoma.

It is good practice to put two clamps on the infundibulopelvic fold.

If the pedicle is of any size it should be secured with three or four ligatures. ------>

MUCINOUS CYSTADENOMA

A unilocular or multilocular cyst of ovary lined by tall columnar epithelium resembling that of the cervix or large intestine. It is usually large and may reach immense proportions, occupying the whole peritoneal cavity and compressing other organs. It may occur at any age. Together with dermoids they are the commonest cystic neoplasms of the ovary.

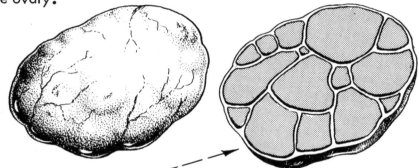

The surface of the cyst is completely smooth and round but may be slightly nodular due to projecting loculi.

The cut surface of the cyst is multilocular and has a mosaic pattern.

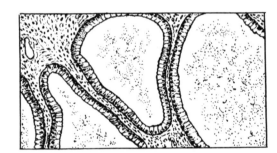

Microscopically the tumour has an outer fibrous capsule from which extend septa supporting the walls of the cysts. The latter are lined by tall columnar epithelium with basal nuclei and contain a gelatinous glycoprotein or mucin.

The signs and symptoms are those generally associated with any non-functioning ovarian tumour. Rupture may occur and seeding of the epithelium on the peritoneal surface will cause pseudomyxoma peritonei.

MUCINOUS CYSTADENOCARCINOMA

This is only a third as common as the serous variety. Malignancy in a mucinous cyst is characterised by the formation of areas of solid carcinoma in the wall. The cells are columnar, show mitoses and tend to form glandular structures.

SEROUS CYSTADENOMA

A unilocular or multilocular cyst lined by epithelium similar to the Fallopian tube. They are common and form 20 per cent of all ovarian neoplasms. In a third of cases they are bilateral. It is uncommon to find them larger than a foetal head. They show one of three structures:−

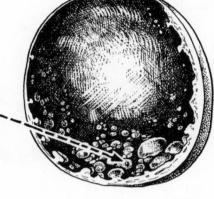

(1) A simple cystic form with smooth surface and smooth lining.

(2) A cystic structure with intra-cystic papillary formations. The latter may be sessile buttons or pedunculated frond-like projections.

(3) An adenomatous form where many of the loculi are small and papillary structures are solid and complex.

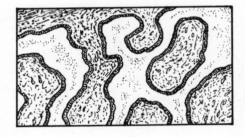

Microscopically the tumour has a fibrous capsule. Septa support the cysts which are lined by cubical epithelium and contain thin serous fluid. They present no distinctive symptoms.

If rupture occurs papillary structures may land on the peritoneal surface where they may grow or lie dormant for years.

SEROUS CYSTADENOCARCINOMA

This is by far the commonest primary carcinoma, accounting for 60 per cent of all cases, and in half the cases it is bilateral. The cysts are always of papillary type and the epithelium burrowing through the capsule produces papillary processes on the serous surface− Extension of the growth to the pelvis and adjacent organs fixes the tumour. Ascites is always present.

The papillomata are always more fleshy than in the simple cysts and microscopically the epithelial cells are several layers thick and show numerous mitoses. When they invade the capsule they frequently take an acinar form.

BRENNER TUMOUR

A benign tumour mainly solid and most common in the 6th decade, composed of fibrous and epithelial elements in varying proportions. It forms 2 per cent of all solid ovarian neoplasms.

It is usually solid and resembles a fibroma. Occasionally there may be microcysts or even an associated large mucinous cyst. Microscopically it is composed mainly of fibrous tissue with small islands of clear epithelial cells of squamous appearance. Sometimes the islands become cystic and the epithelial cells become mucinous.

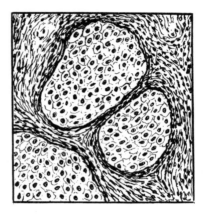

FIBROMA

This is composed of fibrous tissue and resembles fibromata found elsewhere. It is most common in the elderly and accounts for 4 – 5 per cent of all ovarian neoplasms.

The fibroma is believed by many to be a thecoma which has undergone fibrous transformation. It is sometimes associated with Meig's syndrome.

GERM CELL TUMOURS

There are four main types of germ cell tumour:-

(1) Dysgerminoma; (2) Tumours of tissues found in the embryo or adult – the teratomata; (3) Tumours of dysgenetic gonads – commonly a gonadoblastoma; (4) Tumours of extra-embryonic tissues such as choriocarcinoma.

Dysgerminoma

This is the only solid ovarian tumour of characteristic appearance. Usually ovoid with a smooth capsule, it is of rubbery consistency and greyish colour. It is commonest in younger age groups, under 30 years as a rule, and is often bilateral. Sometimes it is found in cases of intersex.

GERM CELL TUMOURS

<u>Dysgerminoma</u> (continued)

Microscopically it consists of masses of large clear epithelial cells with large nuclei, resembling primitive germ cells, in cords or alveoli. Fine connective tissue infiltrated by lymphocytes separates the bundles of epithelial cells. The malignancy varies but many appear to be relatively benign and do not recur. Those in children tend to be more malignant.

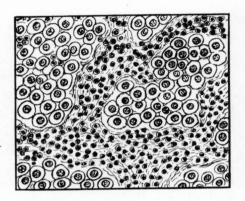

<u>Teratomata</u>

These are broadly divided into (a)cystic and (b) solid forms.

(a) <u>Cystic teratoma or dermoid</u>

This is one of the commonest ovarian tumours and is usually diagnosed during the child-bearing period but may be found at any age and is frequently bilateral.

It is ovoid and unilocular with on one aspect a rounded eminence from which hairs grow and on or in which teeth may be found. The wall consists of dense fibrous tissue lined by stratified squamous epithelium. The eminence may contain sebaceous glands, teeth, hair, nervous tissues, cartilage, bone, respiratory and intestinal epithelium and thyroid gland tissue. Thick yellow sebaceous material fills the cyst.

They are particularly liable to have a long pedicle and easily undergo torsion or interfere with the movement of the pregnant uterus.

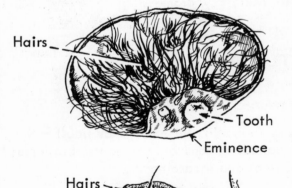

Hairs

Tooth

Eminence

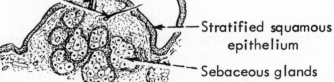

Hairs

Stratified squamous epithelium

Sebaceous glands

GERM CELL TUMOURS

<u>Teratomata</u> (continued)

(b) <u>Solid teratoma</u>

These occur at an earlier age than dermoids, often in childhood. They are solid and may contain any tissue from the three germinal layers, mixed in a completely disorderly fashion. They are particularly liable to undergo malignant change, the malignancy arising in any one of the tissues present.

<u>Gonadoblastoma</u>

This is a tumour associated with dysgenetic gonads, usually streak gonads. The patient is an apparent female and may have a diminutive uterus, tubes and vagina, but usually there is a sex chromosome anomaly such as XO/XY.

The tumour is composed of two types of cell (a) a large primitive germ cell and (b) small cells of granulosa cell type. Call-Exner bodies (small rosettes) may be seen in the latter. These two types of cell form epithelial islands in a stroma which may contain Leydig-like cells. Sometimes the germ cells may undergo rapid proliferation and give rise to a dysgerminoma. Some of the dysgerminomata in children probably arise in this way. Choriocarcinoma may also take origin in a gonadoblastoma. There are frequently some signs of masculinisation and 17-ketosteroid excretion may be raised.

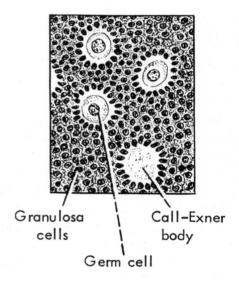

Granulosa cells

Call-Exner body

Germ cell

<u>Choriocarcinoma</u> is mentioned in the succeeding part dealing with hormone-producing tumours.

CARCINOMA OF THE OVARY

Nearly 25 per cent of all ovarian neoplasms are malignant. Approximately 80 per cent of them are primary growths of the ovary, the remainder being secondary, usually carcinomata.

Primary Carcinoma of the Ovary

Eighty per cent of all cases of primary carcinoma of the ovary arise in serous or mucinous cysts. These cysts may however be malignant from the outset. Reference has already been made to these forms of malignancy.

Solid Carcinoma of the Ovary

This accounts for 10 per cent of primary carcinoma. It is commonly bilateral but one tumour is usually larger than the other. The ovarian shape is retained for a time and there is a well marked pedicle but soon the tumours become fixed, secondary deposits occur in the omentum and ascites develops.

Microscopically the growth may take the form of an adenocarcinoma but more commonly it shows solid alveoli or anaplastic epithelial cells in a fibrous stroma.

Endometrial Carcinoma of the Ovary

It is now recognised that carcinoma of the ovary may be of endometrial type, sometimes arising in endometrioma. Attacks of pain, unusual with ovarian cancer, are common. Sometimes there is uterine bleeding in post-menopausal cases.

Usually the lesion is cystic and chocolate brown in colour. If such a cyst ruptures spontaneously malignancy should be suspected. The histology varies as in uterine carcinoma. It may be a well-differentiated adenocarcinoma, an adeno-acanthoma, mucinous adenocarcinoma or clear-celled carcinoma. Like its uterine counterpart it tends to be slow-growing.

Secondary Carcinoma of the Ovary

The ovary may be the site of secondary deposits from growths arising in other parts of the genital tract. These are usually overshadowed by the clinical manifestation of primary growth.

Ovarian metastases from extra-genital tumours are not uncommon. The commonest sites of primary growth are breast, stomach and large intestine. They usually occur in functioning ovaries and their importance lies in the fact that the metastatic growths reach a large size while the primary growth is small and giving rise to no clinical manifestations. They usually reproduce the histological characteristics of the primary cancer. Owing to their rapid growth they tend to be friable and haemorrhagic giving rise to blood-stained peritoneal exudate.

KRUKENBERG TUMOUR

This is a rare secondary carcinoma of the ovary. The primary growth, often clinically silent, is usually in the stomach, less commonly in the large intestine. The ovarian tumours are bilateral, of equal size, smooth and lobulated. They remain freely mobile with no adhesions. Being firm and fibrous in appearance they are frequently mistaken for fibromata, but these are usually unilateral. The patient is usually between 30 and 40, younger than the usual gastric carcinoma patient.

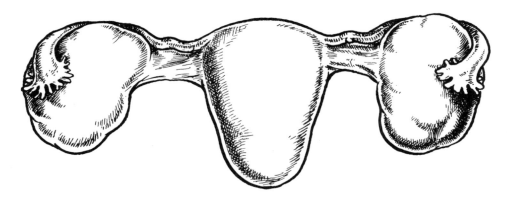

Histologically they have a characteristic appearance. There is a very cellular stroma, resembling a sarcoma, in which are large epithelial cells lying singly or in alveoli. These epithelial cells have a clear cytoplasm with a crescentic nucleus pushed to one side giving a signet-ring appearance which is typical. The cytoplasm is full of mucin.

The majority of patients with this tumour succumb within 1 year of diagnosis.

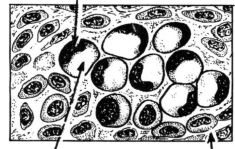

Nucleus of 'signet-ring' cell

Clear mucin-filled cytoplasm

Cellular stroma

CLINICAL STAGING OF MALIGNANT TUMOURS

This has been advocated as a means of allowing comparison of results of treatment between different centres but no system is generally accepted as being useful. The Federation of International Gynaecologists and Obstetricians has drawn up a system which is given here in shortened form with the sub-stages omitted.

Stage 1. Tumour confined to the ovaries
2. Extension to the pelvis
3. Extension to the abdomen
4. Distant metastases

In practice the histological nature of the growth is equally if not more important: the less differentiated the more malignant.

THE PLACE OF RADIOTHERAPY

This is never the primary treatment, and its effectiveness after surgery is a matter of controversy. But it is reasonable to use irradiation in an attempt to destroy as many malignant cells as possible when peritoneal spread is observed at operation.

External irradiation is given to the pelvis or pelvis and abdomen by megavoltage apparatus, and intracavitary radium is used if the uterus has not been removed. Irradiation of large areas often causes radiation sickness which may be so distressing to the patient that the treatment has to be stopped.

RESULTS OF TREATMENT OF MALIGNANT OVARIAN TUMOURS

The most important factor is early diagnosis, when the disease is confined to the ovaries. In practice only about one in four patients survive 5 years.

Stage 1. (confined to ovaries) 70% 5-year survival
2. (spread to pelvis) 30% "
3. (spread to abdomen) 10% "
4. (distant metastases) –

CYTOTOXIC DRUGS

These are substances which prevent the multiplication of cells especially in rapidly growing tissues such as bone marrow, alimentary epithelium, hair follicles.

Side Effects

Bone Marrow: Agranulocytosis, anaemia, thrombocytopoenia leading to local haemorrhages.

Alimentary Tract: Stomatis, glossitis, nausea, vomiting, diarrhoea.

Hair: Baldness, partial or total.

Agranulocytosis may be fatal; but these conditions will normally correct themselves when the drug is withdrawn or given in reduced dosage.

In gynaecology, two groups of cytotoxic drugs are commonly used.

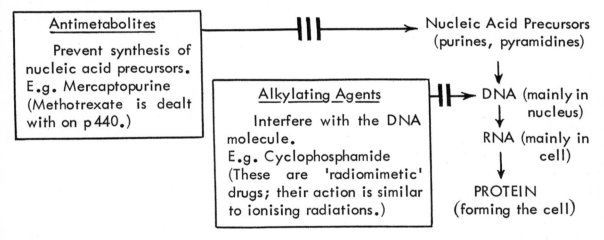

Dosage varies with response and with the leucocyte count, the most sensitive indicator of damage to normal cells. An average daily dose for cyclophosphamide would be 50mg orally for a week at a time.

These drugs are used for palliation only and in gynaecological practice the results are disappointing. Often there is no remission at all; sometimes there is a further lease of six months while ascites and cachexia slowly develop. A good result would be a year of active pain-free life.

HORMONE-PRODUCING TUMOURS

The commonest tumours of this kind are steroid-producing, particularly sex steroids. Both androgenic and oestrogenic effects have been described with every histological variety but certain tumours of well defined histological structures are commonly associated with the production of one type of steroid.

OESTROGEN-PRODUCING TUMOURS

These belong to the granulosa-theca cell group and are found at all ages. They account for 3 per cent of all solid tumours of the ovary.

Oestrogen excess causes:- 1. Hyperplasia of myometrium ➞ enlarged uterus.
2. Hyperplasia of endometrium ➞ irregular bleeding.
3. Hyperplasia of mammary gland tissue ➞ enlargement, tenderness of breasts.
4. Oestrogenic vaginal smear.

In childhood there is accelerated skeletal growth and appearance of sex hair.

5 per cent occur in children ➞ precocious puberty.
60 per cent occur in child-bearing years ➞ irregular menstruation.
30 per cent occur in post-menopausal women ➞ post-menopausal bleeding.

Diagnosis

Granulosa cell tumour in childhood is the usual cause of female precocity and diagnosis is obvious. In child-bearing and post-menopausal years diagnosis is difficult owing to multiplicity of causes of irregular vaginal bleeding. Laparoscopy and ovarian biopsy may be useful.

Pathology

These tumours vary very much in function. Large tumours may be virtually functionless. In childhood and early adult life the tumour is composed mainly of granulosa cells. In later life they are usually theco-mata. The granulosa cell type of growth should be considered as a carcinoma. Recurrence may occur many years after removal of the primary growth. It is not possible to correlate accurately malignancy with histological appearances. In 14 per cent of cases endometrial hyperplasia becomes atypical and carcinoma develops.

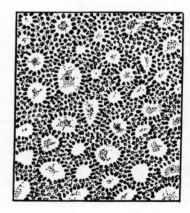

ANDROGEN-PRODUCING TUMOURS

Three distinct types of masculinising ovarian tumour are recognised:–
(a) Arrhenoblastoma, (b) Hilus Cell Tumour, (c) Lipoid Cell Tumour.

ARRHENOBLASTOMA

A rare tumour and forms less than 1 per cent of all ovarian tumours. It occurs in young adult females. Clinically two stages are recognised.

1. Period of defeminisation   2. Period of masculinisation

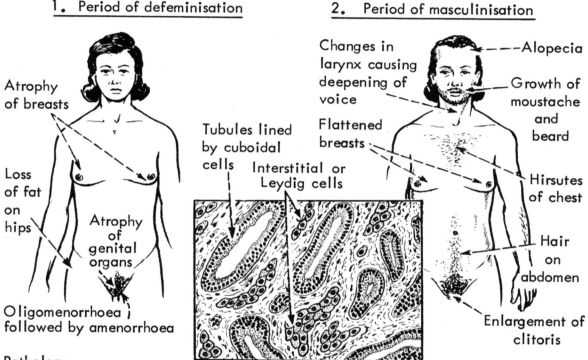

Atrophy of breasts

Loss of fat on hips

Atrophy of genital organs

Oligomenorrhoea followed by amenorrhoea

Tubules lined by cuboidal cells

Interstitial or Leydig cells

Changes in larynx causing deepening of voice

Flattened breasts

Alopecia

Growth of moustache and beard

Hirsutes of chest

Hair on abdomen

Enlargement of clitoris

Pathology

Usually a small white or yellowish tumour within the ovarian substance. Cystic degeneration may occur. In 20 per cent the tumour is malignant and behaves like a carcinoma producing widespread metastases.

Histologically it consists of primitive tubules surrounded by Leydig cells which may contain crystalloids of Reinke. These are rod-shaped structures in the cytoplasm of Leydig cells and said to be diagnostic of these cells.

ANDROGEN-PRODUCING TUMOURS

ARRHENOBLASTOMA (continued)

Biochemistry

The symptoms are due to the secretion of testosterone. The quantities are small and therefore the output of metabolites such as 17–ketosteroids is within the normal range. Direct estimations of blood testosterone can be made but this requires very sophisticated laboratory procedures.

Removal of the tumour results in regression of symptoms in the same order as their appearance. Menstruation returns within a month or two. Voice changes tend to be permanent.

HILUS CELL TUMOUR

This is a very rare tumour found in post–menopausal women. Defeminisation occurs but signs of virilism are usually mild, consisting of hirsutes, alopecia and enlargement of the clitoris.

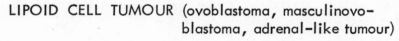

Pathology

Hilus cell tumours are small, brown, simple tumours in the ovarian hilum consisting of polyhedral Leydig cells. Crystalloids of Reinke are occasionally present. 17-ketosteroids are usually within the normal post-menopausal range. Small quantities of androgen are produced.

LIPOID CELL TUMOUR (ovoblastoma, masculinovo-
blastoma, adrenal–like tumour)

This is also a rare tumour causing masculinisation and producing symptoms and signs of hypercorticoidism such as skin striae, obesity, polycythaemia, a diabetic glucose tolerance curve and hypertension.

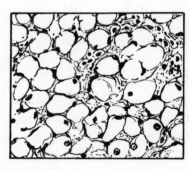

Pathology

The tumour consists of cells with a high content of lipoid and is commonly large and yellowish.

Unlike other virilising tumours the 17–ketosteroid output is greatly increased and the excretion of 17–hydroxycorticosteroids is also raised. ACTH or chorionic gonadotrophin will cause a further increase, but dexamethasone does not diminish the output, thus helping to differentiate the condition from virilism of adrenal origin.

OTHER HORMONE-PRODUCING TUMOURS

Carcinoid (Argentaffinoma: serotonin-producing tumour)

This tumour arises in association with cystic teratoma of the ovary and is derived from respiratory or intestinal epithelium sometimes found in these cysts.

It may give rise to a typical carcinoid syndrome with patchy cyanosis, flushing, diarrhoea, intestinal colic, oedema and cardiac failure due to tricuspid valve lesion. Sometimes the syndrome does not appear until the tumour has metastased to the liver.

Struma Ovarii

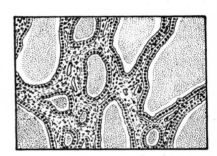

Small foci of thyroid tissue are common in ovarian teratomata but large amounts are rare and functioning thyroid tissue is still more rare. When the thyroid tissue actually proliferates and forms a tumour 5 to 10 per cent become malignant.

Choriocarcinoma of the Ovary

This is an extremely rare tumour of the ovary. Most commonly it is associated with dysgerminoma and both in turn may be derived from germinal cells in a dysgenetic gonad. Syncytiotrophoblast is always present, but sometimes cytotrophoblast is also formed. The hormones produced are those normally associated with chorionic tissue - chorionic gonadotrophin, oestrogens, etc. Metastases may occur as in any choriocarcinoma.

HORMONE-PRODUCTION BY NON-FUNCTIONING TUMOURS

Occasionally the presence of tumour growth in the ovary induces a thecal transformation of the ovarian stroma which in turn produces steroids, sometimes androgenic but more commonly oestrogenic. This has been reported in association with benign and malignant cysts, Brenner tumours, fibroma and secondary carcinoma of ovary. The secretion of steroids results in menstrual upset and in the case of androgens, virilism.

CHAPTER 17
SEXUAL PROBLEMS

INFERTILITY

Infertility occurs in about 10 percent of marriages and may be defined as failure to conceive after two years of unrestricted intercourse.

CAUSES OF INFERTILITY IN THE FEMALE

1. No cause
That is, no cause is found. A third or more of patients who seek advice do ultimately conceive.

2. Age of the woman
There is a natural decrease in fertility from the age of 25.

3. Coital factors
Ovulation time is far from being completely predictable, and conception is more likely if the female genital tract is regularly replenished with an ample supply of active sperms. Conditions preventing this include:

Apareunia
    Vaginismus
    Congenital abnormality

Dyspareunia
    Pelvic inflammation
    Vaginal infection
    Retroverted uterus
    New growths
       (especially vaginal)
    Vulval atresia
       (congenital or acquired)

4. Anatomical abnormality
E.g. Uterus unicornis
     Uterus subseptus

5. Uterine displacement
E.g. Retroversion.
(4 and 5 would only be worth treating if no other cause were found.)

6. Infection
Chronic pelvic inflammation, the organism being unknown.
Tuberculous endometritis.
Gonorrhoea.

7. Endometriosis

8. Endocrine causes
Except for specific conditions such as Addison's disease, endocrine factors are difficult to identify. They manifest themselves as menstrual irregularity, amenorrhoea, and failure of
                  ovulation.

9. Immunological factors
The immunology of conception is as yet only a subject of research. Many species can be immunised against conception by repeated injections of spermatozoa or seminal plasma, and circulating antibodies of this group have been found in women. It has been known for some years that spermatozoa are powerful antigens and the normal female genital tract is presumably endowed with a means of preventing an immune reaction.

INVESTIGATION OF THE WIFE

In about one third of cases some cause will be found in the wife, and in another third the husband will be responsible, while the remaining third will be unexplained. Some infertility clinics make a point of dealing equally with both partners and this calls for the close co-operation of gynaecologist and urologist. However the treatment of male infertility is disappointing, and there may be some advantage in the more unassuming approach whereby the wife is first investigated at an ordinary gynaecological clinic.

Name *Mary Smith*	Age 29	Married 3 yrs.
Menstrual History *Menarche 13 Cycle 5/28 regular. Has occasionally missed a period.* *No dysmenorrhoea*	**Pregnancies** *One ?? abortion 6 months after marriage.* *No curettage.*	
Past Medical *'Shadow on lung' aged 13.* *Father died of hypertension*	**Past Surgical** *Appendicectomy aged 6.*	
Contraception *Sheaths for first 3 months.* *Never on the pill.*	**Frequency** *Now 3/4 times a week.*	
Coital Difficulties *None after first 3 months.* *Occasional orgasm.* *Libido +.*	**Special Notes** *Husband not keen to be investigated.*	

HISTORY TAKING

The usual general medical, surgical and gynaecological information is noted down.

Once a rapport is established, the patient will be able to reply in a relaxed manner to detailed questioning about her sexual life, contraception methods, frequency of intercourse, coital difficulties etc.

Patients with a complaint of infertility are often imbued with a sense of failure, and an attempt should be made to dissipate this. No 'blame' should be attributed to the patient or her husband.

INVESTIGATION OF THE WIFE

The next step is admission to hospital during the second half of the menstrual cycle for examination under anaesthesia, endometrial biopsy and a test of tubal patency.   A secretory endometrium is presumptive evidence of ovulation, and material is also sent for culture for M. tuberculosis: tuberculous endometritis often presents as infertility.   Tubal patency is demonstrated in the first place by the insufflation of CO_2.

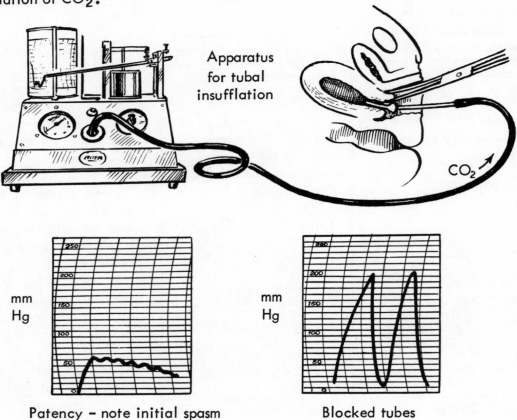

Apparatus for tubal insufflation

CO_2

mm Hg

mm Hg

Patency – note initial spasm

Blocked tubes

The free passage of gas is evidence of patency although not of normal tube function, but blockage may be due only to what is presumed to be spasm, and further tests would be required, either the injection of dye at laparoscopy or a hysterosalpingogram.

TESTS FOR OVULATION

Pregnancy is at present the only incontrovertible proof of ovulation, but there are various methods of providing strong presumptive evidence.

1. Symptoms
Regular menstruation often with mid-cycle discomfort or bleeding, is good evidence.

2. Bimanual Palpation
Daily examinations to detect ovarian enlargement. This is an unreliable method.

3. Endometrial Biopsy
Secretory endometrium is the best sign of ovulation but does not indicate precisely when it has occurred. Repeated biopsies may not be acceptable to the patient but a small biopsy curette can usually be passed without anaesthesia and a small strip of endometrium obtained.

4. Temperature Changes
The temperature is taken every morning by the same route (the axilla is most convenient) before the patient gets up. Ovulation is indicated often by a slight fall and then by a rise of about half a degree above the readings of the first half of the cycle.

This graph shows a well marked response to ovulation. Circles indicate when intercourse has taken place.

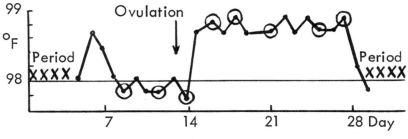

This graph seems to suggest a second half rise, but graphs constructed by patients are often equivocal.

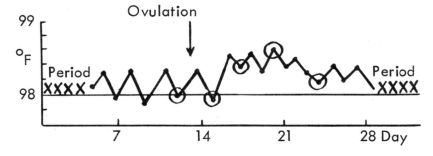

TESTS FOR OVULATION

5. Inspection of Cervical Mucus

The changes described are all due to the increased oestrogen levels preceding ovulation.

(i) Cervical discharge is very much increased (the 'cervical cascade').

(ii) The 'spinnbarkeit' phenomenon should appear. A drop of mucus placed between two slides can be stretched into a thread about 10cm long without breaking.

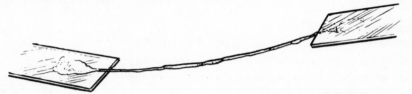

(iii) The Postcoital Test

Microscopic inspection of a drop of mucus 24 hours after coitus should show good penetration by sperms with about 12 active motile sperms in a high-power field.

(iv) Sperm Invasion Test

This test requires a specimen of ejaculate, a drop of which is placed beside a drop of cervical mucus on a warmed slide. Under the microscope the sperms should be seen actively invading the mucus.

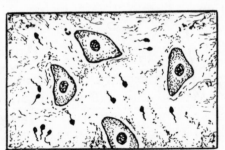

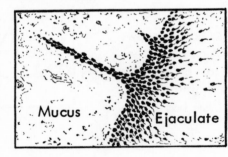

(v) Ferning Test

Cervical mucus when allowed to dry will show a pattern of 'ferning' or arborisation under the microscope. A subsequent increase in progesterone (suggesting ovulation) will abolish this pattern.

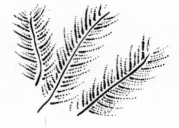

TESTS FOR OVULATION

6. Vaginal Smear

In the first half of the cycle the predominant feature is a large squamous cell with a small nucleus (the pyknotic cell) which is due to oestrogenic influence. After ovulation many of these cells are seen to develop rolled edges and there is a marked 'shower' of leucocytes. This appearance is often confused by the presence of vaginal infection.

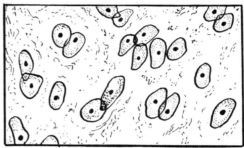

Pre-ovulatory

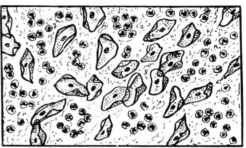

Post-ovulatory

7. Hormone Assays

Daily estimations are required – a considerable strain on laboratory resources. The graph of the urinary excretion rate of oestrogens reaches a peak at ovulation, and the pregnanediol excretion rate is increased in the second half of the cycle.

The excretion rate of gonadotrophins shows wide variations and estimations would only be carried out if treatment with gonadotrophins was being contemplated.

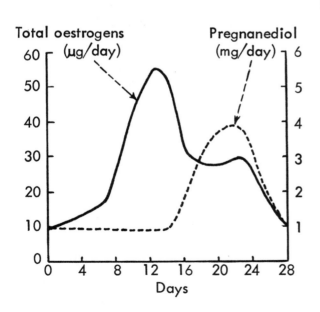

HYSTEROSALPINGOGRAPHY

The radiological visualisation of the genital tract by the injection through the cervix of a radio-opaque fluid. This provides information about intra-uterine abnormalities and is an almost completely reliable indication of tubal patency or blockage; but laparoscopy is to some extent displacing radiology in the diagnosis of pelvic pathology.

Technique

The fluid is usually injected with the conscious patient lying on the X-ray table, but some nervous women will require an anaesthetic. The cervix is exposed with a speculum, the anterior lip grasped with a single-toothed forceps, and the cannula pressed into the cervical canal. Image intensification apparatus is preferable, connected to a television screen. This reduces the amount of radiation to the patient's ovaries, and allows the radiologist to observe the fluid as it flows rapidly through uterus and tubes to the peritoneal cavity. Indeed correct interpretation of radiograph stills may otherwise be impossible.

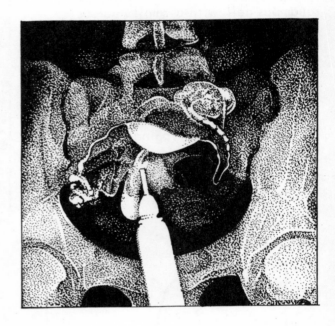

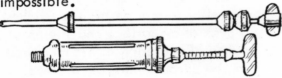

This is the Green-Armytage cannula. The syringe has a screw plunger and one turn delivers 1ml. But any cannula and syringe will serve. Up to 20ml may be needed.

This is a normal hysterosalpingogram. Note:
1. The anteverted uterus is fore-shortened.
2. The long thin tubal outline.
3. The ill-defined shadow of peritoneal spill.
4. Cervico-vaginal leakage.
   Hysterograms often require expert interpretation.

HYSTEROSALPINGOGRAPHY

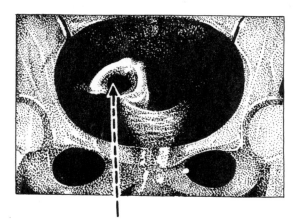

This hysterogram shows a space-filling tumour in the uterine cavity which is in fact a very early pregnancy. The best time to do a hysterogram is in the second week of a cycle, but even then a pregnancy may be disturbed.

INDICATIONS FOR HYSTERO-SALPINGOGRAPHY

1. If tubal insufflation and dye injection at laparoscopy have failed to demonstrate patent tubes.
2. To demonstrate the site of blockage.
3. If some intracavitary anomaly is suspected.
4. If the patient is unsuitable for laparoscopy.

CONTRAINDICATIONS

1. Active pelvic infection.
2. Cervicitis or purulent vaginal discharge.
3. If pregnancy is suspected.

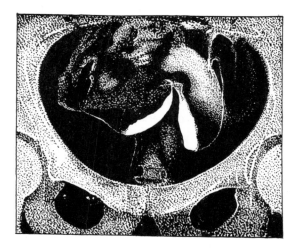

This hysterogram shows the two corpora of a uterus didelphys (foreshortened). This sort of anomaly is better demonstrated by laparoscopy.

COMPLICATIONS OF HYSTERO-SALPINGOGRAPHY

1. In a few cases severe pelvic pain and vomiting may occur an hour or two after injection for reasons unknown. Recovery is within 12 hours but admission to hospital is required for sedation and observation.
2. Infection, or exacerbation of already present infection.
3. With oily radio-opaque media there is a risk of embolism following intravasation. Watery media are safest and are quickly absorbed and excreted.
4. The procedure is something of an ordeal for the conscious patient.

INDUCTION OF OVULATION WITH CLOMIPHENE

Clomiphene (Clomiphene citrate) is a substance which inhibits gonadotrophins in animals but appears to stimulate their production in humans and produce ovulation. It is closely related to chlorotrianisene (Tace) which is a weak oestrogen; yet its clinical use is occasionally complicated by hot flushes, which are an anti-oestrogenic effect. At present the mode of action of clomiphene is not known.

$$OCH_2CH_2N(C_2H_5)_2$$

Clomiphene citrate

$$C_6H_8O_7 \left.\right\} \text{Citric acid radicle}$$

Indications
1. Treatment of ovulatory failure in patients complaining of infertility. The patient's ovaries must have follicles capable of ripening and the pituitary gland must be functioning. Patients with primary ovarian failure, or menopausal symptoms do not respond well.
2. Treatment of the Stein-Leventhal syndrome or the lactation-amenorrhoea syndrome.
3. Postpartum amenorrhoea or post-oral contraceptive amenorrhoea.

The main contraindication is liver disease. Clomiphene is teratogenic in experimental animals, so the possibility of an early pregnancy must be excluded before each cycle of treatment.

Method
A full infertility investigation of husband and wife is first performed and temperature charts kept for several months. Other tests for ovulation will depend on the facilities available.

Dosage
50mg daily from the 5th to 9th day, doubling the dose next month if no ovulation has occurred. Treatment is for 6 months at the most. Temperature charts must be kept and the patient examined regularly.

Unwanted Side-effects

1. Hot flushes in about 10% of cases.

2. Abdominal discomfort due to ovulation in about 5%.

3. Visual blurring - rare.

4. Ovarian enlargement. Gross and dangerous enlargement is almost unknown for the dosage given; but the patient should be examined on completion of each course.

INDUCTION OF OVULATION WITH GONADOTROPHINS

Gonadotrophins are glycoproteins of large molecular weight (between 30,000 and 100,000). All gonadotrophins cause antibody formation and sometimes there is a reaction at the site of injection.

Substances Used

1. HPG (Human Pituitary Gonadotrophin) This substance is obtained from human pituitary glands after death.

2. HMG (Human Menopausal Gonadotrophin) This substance is obtained from the urine of postmenopausal women.

Both these preparations contain FSH and LH and their potency is expressed in international units. Thus the commercial preparation of HMG (Pergonal) contains 75 i.u. each of FSH and LH. (There may be more LH: but FSH is the therapeutic element.)

3. HCG (Human Chorionic Gonadotrophin). This substance is obtained from the urine of pregnant women. It has the same action as LH and is used as a substitute.

Object of Treatment

To induce gradual ripening of one or more follicles by serial injections of HMG (or HPG) and then induce ovulation by the injection of HCG.

Difficulties of Treatment

The amount of FSH required to produce a follicle ripe for ovulation varies with each patient depending on the potency of the preparation used, and the amount of endogenous gonadotrophin produced by the patient herself. This ripeness is measured by observing the increasing oestrogenic effects in cervical mucus and vaginal cytology, and by serial estimations of urinary oestrogen levels which should reach at least 50μmg/24hrs. This requires the resources of a large laboratory.

INDUCTION OF OVULATION WITH GONADOTROPHINS

Results of Overdosage

1. Multiple Pregnancies
   These generally abort; but there have been occasional dramatic survivals.

2. Hyperstimulation Syndrome
   This presents as abdominal pain and nausea due to ovarian enlargement and may proceed to ascites and hydrothorax, leading to hypovolaemia, haemoconcentration, increased blood viscosity and thrombosis. There is also danger of severe haemorrhage from rupture of a large follicular cyst. This complication does not occur until after the injection of HCG. Treatment must include removal of the ascitic fluid and restoration of blood plasma levels by giving concentrated plasma. Transfusion of human albumin has been advised.

Selection of Patients

Repeated failure of ovulation must be established as accurately as possible, but women with complete ovarian failure, primary or secondary, are unsuitable subjects. Such patients will have the high FSH excretion rates characteristic of menopausal women, and an ovarian biopsy by laparoscopy will help to determine whether the patient's ovaries do contain primordial follicles.

Scheme of Treatment

This varies very much indeed. A typical dosage would be:

1. Three injections of HMG on every third day, giving a total dose of anything between 500 and 15,000 i.u. depending on the sensitivity of the patient.

2. Two days later 5,000 i.u. of HCG are injected, provided there has been an adequate oestrogenic response.

3. Intercourse should take place about the day of the HCG injection and on the days following.

CAUSES OF INFERTILITY IN THE MALE

Seminal fluid

The average ejaculate is about 4ml in volume and contains anything between 20 and 200 million sperms per ml. At least 60 percent should be normally formed, and at least 50 percent should show active motility 5 hours after ejaculation. The motility of sperms is more important than sperm count, and reliable seminal analysis requires considerable experience.

Coital Factors

The correct frequency of intercourse to maintain the highest sperm count varies with the individual, and it is probably best to leave the husband to follow his inclination, provided coitus takes place every 48 hours at least during the presumed period of ovulation.

Immunological Factors

At least two types of auto-antibody are known which can either cause azoospermia (autoimmune aspermatogenesis) or agglutinate the sperms after ejaculation and prevent penetration of the cervical mucus.

Gonadal Failure

Congenital hypogonadism.
Cryptorchidism.
Atrophy due to orchitis (pyogenic infection, mumps, gonorrhoea).
Atrophy due to damage to blood supply during hernia operation.

Obstruction of the Vas

Infection, trauma, or congenital defect.

Varicocele of Spermatic cord

Fertility is sometimes restored by varicocele ligation.

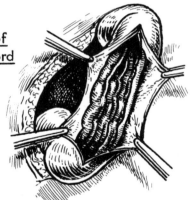

GENERAL EFFECTS OF SYSTEMIC DEBILITATING DISEASE

Pretty well any illness, nutritional disturbance, or emotional upset can depress fertility in male or female, and such conditions must be treated. However if ovulation and spermatogenesis are normal, and coitus feasible, conception is likely to follow.

DYSPAREUNIA

OTHER SEXUAL PROBLEMS

The causes of sexual frustration are not confined to the pelvis and it is the duty of the gynaecologist to ask his patient about her sexual life and so to have her confidence that she will talk freely of her problem to a sympathetic listener. When it comes to treatment however the gynaecologist must remember that he is not a psychiatrist or a marriage guidance councillor but a surgeon, and his primary concern is with the mechanics of copulation.

DYSPAREUNIA – Painful Coitus

Superficial Dyspareunia

This is pain in the vulva or vagina during intromission of the penis. It is usually a genuine complaint (i.e. not simulated with the intention of avoiding coitus for some psychological reason) and the causes include:

1. Painful scar (episiotomy or perineorrhaphy).
2. Acute vulvo-vaginitis.
3. Vaginal cysts.
4. Cyst or abscess of Bartholin's gland.
5. Senile shrinkage.
6. Congenital anomaly of vulva or vagina.

Deep Dyspareunia

This is pain due to pressure by the glans penis on an area of tenderness adjacent to the vaginal vault. The cause is often difficult to identify and there may be no obvious organic disease. Bizarre symptoms are described, and if the gynaecologist cannot reproduce the pain complained of by pressing with his fingers in the vault or moving the cervix, he should consider the possibility of a functional basis for the complaint. Causes include:

1. Retroverted uterus with prolapsed ovaries.
2. Chronic pelvic infection.
3. Endometriosis.
4. Pelvic tumours including the pelvic haematocele of tubal pregnancy.

FRIGIDITY

Absence of sexual desire (libido). If no organic cause is found it is best to refer the patient and her husband to a psychiatrist. None of the steroid hormones has a proven aphrodisiac effect, but it is rational to prescribe small doses of oestrogen say ethinyl oestradiol 0.1mg daily for the first half of the cycle.

APAREUNIA

APAREUNIA   Inability to perform normal coitus

Causes

1. Impotence in the husband
The gynaecologist should ascertain from his patient that her husband:
(a) has normal sexual desire
(b) can sustain an erection.

2. Organic Disease
Vulval atresia, tough hymen, painful scars, acute vulvo-vaginitis, obstructing tumours.

3. Psychological Inhibition
This is by far the commonest cause and manifests itself as a spasm of the vaginal sphincter muscles known as 'vaginismus', which prevents examination.

Treatment

1. The consultations by themselves should allay some of the anxiety and provide hope of cure but a mild tranquillising drug should be prescribed.

2. The patient should be instructed in the use of lubricated vaginal dilators and be seen to pass the smallest size, before going home with a graduated set. After a few weeks she should have enough confidence (the purpose of the dilators) to allow coitus. The husband should understand exactly what is being attempted.

Investigation of Vaginismus

1. The gynaecologist must gain his patient's confidence and get her to talk freely about her problem; and he must even make sure that she and her husband know exactly what they are supposed to be about.

2. An examination under anaesthesia is carried out to exclude organic causes.

3. The patient and her husband should be interviewed by a psychiatrist working in co-operation with the gynaecologist. The causes of vaginismus extend from simple fear and ignorance to profound disturbances of personality, aspects of human behaviour on which the gynaecologist should recognise his ignorance.

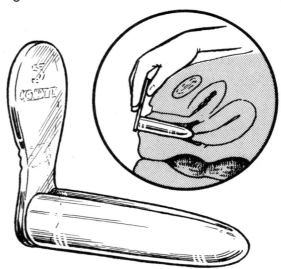

ORAL CONTRACEPTIVES

These are drugs taken daily by mouth which permit the patient to indulge in normal coitus without the risk of conception. Two types of drug are used, an oestrogen and a progestogen combined in one tablet (the 'pill').

Oestrogen   This is either ethinyl oestradiol or mestranol (which is ethinyl oestradiol – 3 – methyl ether) in a dose of 0.05mg.

Ethinyloestradiol

Progestogen   Several compounds are in use: norethisterone, norethynodrel, ethynodiol diacetate. There are many progestogens, all synthetic drugs with a progesterone action.

Norethisterone

Administration

One tablet is taken daily for 21 days from the 5th to 25th day of the cycle. Withdrawal bleeding occurs at the expected time of the period and the tablets are begun again on the 5th day. The combined oestrogen–progestogen tablet is 100% effective, but 'sequential' dosage schemes – 14 days of oestrogen followed by 7 days of the combined tablet – are less reliable although they reduce the amount of steroid taken. Tablets containing progestogen alone avoid oestrogen side-effects but are not completely reliable.

Action of Oral Contraceptives

Ovulation is suppressed by inhibition of the hypothalamic releasing factors, HRF (for FSH) and HRL (for LH). Oestrogens may also directly inhibit FSH on the feedback principle.

Endometrium   Cyclic changes are depressed and menstrual loss much reduced. This effect prevents implantation if ovulation and fertilisation should occur.

Cervix   The cervical mucus remains hostile to sperms.

The exact mechanism of action of oral contraceptives is not yet known. Each drug taken by itself is not a reliable contraceptive and results in considerable menstrual irregularity.

ORAL CONTRACEPTIVES

CHANGES IN GENITAL TRACT

Ovary

Prolonged dosage results in slight shrinkage in size. The follicles are as numerous as before but never enlarge beyond 2-3 millimetres, and the stroma is less vascular. This pattern is reversible.

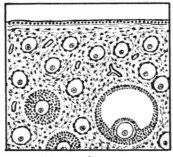

Normal ovary

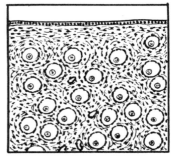

After prolonged dosage

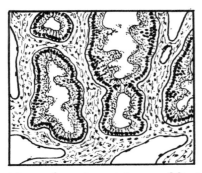

Normal endometrium – 22nd day

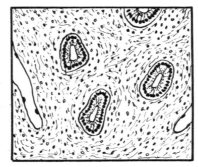

'Pseudo-atrophy'

Endometrium

A 'pseudo-atrophy' develops. The glands although showing secretory activity are much less numerous. The stroma is less vascular.

Cervix

There is an increased vascularity (often seen as a 'pill erosion') and the mucus is thick and tacky and hostile to sperms.

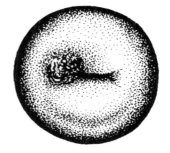

These effects are on the whole favourably received by the patient. The menstrual cycle is regularised, the loss of blood reduced and the period is free of pain and discomfort.

ORAL CONTRACEPTIVES

METABOLIC EFFECTS

Oral contraceptives (OC) act on every system and cause-and-effect relationships are difficult to prove. Most of the undesirable effects are due to the oestrogen.

Effect on the Liver

Liver biopsies sometimes show minimal amounts of cellular degeneration and necrosis and liver function tests are impaired. Jaundice is rare and as a rule the only symptoms are some nausea and vomiting when OC are started. There is however a general increase in the circulating level of the various globulins used as carrier proteins and enzyme substrates. This affects every system and is due either to increased synthesis in the liver, or decreased rate of breakdown.

Hypertension

The increase in circulating renin substrate leads to an increase in angiotensin and the blood pressure rises. There is also sodium retention and increased aldosterone secretion.

It is difficult to estimate the incidence of OC-induced hypertension, because it is such a common condition anyway in pre-menopausal women; but a significant number do develop a mild rise which subsides when OC is stopped.

Thrombosis

1. The level of substrate used in the coagulation and fibrinolytic systems is increased.
2. The level of plasma lipoproteins is increased, and one of these, lecithin, is associated with an increase in platelet sensitivity.

These factors may contribute to an acknowledged although very slight increase in the incidence of thrombophlebitis in women taking OC.

Carbohydrate Metabolism

There is some impairment of glucose tolerance in spite of increased plasma-insulin levels, and some women develop a chemical diabetes. OC are not a cause of diabetes mellitus.

Anaemia

Serum transferrin levels are increased without apparently affecting the haemoglobin content. But serum folate levels are lower and some women will develop a severe folic acid deficiency.

Immunological Disease

Immunoglobulin levels are raised and positive L.E.-cell tests have been reported which became negative when OC was stopped.

ORAL CONTRACEPTIVES

METABOLIC EFFECTS

Adrenal glands

There is an increase in the blood level of corticosteroid-binding globulin (transcortin), but no evidence of impaired adrenal function under stress.

Central Nervous System

Some neuro-ophthalmic disorders (neuritis, blurring) have been reported in association with OC. If such symptoms occur the drug must be stopped at once, whether or not there is any relationship. Headache is not uncommon during the first month.

Psychological Effects

Mood changes are often reported by patients, but such observations are of course very subjective. There is no definite or predictable alteration in libido.

Thyroid Gland

Thyroxin-binding globulin is increased and some thyroid function test may be impaired. Thyroid function is not affected and the basal metabolic rate is not increased.

Skin

Some pigmentation may occur and is most marked with brunettes. It usually takes the form of freckles, and it is not possible to diagnose OC consumption by the facial appearance. Acne and skin greasiness are variably affected, sometimes diminished, sometimes increased.

Carcinogenesis

There is no evidence of any relationship between OC and human cancer, but such a possibility must be considered. One progestogen, chlormadinone acetate, has been found to produce benign tumours in bitches; and there is some suggestion that the activity of cervical epithelial cells is increased.

In spite of the fundamental emancipation which OC make possible, many women are still frightened to take them, saying simply 'I don't believe in the pill'. This uncertainty is communicated by their doctors who must themselves be still uncertain. At present it may be said that there is no medical objection to OC provided the woman has no tendency to thrombophlebitis and is not suffering from liver disease or carcinoma.

Once embarked on OC the patient should ideally undergo an annual test of her blood pressure, urine and haemoglobin level, and have a cervical smear taken.

INTRA-UTERINE CONTRACEPTIVE DEVICES (IUCD)

A polyethylene spiral or coil is inserted into the uterine cavity and effectively prevents conception although the mode of action is not known. Ovulation is not prevented and no recognisable characteristic changes occur in the endometrium.

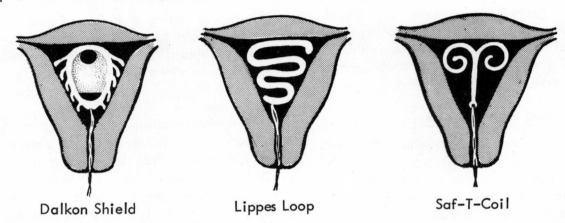

Dalkon Shield   Lippes Loop   Saf–T–Coil

IUCDs are flexible and can be straightened out and held inside a straight cannula for insertion into the uterus. When ejected the coiled shape is resumed, provided the device has not been kept straight for more than 2 or 3 minutes.

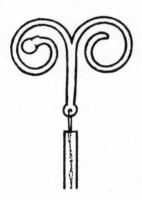

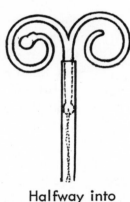

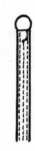

IUCD with nylon thread attached, about to be pulled into introducer.

Halfway into introducer

Completely inside the introducer. Note how the protruding end of the IUCD acts as an obturator.

INTRA-UTERINE CONTRACEPTIVE DEVICES

Insertion of the IUCD

This may be done in the outpatient department or surgery but must be a sterile procedure. About 1 in 4 women is likely to require an anaesthetic either because of nervousness or difficulty in insertion.

1. The cervix is grasped with a tenaculum forceps and the introducer passed through the canal as far as the mark indicates.

2. The IUCD is slowly expelled into the cavity. The thread is pulled gently to make sure the device is properly seated.

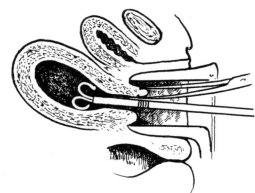

Complications

1. Bleeding.   Heavy and irregular bleeding is the chief disadvantage, and in about 10% of patients the coil must be removed. As a rule the periods become normal after the second month, although the loss is always a little heavier. The haemoglobin level should be checked every 6 months.

2. Pain   Cramping pain is common for the first 48 hours but not thereafter.

3. Expulsion   There is a 5 to 10% incidence nearly always in the first 6 months. The coil is best inserted just after a period when the uterus is said to be less 'irritable' and pregnancy almost impossible.

4. Infection   The coil should not be inserted through a grossly infected cervix or where pelvic inflammation is suspected.

5. Perforation   This presumably occurs during insertion and is a failure of technique. Unexpected pain or resistance during insertion should arouse suspicion, and the exact position of the coil can be checked by X-rays with a sound in the uterine cavity to act as a marker. Polyethylene coils are symptomless in the peritoneal cavity but should be removed.

Pregnancy   IUCDs are not quite so effective as oral contraceptives and the pregnancy rate in a year is about 1-2%. Unnoticed expulsion is a common cause.

THE VAGINAL DIAPHRAGM

THE VAGINAL DIAPHRAGM ('Dutch Cap')

This is a rubber diaphragm which when smeared with spermicidal cream will prevent sperms from reaching the cervical canal. It is less efficient than oral contraceptives or IUCDs unless used strictly according to instructions; but it has no side-effects.

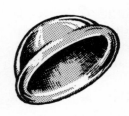

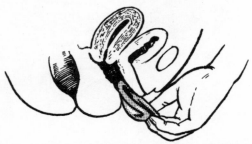

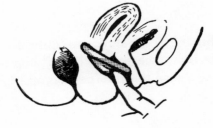

1. The diaphragm is smeared with spermicidal cream round the edges and on both sides, and guided into the posterior fornix.

2. The front end is tucked up behind the symphysis.

The diaphragm must not be removed until six hours after intercourse, and if intercourse is repeated in that period more cream must first be injected with an applicator.

VAGINAL SPERMICIDES

Spermicidal creams, gels, pessaries or aerosols can be inserted directly into the vagina. One dose of spermicide must be injected before each act of coitus, and the method is not completely reliable, but simpler in practice than the diaphragm.

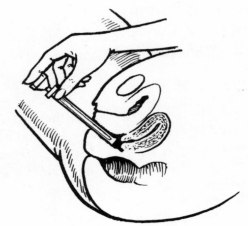

RHYTHM METHOD

RHYTHM METHOD ('The Safe Period')

This means the avoidance of coitus around the time of ovulation. The woman must take her temperature every morning, watching for the sustained rise which indicates ovulation.

Once she has established her normal rhythm she may assume that ovulation occurs between say the 12th and 14th days. Another day is added to allow for ovum survival, and as sperms may live for at least 3 days, coitus must be avoided from the 9th to the 18th day; and the 7th to 20th day would be safer.

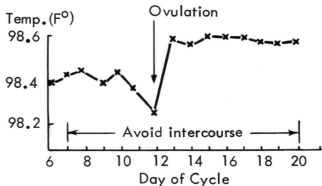

Even this semi-celibacy is unreliable because it depends too much on regularity of ovulation.

Contraception by the Husband

Sheath ('Condom', 'French Letter')

A thin rubber sheath (for the rich man a lamb's caecum) is placed over the erect penis. This is a very efficient method but it interferes with the coital sensations.

Coitus Interruptus (Withdrawal)

The husband withdraws his penis just prior to ejaculation. This method is widely practised, but is unreliable as some sperms are bound to enter the vagina and the act of withdrawal at that point is unnatural.

Vasectomy

About an inch of vas deferens is excised and the ends turned back and sutured. If done properly this operation is not reversible and it is being advocated in many countries as an alternative to tubal ligation, chiefly on the ground of convenience as it can be done as an out-patient procedure. About 4% of cases are followed by some complication such as infection or haematoma, and a case of scrotal gangrene has been reported. There is still some doubt about its legality (as about tubal ligation) and the psychological implications must be given thought.

Two tests for the absence of sperms must be carried out over a month before the man can be regarded as sterile.

MEDICO-LEGAL PROBLEMS

RAPE

The doctor may on occasion be asked to examine a victim of alleged rape. This crime has heavy penalties and examination must be thorough and careful. The following preliminary notes should be made :-
1. Authority for examination.
2. Consent for examination.
3. General appearance of person and clothing.
4. History of circumstances of crime.

Rape is defined as unlawful sexual intercourse with a woman by force and against her will.

Sexual intercourse is described as the slightest degree of penetration of the vulva by the penis and entry of the hymen is therefore not necessary. (Use of vaginal tampons by the unmarried may confuse the issue.)

The vulva should be inspected for signs of bruising, scratching or tearing. The hymen may be torn and bleeding.

When the orifice is small or the hymen vestigial, bruising may be present because of the force needed to penetrate against the resistance of the victim. The presence of seminal fluid in the vagina and cervix may be the only sign. This fluid is removed and examined microscopically.

General examination of the patient may show injuries and bruising confirming a story of resistance overcome by violence.

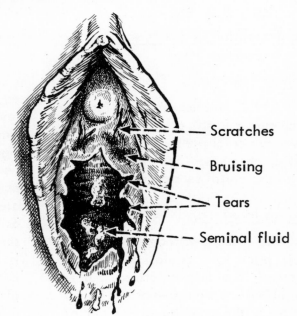

— Scratches

— Bruising

— Tears

— Seminal fluid

MEDICO-LEGAL PROBLEMS

SIGNS OF RECENT DELIVERY

Pregnancy and birth have usually been concealed when a medical opinion is sought.   The patient is usually primiparous and looks exhausted and pale.   The breasts, their veins prominent, are enlarged, tense and knotty, and pressure will express milk and colostrum.

The abdomen is lax and there may be fresh striae gravidarum – especially in the flanks.

The uterus is firm and rises 5–6 inches above the pubis in the first day or two, is behind the pubis by the tenth day and in six weeks is completely involuted and of normal parous size.

The labia and perineum may be lacerated and bruised.

The cervical os is torn and soft and will admit two fingers for a few days and one finger for another week or so.   At two weeks the os is closed.

The lochial discharges are of blood and mucus for about five days, becoming brown, yellow and finally serous, and drying up in four weeks.

A pregnancy test is normally positive for a few days in the puerperium.

CRIMINAL ABORTION

Expulsion of the uterine contents by unlawful means is a crime in Scotland and in England and Wales.   If death occurs the crime becomes at least culpable homicide (manslaughter in England and Wales) and may be murder.

The history may help.   Examination of the woman is important.   The cervix is soft and partly patent with recent abortion.   The abortion may be incomplete.

Visual examination of the cervix may show signs of injury, e.g. forceps marks. There may be signs of uterine infection or of peritonitis.

If it is considered that death is likely then the police should be notified.

CHAPTER 18
ABORTION

ABORTION

ABORTION

The termination of a pregnancy before the 28th week.

The causes and prevention of abortion are matters of obstetrical concern, but gynaecological units often admit abortion patients for treatment.

THREATENED ABORTION

Technically this refers only to bleeding from the placental site which is not yet severe enough to terminate the pregnancy. In practice any case of bleeding before the 28th week may be classed as a threatened abortion in the absence of other explanation. The patient is confined to bed and urine sent for a pregnancy test. After 48 hours a gynaecological examination is carried out.

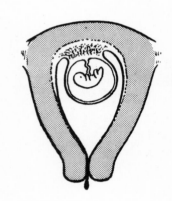

__Threatened abortion__

Bleeding is slight, not retro-placental and the cervix is closed. Pregnancy is likely to continue.

INEVITABLE ABORTION

Here bleeding is also slight and the cervix is closed. Clinically the patient has a threatened abortion, but bleeding is retroplacental and the ovum is already dead.

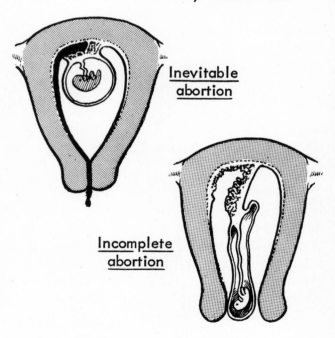

__Inevitable abortion__

INCOMPLETE ABORTION

The foetus and membranes are expelled but the placenta remains attached and bleeding continues. This abortion must be completed by curettage.

__Incomplete abortion__

ABORTION

MISSED ABORTION

The retention of a dead ovum for several weeks. The normal reaction of the uterus to the death of the ovum is to expel it, but for some unexplained reason this may not occur.

Up to about 12 weeks, the whole pregnancy is gradually absorbed and often presents gynaecologically as an unexplained amenorrhoea. After about 12 weeks, the formation of a carneous mole is likely, and after 18 weeks a macerated foetus is usually expelled.

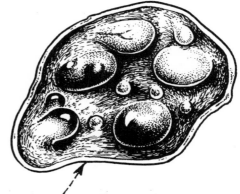

A carneous mole is a lobulated mass of laminated blood clot. The projections into the shrunken amniotic cavity are caused by repeated haemorrhages in the choriodecidual space.

Treatment

If left alone spontaneous expulsion is likely, but if the uterus is no larger than about 10 weeks size, it may be emptied by curettage. This operation requires experience as bleeding is free until the uterus is emptied. If the uterus is too large for the curette the patient is better managed in an obstetric unit. Prostaglandins (p 423) may turn out to be the treatment of choice for this condition.

THERAPEUTIC ABORTION

A termination of pregnancy carried out under the provisions of the Abortion Act of 1967.

The term 'therapeutic' was previously used to imply that the pregnancy was being terminated to save the life or reason of the mother. In practice, various socio-economic factors are also given consideration: the woman has no husband, or cannot afford another baby, or does not want another baby.

CRIMINAL ABORTION

A termination of pregnancy not carried out under the provisions of the Abortion Act. Such abortions concern gynaecologists because of the likelihood of their being done by unskilled hands which introduce trauma and sepsis.

SEPTIC ABORTION

Any abortion which becomes infected. Such infection carries a risk of septic shock.

CLASSIFICATION OF ABORTION

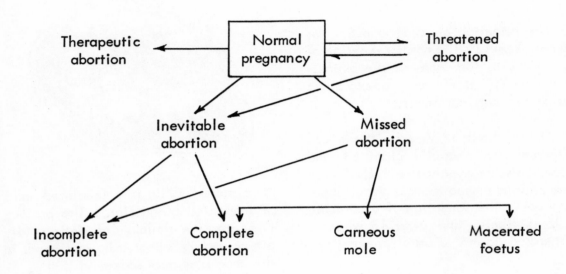

Indications for Therapeutic Abortion under the Abortion Act (1967)

1. the continuance of the pregnancy would involve risk to the life of the pregnant woman greater than if the pregnancy were terminated;
2. the continuance of the pregnancy would involve risk of injury to the physical or mental health of the pregnant woman greater than if the pregnancy were terminated.
3. the continuance of the pregnancy would involve risk of injury to the physical or mental health of the existing child(ren) of the family of the pregnant woman greater than if the pregnancy were terminated;
4. there is a substantial risk that if the child were born it would suffer from such physical or mental abnormalities as to be seriously handicapped.

DILATATION AND CURETTAGE ('D and C')

The uterus is best emptied by curettage and it is often necessary to dilate the cervix further to allow passage of the instruments.

DILATATION is achieved by the application of the mechanical principle of the wedge. Each dilator is a steel tube with a conical tip which is 3mm diameter less than the shaft. Dilators are graduated in size going from 3/6mm up to at least 14/17mm.

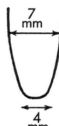

7 mm

4 mm

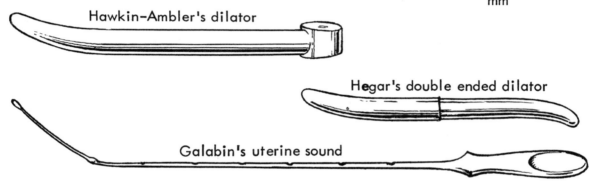

Hawkin-Ambler's dilator

Hegar's double ended dilator

Galabin's uterine sound

Technique

The dilator must be held firmly in the hand and pressed into the cervical canal against the pressure exerted by the other hand.

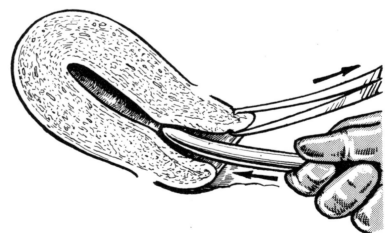

COMPLICATIONS OF DILATATION

1. Tight Cervix
   Resistance can be much reduced by lubricating the dilators with antiseptic cream.

2. Splitting the Cervix
   This may occur without warning at the hands of an experienced operator, but clumsiness is usually a factor. Dilatation should be stopped and the uterus emptied by abdominal hysterotomy. At the same time the broad ligament can be opened up and the cervical tear repaired.

   Bleeding is often slight and there is a greater risk from passing a curette through the unrecognised tear and injuring vessels or bowel.

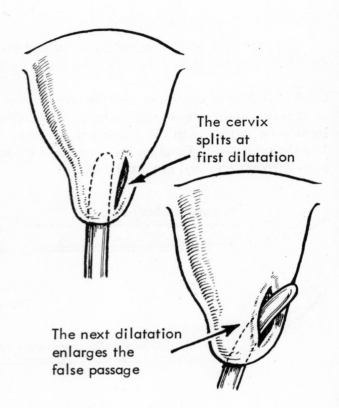

The cervix splits at first dilatation

The next dilatation enlarges the false passage

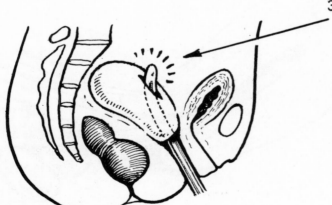

3. Perforation of the Uterus
   This may be the result of clumsiness especially if the existence of a retroflexion has not been noted. The operation must be continued by the abdominal route and any damage repaired.

   (When the uterus is damaged during dilatation and curettage for diagnostic purposes only, it is usually safe to leave the patient alone and observe her for 24 hours.)

INCOMPLETE ABORTION

INCOMPLETE ABORTION - Curettage

Once dilatation is sufficient the bulk of placental tissue may be removed with ovum forceps.

The remnants of tissue are removed with the curette. A blunt curette is ineffective and a large sharp one should be used, always with care.

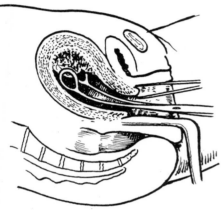

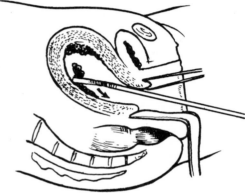

Before using any instrument inside the uterus, oxytocin 5 units should be given to thicken the uterine wall.

The concave side of the curette loop is pressed against the uterine wall and pulled down. A 'clean' uterine wall gives a characteristic sensation to the operating hand.

Packing the Uterus

This is necessary if bleeding continues from an empty uterus and oxytocics are ineffective. Dry sterile gauze is used and the cervix should be dilated up to about 20mm to make it easier to get packing into the whole cavity.

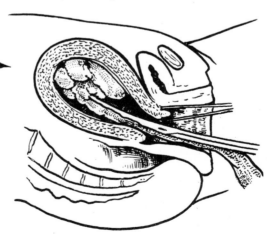

ABDOMINAL HYSTEROTOMY

This operation is for pregnancies of over 12 weeks maturity. The surgical risk is very small but a scar is left on the uterus.

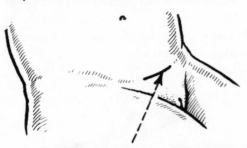

A small transverse suprapubic incision is made below the hair line. There is no need to catheterise the bladder.

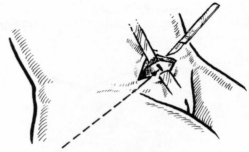

A stab wound is made in the uterus.

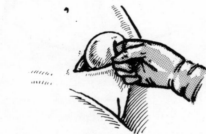

A finger hooked through the stab wound delivers the uterus. Quite a large uterus can be eased through a small wound.

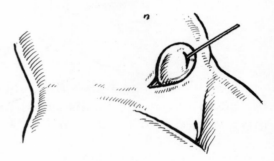

Once the foetus and placenta are extruded the cavity is curetted.

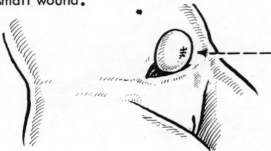

The uterus is closed with continuous catgut sutures. Once it is returned to the pelvic cavity it will contract satisfactorily and bleeding will stop. It is wise however to inject ergometrine just before opening the uterus.

THERAPEUTIC ABORTION

VACUUM ASPIRATION

Evacuation of conceptus by suction. This is now the commonest method of carrying out termination up to 12 weeks.

1. As the suction tube does not need to be pressed so close to the uterine wall there is less risk of perforation than with ovum forceps and curette.

2. In practice it is easier to separate the placenta by suction than with the ovum forceps.

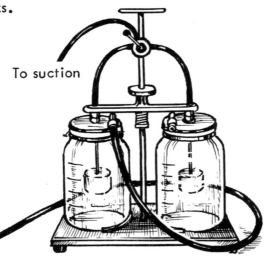

To suction

Technique

The cervix is dilated up to 15mm, ergometrine is injected and the suction tube inserted. A negative pressure of about 20lb/sq.in. is required and a gentle 'curetting' movement is made to dislodge the placenta and foetus which will either pass into the bottle or appear at the cervical os where they can be picked off. It is usual to check that evacuation is complete with a sharp curette.

Complications

1. Haemorrhage is the same as with curettage. About 250ml will be lost at 10 weeks, upwards of a pint at 12 weeks.

2. Perforation. As with all instruments passed blindly into the uterus, there is a risk of perforating the uterine wall. If this injury is suspected suction must be stopped at once and the cavity carefully probed with a sound.

3. Sepsis Incomplete evacuation is not uncommon and antibiotics should be given if this is suspected. It is not always easy to say from an inspection of the material removed, whether the abortion is complete.

THERAPEUTIC ABORTION

Induction of abortion by INTRA-AMNIOTIC INJECTION of hypertonic saline

Mechanism of Action
As in surgical induction of labour, the mechanism has not been explained.

Theories ─ ► But:

1. Foetal death naturally leads to abortion.
2. Placental function is affected and the progesterone level falls.
3. Osmotic attraction causes sudden mechanical distension of the uterus, by increasing volume of liquor.
4. Direct effect of sodium on the myometrium.

Abortion is much quicker than after a natural intra-uterine death.

The most effective method of obstetrical induction is to reduce the volume of liquor.

Dextrose is as effective.

Technique
Dextrose is likely to encourage infection, possibly fatal, and 20% NaCl is now the fluid of choice although urea is also being tried.

1. The gestation must be at least 16 weeks i.e. big enough to allow safe amniocentesis. About 100ml liquor are withdrawn and an equivalent amount of saline injected.
2. If there is any doubt about the needle being in a vessel or not completely in the sac saline must not be injected. The injection should stop if the uterus appears to be distending.
3. Abortion should occur within 48 hours.

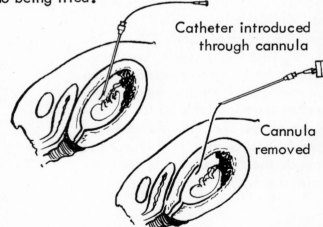

Catheter introduced through cannula

Cannula removed

The safest method is to introduce a plastic catheter through a wide bore needle.

THERAPEUTIC ABORTION

INTRA-AMNIOTIC INJECTION (continued)

Complications

1. The procedure like surgical induction cannot be relied upon completely. A proportion of patients will need oxytocin infusion, and curettage may be required to make sure that the uterus is empty.

2. It is not always possible safely to carry out amniocentesis. The number of technical failures should be reduced by experience and by dealing only with pregnancies of 16 weeks or over.

3. The contractions produced are stronger than those of a normal full-time labour and there is a risk of uterine rupture or of cervical damage.

Dangers

1. Sepsis   This is a well recognised risk with all operations on the pregnant uterus. A mild pyrexia is normal but should not persist after abortion is complete.

2. Systemic Infusion of Hypertonic Saline.
   If this happens to any extent it will kill the patient. It can occur either by direct injection into a uterine vein, by transperitoneal absorption, or possibly by intravasation when too great a volume of fluid is injected.

   Symptoms: 1. Intense thirst. (Some degree of thirst is always present.)
   2. A burning sensation in the hands and arms.
   3. Headache and convulsions. Death is from cerebral haemorrhage caused by sodium intoxication.

The advantage of the method is the avoidance of uterine and abdominal wall wounds, but it seems unlikely to become the method of choice for therapeutic abortion until some fluid is discovered which can be guaranteed to start labour and is harmless if injected systemically.

THERAPEUTIC ABORTION

INJECTION OF PASTE

through the cervix. The injection of abortificient material must be a very ancient practice: at a modern ethical level it has been employed for the last 40 years.

Mechanism of Action

This has not been explained. The uterus normally reacts to the presence of a foreign body by attempting to expel it; yet injection of paste does not invariably bring about this reaction.

Material

All pastes consist of soft soap mixed with small quantities of iodine and some aromatic tinctures, but probably the soap alone would be effective. The one in use today is called Utus paste.

Technique

No anaesthetic is required. About 20ml of paste is injected through a suitable cannula into the uterine cavity over a period of about 10 minutes. Abortion should follow within 48 hours in 75% of patients.

Complications

1. Failure of method
   About 1 in 5 will need curettage to make the abortion complete. Some will need oxytocin and may not abort for several days.

2. Sepsis
   Some degree of sepsis may well be essential, but about 10% will develop a pyrexia. It is known that uterine contractions force some of the paste through the tubes and peritonitis or septicaemia may result.

3. Bleeding
   Some patients lose enough blood to require transfusion.

4. Spread of paste in the blood stream
   This does occur and may present in mild form with haemolysis and jaundice; or as pulmonary or cerebral embolism.

THE RISKS INVOLVED IN THERAPEUTIC ABORTION

Fatalities have been reported with every method and the surgeon must not sacrifice the patient's safety to her convenience or future advantage. The operation must be done in a fully equipped theatre and blood must be available. It is naturally preferable to avoid opening the uterus in a young unmarried girl; but if the surgeon feels that hysterotomy would be the safest method in the circumstances prevailing, then hysterotomy should be done.

THERAPEUTIC ABORTION

PROSTAGLANDINS

Prostaglandins are of interest to the gynaecologist because of their powerful oxytocic effect even in early pregnancy when posterior pituitary hormone is in-effective.

1. Prostaglandin was the name given (in 1935) to a substance found in human seminal fluid which caused smooth muscle contractions and was thought perhaps to be a hormone sec-reted by the prostate.

3. Classification
Prostaglandins must still be re-ferred to as 'substances'. They are not hormones or enzymes and their biological purpose is not known.

4. Chemical structure
They are all derived from a fatty acid - prostanoic acid. There are four main groups A, B E and F which differ in the car-bon ring, and all active pros-taglandins have one or more double bonds in the side chains.

2. Composition of Prostaglandin
It is now known to consist of at least 13 related compounds some of which may be unstable precursors. They are found in many parts of the body including the male and female genital tracts, brain, thyroid, in-testine, amniotic fluid. They may be a constituent of all living matter.

Prostanoic acid

Clinical Use

Two prostaglandins PGE_2 and $PGF_{2\alpha}$ are particularly effective and are at present under experiment. An intravenous injection of E_2 at $5\mu g/minute$ will induce abor-tion within 15 hours as a rule, and the success rate is high if the method is confined to pregnancies of more than 12 weeks duration. Some nausea and vomiting is common and curettage may be required. Prostaglandins have also been given as vaginal pessaries with the same success.

HABITUAL ABORTION

This condition is said to exist in a woman who has had three consecutive abortions.

<u>Causes</u>

Early abortion before 14 weeks suggests an endocrine or genetic cause. Late abortion is more likely to be due to some local uterine condition, and more likely to be susceptible of cure. In practice a definite cause is seldom found but some investigations should be done if the patient intends to start a fourth pregnancy.

1. <u>Curettage and Laparoscopy</u>

This will reveal any mechanical cause such as congenital uterine anomaly, fibroids, acute retroflexion, cervical laceration.

2. <u>X-ray hysterography</u>

This will reveal any abnormality of the uterine cavity and may help to confirm the suspected presence of a torn and overstretched cervix ('incompetent cervix').

3. General examination should include an X-ray of lung fields, a blood count, a check of the blood pressure and blood urea level, inspection of the urine, and tests of thyroid, adrenal and ovarian function. Blood grouping, tests for syphilis and a chromosomal analysis are carried out on both partners, and on fresh aborted material if it is available. The husband should be asked to provide a specimen of seminal fluid for analysis.

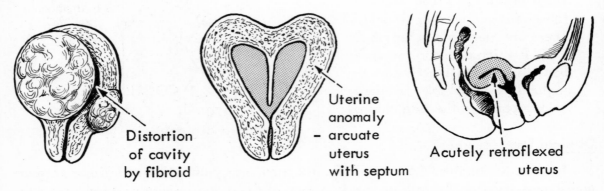

Distortion of cavity by fibroid

Uterine anomaly – arcuate uterus with septum

Acutely retroflexed uterus

These three conditions are shown as possible causes of habitual abortion; but in each case adaptation to the state of pregnancy is possible and abortion is not inevitable.

HABITUAL ABORTION

Treatment

It is rare for any hitherto unknown systemic cause to be uncovered but uterine abnormalities should if possible be dealt with. Fibroids should be removed and congenital defects such as a uterus septus may be corrected by plastic operations. A cervix made incompetent by previous trauma may be repaired by insertion of a suture at the level of the interior os (Shirodkar's suture).

Diagnosis of this condition is made on a history of late abortions and by palpation or occasionally by hysterography.

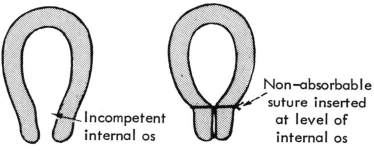

Incompetent internal os

Non-absorbable suture inserted at level of internal os

If the cervix is much torn a formal plastic repair can be carried out (Shirodkar's operation).

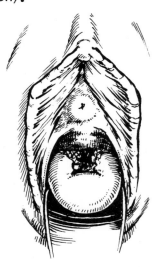

Incompetent cervix. The anterior wall has been torn right through.

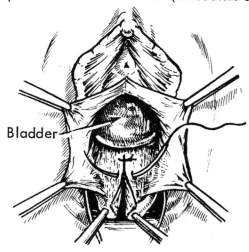

Bladder

Shirodkar's repair. The vagina is opened, the bladder pushed up and the cervical edges trimmed and re-apposed.

SEPTIC ABORTION

Uterine infection at any stage of an abortion

Causes

1. Delay in evacuation of the uterus. Either the patient delays seeking advice, or the surgical evacuation has been incomplete. Infection occurs from vaginal organisms after 48 hours.

2. Trauma, either perforation or cervical tear. Healing is delayed and infection is more likely to be a peritonitis or cellulitis. Criminal abortions are of course particularly liable to sepsis.

Infecting Organisms

These are usually the vaginal or bowel commensals.
1. Anaerobic streptococcus
2. Coliform bacillus
3. Clostridium Welchii
4. Bacterioides necrophorus.

Any of these organisms but particularly the last two may be the cause of septic shock.

Clinical Features

Slight bleeding continues with pyrexia and a raised pulse rate. Examination reveals pelvic tenderness and the patient displays anxiety.

Treatment

This should be active to minimise the risk of septic shock. Cervical and high vaginal smears, and several blood cultures are taken and a broad spectrum antibiotic such as cephaloridine exhibited forthwith. Curettage should be carried out as soon as possible; there is nothing to be gained by leaving infected material in utero. Perforation of a septic uterus is easily done, and in a few cases hysterectomy must be resorted to.

SEPTIC SHOCK

Circulatory failure associated with septicaemia.

The precipitating factors are the endotoxins released by Gram negative organisms and the exotoxins from Gram positive ones. C. Welchii, the organism classically associated with septic abortion produces several necrotising and haemolytic toxins.

Clinical Appearances

These vary, but in a well developed case the patient is fevered, pale, sweating and confused. Blood pressure falls below 100mg Hg. and the pulse is racing. The extremities gradually become cold and cyanosed.

Treatment

Prophylaxis is best of all, with early recognition of the infection. If shock has appeared, large doses of antibiotics must be given at once e.g. kanamycin 0.5g six hourly for Gram negative organisms and cephaloridine in the same dose for Gram positives. (Kanamycin has a toxicity similar to streptomycin.) Smears from the genital tract and throat, urine specimens and repeated blood cultures are sent to the bacteriologist and the antibiotic changes as indicated.

SUGGESTED MECHANISM OF SEPTIC SHOCK

1. The bacterial toxins either directly or by causing the release of vaso-active compounds such as histamine and bradykinin, produce an arteriolar constriction which leads to pooling of blood in the veins and a resultant fall in cardiac output.

2. The fall in output is opposed by the carotid and aortic arch reflexes and there is further release of adrenaline and noradrenaline with further vasoconstriction most marked in the viscera and skin. By this means the blood pressure is maintained and the cerebral circulation protected.

3. But eventually the peripheral anoxia so damages the capillaries and the arterioles themselves that fluid is lost into the tissues with a further and perhaps irreversible fall in blood volume. The heart muscle itself affected by the prolonged toxaemia and ischaemia, goes into fibrillation and cardiac arrest follows.

POSSIBLE MECHANISM OF SEPTIC SHOCK

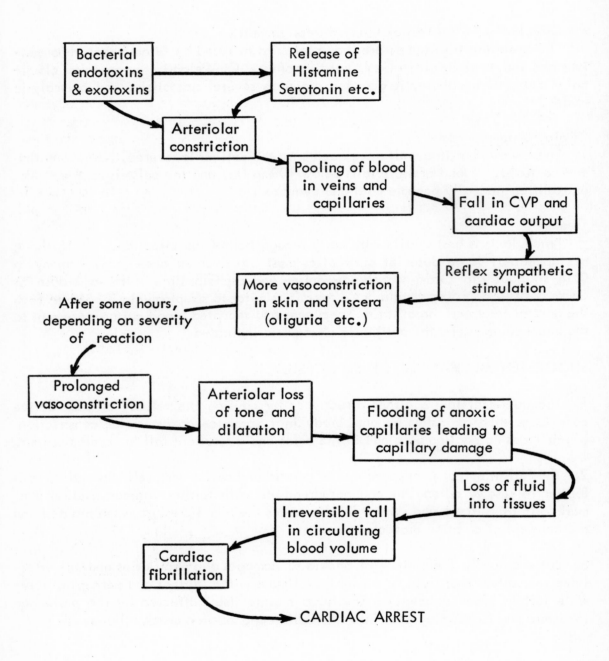

TREATMENT OF CIRCULATORY FAILURE

There is at present a general agreement that in the presence of acute peripheral circulatory failure, management is made easier by passing a catheter into a vein near the heart and monitoring the Central Venous Pressure (CVP).

CVP is technically the pressure in the right or left atrium, but for practical purposes it is taken as the pressure recorded in one of the great veins, preferably the superior vena cava.

CVP is an indicator of the amount of blood returning to the heart and continuous monitoring is necessary. Pressure at the right atrium varies between 0-15cm.H_2O in the normal state and 2-15cm. at the antecubital vein. In shock, if the pressure is persistently below say 5cm. then rapid transfusion is required.

Technique

A special manometer set is used. Once the catheter is in the vein, the manometer connected to it is attached to a drip-stand and the calibrated tape is adjusted so that zero cm. H_2O is at the level of the right atrium.

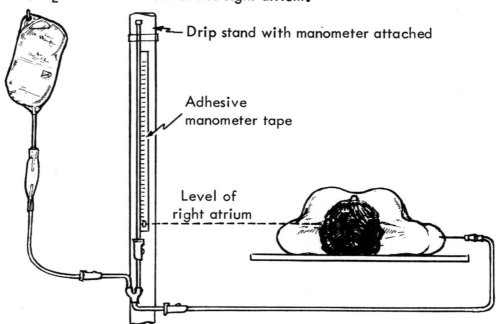

Drip stand with manometer attached

Adhesive manometer tape

Level of right atrium

TREATMENT OF CIRCULATORY FAILURE

CVP monitoring – continued

Level of the Right Atrium

The right atrium lies half way between the back and front of the patient in the plane of the 4th costo-chondral junction.

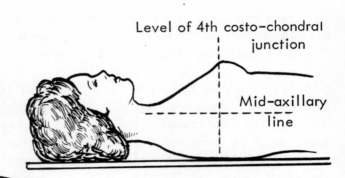

Level of 4th costo-chondral junction

Mid-axillary line

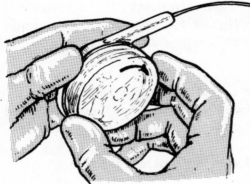

The flexible catheter is 'paid out' like a fishing line.

Inserting the Catheter

This may be passed via the sub-clavian or internal jugular veins if the operator possesses the special technique. The gynaecologist will find it easier to use the external jugular vein, or most familiar of all the antecubital vein, through which a flexible catheter can usually be passed quite easily at least to the subclavian vein.

Complications of CVP Monitoring

1. Central venous transfusions must be given carefully to avoid overloading and pulmonary oedema.
2. The catheter may break off. Only radio-opaque catheters should be used.
3. Thrombosis and embolism may occur especially if the femoral vein is used.
4. The subclavian vein passes over the lung apex and damage there may cause pneumothorax or haemothorax. Other structures in that area which must be avoided are the subclavian artery, the brachial plexus, and on the left side the lymphatic duct.

CVP monitoring is potentially more dangerous than peripheral venous monitoring and transfusion, and its use is not justified in cases of simple haemorrhagic shock.

TREATMENT OF CIRCULATORY FAILURE

Oxygen
The oxygen carrying capacity to anoxic tissues is much reduced and the patient should be nursed in an oxygen tent.

Blood
For the same reason blood is needed, apart from the need to maintain blood volume. Septicaemia of this degree is often accompanied by haemolysis and intra-vascular clotting, and haematocrit figures are required.

Urine Output
Output will be very low and there is often haematuria. If oliguria persists after adequate fluid replacement 100 ml of 10% mannitol should be given and if there is no diuresis renal failure must be considered.

Cardiac stimulants
Circulatory failure from any cause must affect the heart and digitalis should be given without waiting for signs of cardiac failure. Isoprenaline, a β-receptor stimulant which increases cardiac output without any peripheral constriction may have a place in treatment of shock.

Steroids
Large doses of hydrocortisone have been used (up to 2g in 24 hours) to obtain vasodilatation, although it is known that adrenal failure is not always a complicat-ion of septic shock. The value of this treatment is uncertain, and such large doses of steroid have misleading anti-inflammatory and fluid-retaining effects.

Vasodilator drugs
Phenoxybenzamine has an adrenergic-blockading effect and has been used in an attempt to reduce the intense peripheral constriction and thus increase cardiac out-put and achieve a return to normal circulation. One of its immediate effects is to lower the blood pressure and therefore the CVP by about 30% and it must be given with extreme care at the rate of about 1mg/minute, with constant monitoring of the CVP. This treatment like the use of steroids has still to obtain general acceptance, but it would be justified as a last resort.

HYDATIDIFORM MOLE

This is a conceptus lacking an intact foetus, showing swelling of the villi. Aetiology is unknown. Three changes are found in the villi.

1. Trophoblastic proliferation of both the cytotrophoblast (Langhan's cells) and syncytiotrophoblast.
2. Hydropic changes in the stroma.
3. Absence of blood vessels.

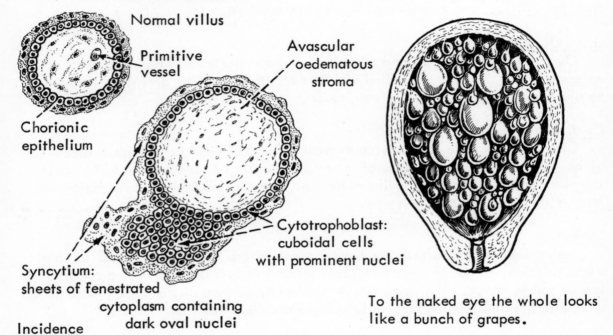

Normal villus

Primitive vessel

Avascular oedematous stroma

Chorionic epithelium

Cytotrophoblast: cuboidal cells with prominent nuclei

Syncytium: sheets of fenestrated cytoplasm containing dark oval nuclei

To the naked eye the whole looks like a bunch of grapes.

Incidence

True incidence is unknown. In the United Kingdom reports vary from 1 in 1,200 to 1 in 2,000 pregnancies.

U.S.A.	1 in 1,000 to 1 in 2,500
Russia	1 in 333
Mexico	1 in 200
Phillipines	1 in 173
Formosa	1 in 120

HORMONAL EFFECTS OF MOLE

The hyperplastic chorion secretes large quantities of gonadotrophin (HCG) and this can usually be detected in the urine. Positive reactions may be obtained with urine diluted up to 1 in 500 in the so-called quantitative pregnancy tests.

The high concentration of chorionic gonadotrophin in the blood may stimulate the ovaries and cause multiple lutein cysts. Enlargement of the ovaries results and they can be easily palpated. The cysts regress after delivery of the mole.

Excessive morning sickness has been attributed to the high oestrogen levels which may be related to the stimulating effect of the gonadotrophin.

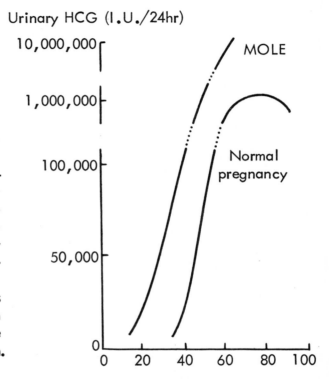

Urinary HCG (I.U./24hr)

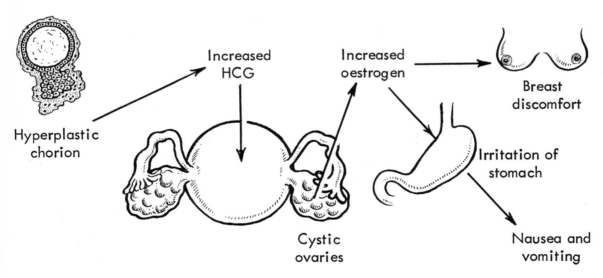

CLINICAL FEATURES OF MOLE

There is a higher incidence of hydatidiform mole below the age of 20 and above 40.

The condition may recur in a second pregnancy and the risk of this is 4-5 times the risk of a mole in a first pregnancy.

The signs and symptoms are the result of rapid enlargement of the uterus, absence of foetus, hormonal changes and bleeding.

1. Morning sickness is excessive.

2. Breast discomfort is exaggerated.

3. The uterus enlarges rapidly and at a non-uniform rate.

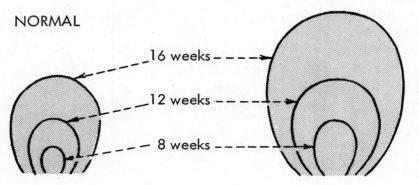

NORMAL

16 weeks

12 weeks

8 weeks

HYDATIDIFORM MOLE

4. The uterus feels boggy and despite its size no foetal parts can be felt.

5. Liquor is absent and ballottement cannot be elicited.

6. By the 12th week external haemorrhage usually occurs. Blood clot is retained in the uterus and anaemia may be quite severe.

7. The retained blood clot may cause cramp-like pains in the back and pelvis.

8. Signs of pre-eclampsia may appear.

CLINICAL FEATURES OF MOLE

<u>Diagnosis</u> may be difficult and the condition confused with incomplete abortion.

1. There may be a haemorrhage or serous discharge containing vesicles.
2. Abnormally large uterus.
3. Absence of foetal parts on X-ray.
4. No foetal heart heard with Doppler flowmeter.
5. High urinary output of CGH.
6. Ultrasonoscopy can often confirm the diagnosis.
7. Curettage may be the only means of diagnosis.

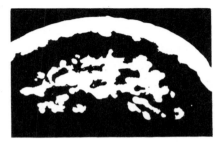

Treatment

1. Because of the invasive nature of trophoblastic tissue, there are always risks of severe haemorrhage and uterine perforation.
2. If abortion has not begun spontaneously, medical induction with stilboestrol and oxytocin should be tried.
3. If unsuccessful, dilatation and curettage must be performed. This is done in theatre with facilities for laparotomy if necessary. Blood and oxytocin infusions should be in position and 4 pints of blood should be available.
4. The techniques vary, but one method is to dilate the cervix with great care until an ovum forceps can be introduced. Molar tissue is removed with forceps and blunt curette until the cavity feels fairly empty and bleeding is slight. The uterus is packed and curettage repeated in 48 hours.
5. Recently the suction curette (see p 86) has been used with considerable success. This reduces the possibility of rupturing the uterus.

Follow Up

The greatest danger is that a hydatidiform mole will undergo malignant change. For this reason the patient must be watched for a year. In 25 per cent of cases there are sequelae in the form of invasive mole or true choriocarcinoma.

Following evacuation of a mole, urinary gonadotrophin should be estimated at weekly intervals for 3 months. It should disappear from the urine in 6 weeks but in some cases a low level may persist for several months. 21 per cent still excrete chorionic gonadotrophin at the end of 2 months but two thirds of these are negative within 8-9 months. The test should be repeated at 3-monthly intervals even if it becomes negative. At any time after evacuation of the mole a rising titre of urinary gonadotrophin is of serious import indicating invasive mole or choriocarcinoma.

The patient should be warned not to start another pregnancy during the follow-up period so that the significance of positive tests is not obscured.

INVASIVE MOLE

INVASIVE MOLE (mola destruens, chorio-adenoma destruens)

In this condition the hydatidiform mole invades the myometrium. It retains its villous structure and is usually confined to the uterus but villi may metastasise to the vagina, parametrium and even to the lungs and brain.

The mole may be of this nature from the beginning or follow on an apparently simple mole. The condition is difficult to diagnose since it may be confused with simple mole or choriocarcinoma. As a result the true incidence is unknown.

Clinical Features

After evacuation of a seemingly simple mole there may be no symptoms or signs of disease for several weeks or even months. Episodes of irregular vaginal bleeding then occur, usually accompanied by pain.

Examination shows that the uterus is still enlarged and cystic ovaries may be felt.

Sometimes the presenting symptom may be dysuria, due to local extension, pleuritic pain or dyspnoea due to pulmonary emboli, or headache and visual disturbance due to cerebral metastases.

Diagnosis

This is always in doubt since differentiation from choriocarcinoma may be impossible.

The urinary output of gonadotrophin is usually high. Curettage reveals a friable, haemorrhage growth with a villous structure. The histological structure is generally benign even in cases with metastases.

Treatment

This tends to be a self-limiting disease and the mole generally dies within the normal gestation period but there are three dangers which make it imperative that active treatment be employed.

1. Haemorrhage may be severe and prove fatal. With extension to the parametrium the haemorrhage may be intra-abdominal.
2. Extension of growth and embolisation. Large pulmonary emboli may occur. Pulmonary and cerebral manifestations must be considered as serious problems requiring urgent treatment.
3. Conversion to choriocarcinoma.

In older women who already have children treatment is total hysterectomy. If the patient is young and desires children or if there are signs of extension of the growth beyond the uterus chemotherapy should be employed as for choriocarcinoma.

CHORIOCARCINOMA

Incidence

In Europe and North America this is a rare disease, the incidence being roughly 1 in 13,850 pregnancies.   The incidence is said to be high however in Asia, 1 in 250 pregnancies, and in Hong Kong 1 in 114.

The condition is preceded by mole in one third of the cases.

Age

It commonly occurs in the third decade (21-30) in Europe and North America but in Asia the highest incidence is at a later age, 31-40.

Time of Occurrence

The tumour usually follows immediately on a mole, abortion or normal pregnancy but may first appear many years after the last pregnancy and cases have apparently occurred after the menopause.

Pathology

Villus formation is absent.   The tumour consists of masses of syncytium and cytotrophoblast.   It invades and destroys the surrounding tissues and causes gross haemorrhage owing to its ability to erode blood vessels.

The cells are irregular with hyperchromic nuclei.   Mitotic figures are frequent.   The syncytial masses are usually fenestrated.

Myometrium invaded by cytotrophoblast cells and syncytial cells

Extension may occur to the vagina or parametrium but metastases to the lungs and other organs by the general and portal circulations are common.   The neoplasm may be wholly outwith the uterus, possibly arising from fragments of chorionic epithelium which have migrated to other sites.

CHORIOCARCINOMA

Clinical Features

These are very variable.

The primary uterine growth may cause haemorrhage and gross anaemia. Metastases give rise to cardio respiratory troubles, or even cerebral symptoms. Positive diagnosis may be impossible although the patient may exhibit clinical choriomatosis i.e.

1. A pregnancy test positive in high dilution.
2. Irregular bleeding.
3. Haemoptysis.
4. Pulmonary shadows on X-ray examination.

Radical treatment may be necessary without the certainty of diagnosis.

Pulmonary X-ray patterns.

1. Discrete. A large round shadow, the so-called cannon ball metastasis may be seen.

This type of metastasis is remarkable for its clinical silence. Dyspnoea is usually absent and lung function tests are normal. Cough with haemoptysis and pleuritic pain may arise as the lesion advances.

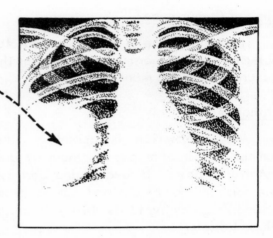

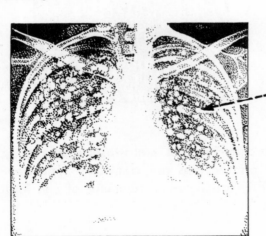

2. Snowstorm. This is uncommon and is due to numerous small tumour emboli of a similar size arising at the same time.

The patient usually has an unproductive cough, moderate dyspnoea and palpitations.

CHORIOCARCINOMA

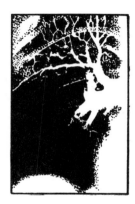

3. Pulmonary Embolus. X-ray shows enlargement of the right ventricle and prominence of the pulmonary artery. This is due to an embolus in the pul- Arteriography provides a more positive diagnosis.

The patient is greatly distressed with dyspnoea, pleuritic pain, unproductive cough, haemoptysis and cyanosis. The patient may die in cardiac failure. Hyperventilation reduces the pCO_2 of the blood but despite this there is anoxia.

Diagnosis

As stated above this may be impossible and only a tentative clinical diagnosis can be made.

1. Curettage usually provides the diagnosis. It must be deep enough to include myometrium so that invasion by the growth may be demonstrated. The results may be negative.

2. Pelvic arteriography. This may be attempted if the diagnosis is in doubt. A catheter is passed up the femoral artery until the bifurcation of the aorta is reached. Radio-opaque material is injected very rapidly. X-ray photographs are taken in rapid succession roughly at 0.5 second intervals for 10-12 seconds.

Results

1. Large uterus outlined.
2. Dilated uterine, myometrial, ovarian and other pelvic arteries.
3. Increased branching of myometrial arteries.
4. General uterine hypervascularity, with a central area of hypovascularity due to necrotic growth.
5. Vaginal metastases may show up due to increased vascularity.

TREATMENT OF CHORIOCARCINOMA

Chemotherapy is the treatment of choice. Treatment is monitored by repeated estimation of the amount of chorionic gonadotrophin excreted per day, and is continued until the amount of luteinising hormone in the urine has fallen to the levels found in non-pregnant females. The assays are carried out by radio-immuno-assay methods which detect as little as 0.005 International Units chorionic gonadotrophin per ml.

The drugs used are all of a type which interferes with either the formation of DNA of nuclei or its function.

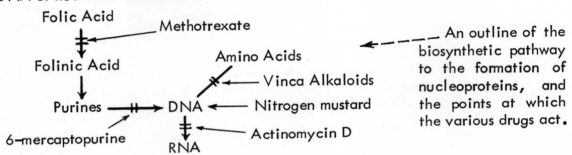

An outline of the biosynthetic pathway to the formation of nucleoproteins, and the points at which the various drugs act.

The drugs most commonly used are methotrexate, 6-mercaptopurine and actinomycin D, but some tumours become resistant under treatment and the drug has to be changed.

Methotrexate may be given orally or parenterally. Approximately 25mg. should be given daily in divided doses to maintain a constant blood level. Folinic acid is given some hours after each dose of methotrexate to counteract the toxic effects of the drug on the normal tissues of the body. A typical regime would be:- 5mg methotrexate by mouth 6 hourly for 3-5 days. 50mg 6-mercaptopurine may be given in combination. Allow 7 days to elapse before repeating course.

Actinomycin D. This drug is given intravenously 0.01mg per kg. body weight daily for 3-7 days. Interval between courses not less than 9 days. Toxicity increases with successive courses.

All of these drugs are extremely toxic. The main effects are on those tissues which have a rapid turnover of cells – haemopoietic system and gastro-intestinal tract. Nausea, vomiting and ulcerations of the intestinal tract may occur, and haemorrhage and infection due to depression of the bone-marrow.

TREATMENT OF CHORIOCARCINOMA

Precautions

1. Prior to treatment renal function must be assessed. Poor function will result in accumulation of the drugs within the body and toxicity.
2. Liver function should be assessed weekly.
3. A full blood investigation should be carried out thrice weekly.
4. Due to susceptibility to infection patients should be isolated.
5. Treatment should be carried out in a centre where facilities for monitoring of treatment are available.

Results of Chemotherapy

If interval between pregnancy giving rise to tumour and start of therapy is less than 3 months the cure rate is 100 per cent. With increase of the interval to 6 months the death rate is 5 per cent; 12 months, 30 per cent; 2 years, 40 per cent; more than 2 years, 64 per cent.

Patients excreting more than 1 million units of chorionic gonadotrophin per day have a poor prognosis.

Subsequent pregnancy.

This should be avoided for not less than 1 year after completion of treatment.

Surgery

If this is contemplated chemotherapy should be given prior to operation if possible. It may be necessary, however, to carry out an emergency hysterectomy because of bleeding.

The last course of chemotherapy should be given 7–10 days before surgery. An even longer period should elapse, 10–15 days before resuming full doses of chemotherapy after operation. The anti-mitotic agents used depress healing and if given too near to operation may produce disastrous results, especially actinomycin D.

CHAPTER 19

ENDOMETRIOSIS AND PELVIC INFLAMMATION

ENDOMETRIOSIS

Tumours arising from ectopic endometrium;   e.g. adenomyoma is endometriosis in the uterine wall.

An endometriosis is functioning endometrial tissue.   It proliferates, becomes secretory and then breaks down and bleeds in time with the normal menstrual cycle.

If the blood can drain away (as in an adenomyoma) or be readily absorbed then little unusual is noted.

If the blood cannot escape or be readily absorbed it will form a tumour or nodule which becomes bulkier in the later stages of each cycle.   If the nodule is palpable it will be tender about the time of menstruation.

Dense adhesions develop around the lesion and much distortion can occur.

The menstrual blood is entrapped and becomes inspissated.   It may contain nodules and flakes of haematin.   The colour of the fluid is like chocolate so the term 'chocolate cyst' or 'tarry cyst' is often used.

There is benign invasion of the surrounding tissues with much distortion.

Malignant change, usually adenocarcinoma, does occur sometimes.

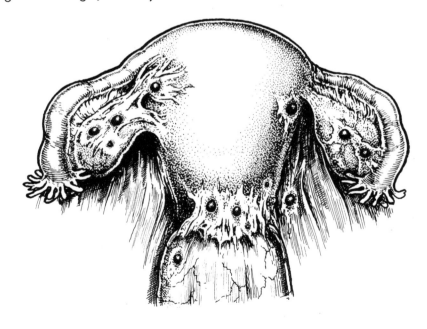

ENDOMETRIOSIS

THEORIES OF CAUSE

1. Retrograde flow of menstrual tissue with pieces of viable endometrium which establish parasitic growth.
2. Transplanted endometrial tissue into wounds.
3. Epithelial tissue which undergoes metaplastic change.
4. Lymphatic or vascular spread by embolism.
5. Metamorphosis of atretic ovarian follicles.

No single theory can explain all the varieties of site.

Less Common Sites

Appendix, Ileum, Abdominal wounds, Umbilicus, Bladder, Lungs and Pleura, Breasts, Limbs.

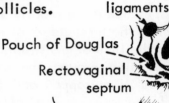

COMMONEST SITES

Ovary

Uterine wall

Uterosacral ligaments

Pouch of Douglas

Rectovaginal septum

The deposits are purple ranging to black spots with surrounding fibrosis.

CLINICAL DIAGNOSIS

1. History
   (a) Growing pain and tenderness synchronous with periods.
   (b) Dysmenorrhoea - increasing in severity.
   (c) Dyspareunia.
   (d) Infertility - a combination of ovarian dysfunction and dyspareunia.
   (e) Menstrual haematuria.

2. Appearance
   The lesion may be at a visible site (e.g. an abdominal wound) or seen by laparotomy or laparoscopy. Dense adhesions are often present.

3. Palpation
   There is tenderness at the site of the lesion and is most marked at time of menstrual flow. There is limitation of mobility in the region of the lesion and masking of details.

ENDOMETRIOSIS

DIFFERENTIAL DIAGNOSIS

(a) Pelvic inflammation is usually bilateral.   There may be pyrexia.
The white blood count is raised.

(b) Malignant disease is not usually associated with pain in the earlier stages
and there is not a menstrual rhythm for the discomforts.

(c) Diverticulitis is not linked with menstrual flow but is erratic in times of
discomfort and inflammatory in type.   The bowel activity is often greatly
increased resulting in diarrhoea at times.

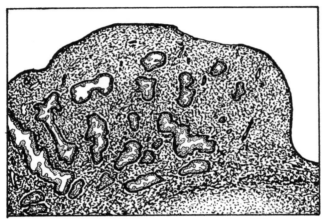

Endometrial deposition on pouch of Douglas

TREATMENT

. Treatment of the lesion is primarily by excision.   This may be difficult or incomplete because of adhesions and the destruction of tissue definition.

Endometriosis ceases to function at the menopause and during pregnancy.

Suppression of the natural oestrogen effects may be used when complete excision
of the tumour is undesirable or uncertain.   Progestogens are used for this such as
Dydrogesterone (Duphaston) or an oral contraceptive for a period of 9–12 months to
create a pseudo pregnancy.

Adhesions may cause trouble and symptoms after the endometriosis has died down.

PELVIC INFLAMMATION

Endometritis

Acute inflammation may develop in response to infection following childbirth or abortion, or the insertion of a contraceptive device; or as part of a gonorrhoeal infection.

Chronic Endometritis is a rare condition because of the frequency with which the endometrium is shed.   The diagnosis is histological and there are no specific signs or symptoms, but the microscopic appearances are of infiltration mainly by plasma cells and lymphocytes.   (For TB endometritis see p461).

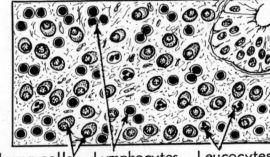

Plasma cells   Lymphocytes   Leucocytes

Senile Endometritis

Postmenopausal endometrium has little resistance to infection, and endometritis may arise from cervicitis or from tumour. If the cervix is stenosed by infection or growth, the uterus becomes distended with pus and the condition is known as pyometra.   Cervical dilatation will release the pus but curettage must be done to exclude malignancy and in such a situation it is very easy to perforate the uterus.

Metritis

Acute inflammation of the myometrium is a serious condition resulting from infection introduced during childbirth or abortion (see septic abortion p426).

'Chronic Metritis'
'Fibrosis Uteri'
'Chronic Subinvolution'
'Myohyperplasia'

Many patients at gynaecological clinics are found to have an enlarged mobile 'flabby' uterus, often retroverted and sometimes associated with general pelvic inflammation.   Menstrual irregularities and congestive discomfort or pain are complained of and the cause is not known.   The histological appearances are normal unless there is other infection.

Treatment   If there is no organic cause, the menstrual irregularity may respond to steroid hormones.   In the woman over 40 who wishes no more family, there is much to be said for simple hysterectomy.

PELVIC INFLAMMATION

CLINICAL FEATURES AND TREATMENT

ACUTE INFLAMMATION

The history is often of a prolonged period followed by the gradual onset of pelvic pain and irregular bleeding. There is abdominal tenderness and guarding, and pelvic examination reveals extreme tenderness in the fornices. The patient is fevered.

Diagnosis may be impossible without laparotomy.

Appendicitis   Signs are mainly in the right iliac fossa and the menstrual cycle is undisturbed.

Diverticulitis   This is a disease of older women and the signs are mainly in the left iliac fossa.

Torsion of pedicle of a cyst.   There may be a history of intermittent pain over several months. A cyst should be palpable.

Tubal Pregnancy   The history may be helpful, but in young women in whom salpingitis and tubal pregnancy may co-exist, the distinction may be very difficult.

Treatment

Smears should be taken from vagina and cervix, bearing in mind the possibility of acute gonorrhoea and an antibiotic such as cephaloridine is given. If the patient does not respond, laparotomy must be carried out, but if only salpingitis is found the abdomen should be closed. All abscesses must be opened and drained.

CHRONIC INFLAMMATION

The patient's complaint is of pelvic pain aggravated by menstruation. The periods are irregular and heavy, and dyspareunia is common.

Examination

A swelling may be felt but often there is little to be found except tenderness in the fornices. A large mass suggests adhesions between bowel and pelvic organs. An exact diagnosis and estimate of the extent of the disease cannot be made without laparotomy or laparoscopy.

Treatment

Examination under anaesthesia and curettage are first done to exclude malignant conditions and tuberculosis. The course of pelvic inflammation is not predictable. In many cases it resolves itself, so conservative treatment is justified. Distensions due to blood etc. must be relieved by drainage or excision of the tubes, and in the woman over 45 the best treatment is total hysterectomy and salpingo-oophorectomy. Retroversion should be corrected if the patient complains of dyspareunia.

Physiotherapy in the form of pelvic diathermy, and courses of antibiotics are empirical treatments which sometimes help the patient. They should be tried in young women before surgery is offered.

SALPINGO-OOPHORITIS

Infection of the tubes usually involves the ovaries and the peritoneum as well, and the combined conditions are described as pelvic inflammation. All degrees are met with from mild thickening and oedema of the tubes, to a widespread inflammatory reaction involving tubes, ovaries, peritoneum, uterus, omentum and bowel.

Acute infections are caused by the gonococcus or a pyogenic organism such as E.Coli. When the infection is chronic it is very rare to identify any organism except in the case of tuberculosis. Even pus from an abscess is sterile.

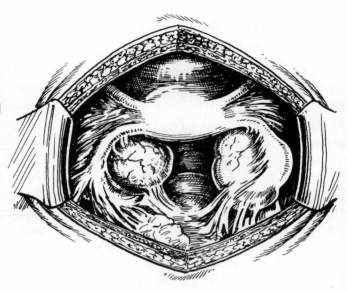

Pathology

The infection must often spread directly from the vagina, but blood borne and lymphatic spread are possible. The tubes are sealed

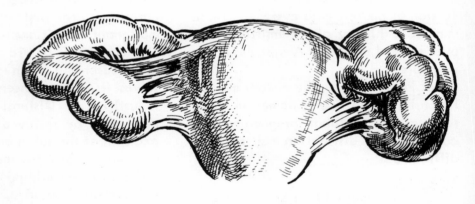

off quickly by oedema and adhesions, and they either swell up, filling with watery exudate – hydrosalpinx: or blood – haematosalpinx: or pus – pyosalpinx: or they become convoluted and thickened and very adherent to the ovary – chronic salpingo-oophoritis. The ovary can also be the seat of abscess formation, or can develop a 'chocolate' cyst full of altered blood, often described wrongly as an 'endometrial cyst'.

PELVIC CELLULITIS

Infection of the fibro-fatty connective tissue of the pelvis (the 'visceral layer' of the pelvic fascia - p 25).

	Acute Cellulitis	Chronic Cellulitis
Primary Follows injury to vagina or cervix at childbirth or abortion. Follows pelvic surgery. Associated with radiotherapy for carcinoma of the cervix.	Secondary Simply an extension of pelvic inflammatory disease.	Mainly inflammatory thickening of the uterosacral and transverse ligaments of the uterus.

The classical identifying sign is a hard inflammatory mass somewhere in the pelvis.

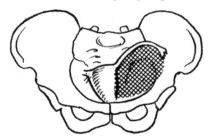

1. A lateral swelling in the tissues below the broad ligament. Note the displaced uterus.

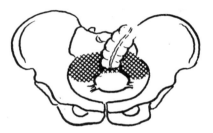

2. Posterior swelling in the tissues round the rectum (the 'horseshoe swelling').

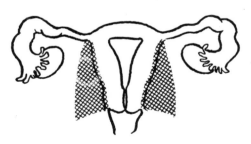

3. Bilateral swelling alongside the uterus.

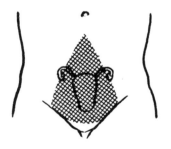

4. Anterior swelling in Scarpa's fascia of the abdominal wall.

451

PELVIC CELLULITIS

CLINICAL FEATURES

1. The condition presents with fever, irregular bleeding and pelvic pain. Examination reveals the characteristic hard swelling in the pelvis and often in the abdomen as well. Tenderness is marked but the pain seems to be much less severe than might be expected from the clinical signs.

2. Diagnosis is made on these findings and on the recent history of childbirth or abortion or pelvic operation. For reasons not known there is often a delay of 10-14 days before symptoms appear in puerperal patients.

Treatment is conservative unless suppuration is suspected. The infecting organism can be any pathogen (commonly a streptococcus such as Str. Faecalis) but it is usually impossible to identify it unless pus forms, so a broad spectrum antibiotic such as ampicillin should be exhibited. Complete resolution is usual and persistent pyrexia suggests abscess formation.

Complications of cellulitis

These are rare, as is the disease itself.

1. Suppuration. (See below)

2. Thrombosis of the pelvic and femoral veins with the risk of pulmonary embolism

3. Development of chronic cellulitis.

Chronic cellulitis

This condition leaves the patient with thickened and tender uterine ligaments and often with scarring and displacement of the genital tract. It is associated with irregular bleeding, backache and deep dyspareunia which is difficult to treat. Courses of antibiotics and pelvic diathermy may be tried, but if the woman is old enough, hysterectomy is often the best treatment.

Chronic cellulitis is nowadays most often seen as a complication of radiotherapy for cervical carcinoma. Like the other side-effects of radiation it tends gradually to resolve but there is often considerable thickening of the tissues especially if there has been spread to the fascia of Scarpa.

ABSCESS FORMATION IN PELVIC CELLULITIS

This is strongly suggested by a persistent pyrexia and tenderness. It is advisable to wait for signs of localisation before attempting drainage.

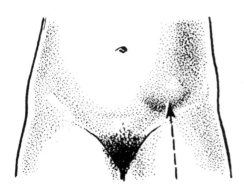

1. The commonest site for pointing is above the inguinal ligament.

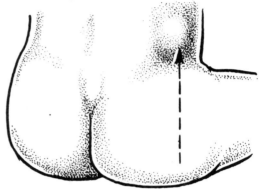

2. Pus may track along the path of the ureter and point in the loin...

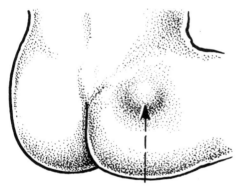

3. ...or through the sacrosciatic notch to point in the buttock.

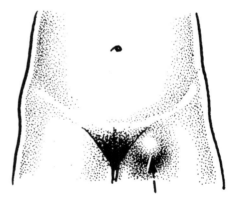

4. ...or through the femoral canal.

Other possible sites for pointing are the rectum, the vagina (through the posterior fornix), the inner aspect of the thigh (through the obturator foramen) and the ischiorectal fossa (through the hiatus of Schwalbe between levator ani and obturator internus).

453

GONORRHOEA

GONORRHOEA is increasing in incidence and should be suspected when there is a history of urinary frequency and burning dysuria plus a thick deep yellow discharge. The acute phase is often of only a few days duration followed by a chronic stage when discharge is the main complaint. This then lapses into a carrier state where the symptoms are minimal but the ability to infect is present for many weeks.

Many women have no acute phase especially if the cervix is the primary source of infection.

The incubation period of gonorrhoea is three to ten days from infection. Neisseria gonorrhoea is a delicate organism and does not survive easily outside the body. Gonorrhoea is acquired by intercourse with an infected person, though it may be spread by clothing or towels, especially in young children.

Recovery from the disease does not confer immunity.

<u>Diagnosis</u> is confirmed by the presence of intracellular diplococci and by culture of the organism.

<u>Skene's glands</u> may harbour the organism. They should be 'milked' as shown in the diagram. This also discharges the urethral glands and the pus is examined by spreading immediately on a slide and also by placing a swab in Stuart's transport medium for culture.

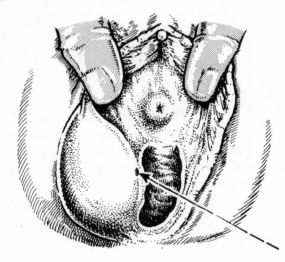

<u>Bartholin's glands</u> may be affected leading to abscess formation. The duct may show as a bright red spot.

GONORRHOEA

The <u>Cervical glands</u> are affected also giving a purulent cervicitis.

Smears for microscopic examination and culture should be taken from the urethra (Skene's and urethral glands), Bartholin's gland duct and the endocervix.

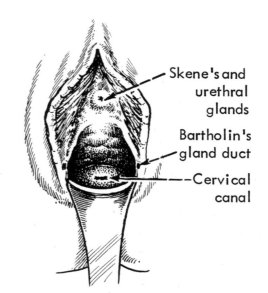

Skene's and urethral glands

Bartholin's gland duct

Cervical canal

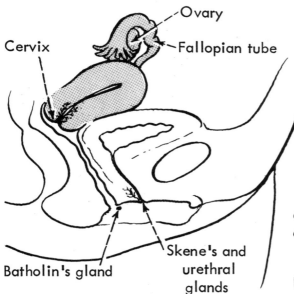

Ovary

Fallopian tube

Cervix

Batholin's gland

Skene's and urethral glands

The infection may spread to the uterus and fallopian tubes leading to salpingo-oophoritis causing sterility.

Metastatic lesions are now rare but purulent arthritis is seen on occasion.

TREATMENT

(This is best carried out at a Venereal Disease Clinic which has facilities for following up the patient and tracing her contacts.)

A single injection of procaine penicillin 2-2.5g (2,500,000 units) is usually sufficient in uncomplicated cases. If symptoms persist or relapse in a few days then the patient should be given 1.5g procaine penicillin + benzyl penicillin 0.5g (procaine penicillin, fortified B.P.). A single injection of streptomycin 1g may be effective.

Unfortunately many of the strains of gonococcus are now penicillin resistant. The treatment of gonorrhoea may suppress a syphilitic lesion and serological tests for syphilis should be carried out in three and six months' time.

SYPHILIS

The incubation period is about three to four weeks.

The primary lesion is the chancre and is found as an indurated nodule about 1cm in size with an ulcerated surface and oedema of the surrounding tissues. It is usually found on the inner surface of the labium (minus or majus) and occasionally on the clitoris.

It is accompanied by inguinal adeno-pathy – the glands are hard and enlarged but not tender – an inguinal bubo.

The primary chancre may be on the cervix and will cause few symptoms. Sometimes the primary lesion is extra-genital. Diagnosis of syphilis is confirmed by examining the discharge from the lesion by dark ground illumination and watching the movements of the treponema.

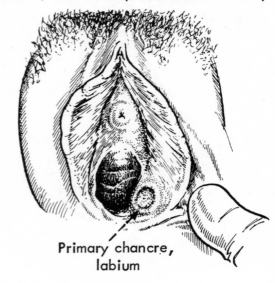

Primary chancre, labium

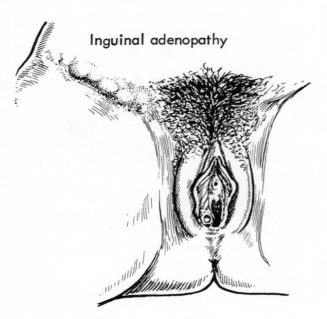

Inguinal adenopathy

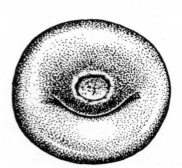

Cervical chancre

456

SYPHILIS

SECONDARY SYPHILIS appears a few months, usually two or three, after the primary stage. It is a systemic infection with various skin rashes – usually symmetrical and of a copper-brown colour like "raw ham" and without irritation.

"Snail track" ulcers, painless shiny grey patches, appear in the mouth. There may be sore throat, generalised lymph node enlargement and low fever.

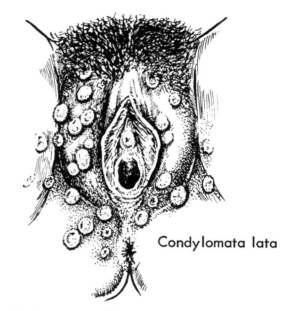

Condylomata lata

The gynaecologist however is usually consulted because of the vulvar and perineal condylomata – multiple round and oval shaped, only slightly raised, warts.

The lesions are highly infective. Dark ground illumination is positive and the serological tests are now positive.

TERTIARY SYPHILIS appears years (often many) after infection. The lesion is a localised swelling called a gumma (Latin; gummi – the gumma has the consistency of rubber).

The gumma does not contain treponemata and is not infective. Gummata are irregular in distribution and may be found anywhere in the body.

A gumma may break down and give a punched out ulcer.

TREATMENT

If possible the patient should be under the care of a venereologist.

Procaine penicillin 600mg daily for ten days or 2.5g benzathine penicillin by a single intra-muscular dose.

Regular clinical and serological examinations should be carried out for at least two years.

CHANCROID

CHANCROID (Soft Sore) is a venereal disease and is rare in Britain. It is caused by Ducrey's bacillus (Haemophilus Ducrei – gram negative 1–2μ in length). The incubation period is two to fourteen days. The ulceration is irregular and ragged in outline. The edges are undermined and the base is granulomatous and purulent. There is little or no surrounding induration but there is erythema and oedema especially if the lesion is in the labia majora. Pain is a common feature. The inguinal lymph nodes enlarge and may suppurate.

   Diagnosis is by identification of Ducrey's bacillus in scrapings from the ulcer.

   Treatment is by sulphadimidine or other sulphonamide.

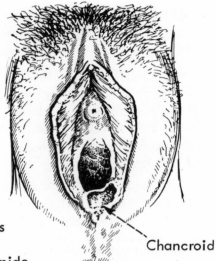
Chancroid

LYMPHOGRANULOMA INGUINALE (Lymphogranuloma Venereum or Lymphopathia Venereum)

   This disease, caused by a large virus, is rare in Britain but not uncommon in America, affecting negroes more than others.
   The incubation period is 5–21 days.
   Initially there is a small vesicle or ulcer on the labia with inguinal adenitis and this progresses to large tumour-like masses which suppurate and discharge through many sinuses (esthiomene) extending into the perineum and rectum and can cause elephantiasis of the vulva and stricture of the rectum.
   Diagnosis is by Frei's Intradermal Test. The test is negative until several weeks after infection and once positive remains so for life. A person who has had the disease is sensitive to an antigen prepared from the virus. Control material is prepared too. The reaction is positive in 48–72 hours.
Treatment may be successful with sulphonamides or tetracylines.

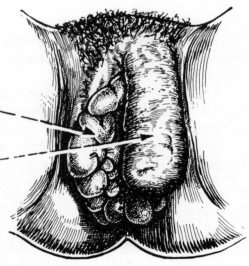

GRANULOMA INGUINALE

GRANULOMA INGUINALE   (Donovania Granulomatosis)

This is a separate disease from Lympho-granuloma Inguinale. It has a venereal spread and the primary lesion is usually on the external genitalia but may be seen on vagina, cervix or groin. It is found in tropical and subtropical regions.

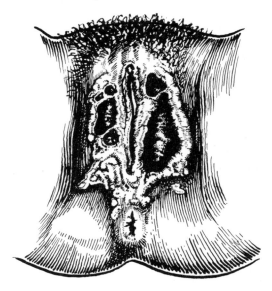

The lesion is of the cutaneous and subcutaneous tissues. It is primarily a nodule which ulcerates and joins with other papules and ulcers to form a large raw area with rolled edges.

<u>Diagnosis</u> is by recognition of "Donovan Bodies", small oval organisms contained in macrophages in the granulation tissue.

The disease progresses by fibrous healing so scarring and ulceration are present together. Lymphatic blockage and vulvar elephantiasis can occur.

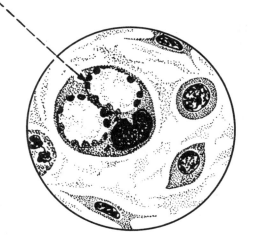

Treatment

Large dosage of chloramphenicol, 1000 mg. daily for a month should cure. (The possible depressant effect of chloramphenicol on the bone marrow must be remembered.)

DIAGNOSIS OF SYPHILIS

Positive identification of T.Pallidum is difficult for various reasons including the failure, so far, to grow the organism in vitro. The usual method of diagnosis is by serological tests which become positive 4–6 weeks after infection.

Reagin This is a non-specific antibody which appears in the tissues after infection with syphilis and many other bacteria and viruses. Its presence is detected by complement-fixation tests which are modifications of the original Wasserman reaction (WR) or by flocculation tests in which a reaction is observed under the microscope between infected serum and cardiolipin antigen.

False Positives are usually weaker than a reaction due to syphilis, but if a positive result is obtained further tests are made.

Reiter's Test is a complement-fixation test using a non-syphilitic treponeme as the antigen. A positive result means that the reagin is present because of a treponeme, and of course probably T. Pallidum.

Treponemal Immobilisation Test (TPI). This is specific for syphilis but is expensive. Live T.Pallida are used (from a rabbit chancre) and are seen to be immobilised if combined with syphilitic serum.

Fluorescent Treponemal Antibody Tests are becoming very widely used for verification of the 'positive WR'.

Principle of Fluorescent Tests (FTA)

1. Anti-human globulin is combined with fluorescein.

2. Dead treponeme is combined with test serum. If infected, the treponeme acquires a coating of globulin antibody.

3. 1 and 2 are combined and the treponeme becomes fluorescent.

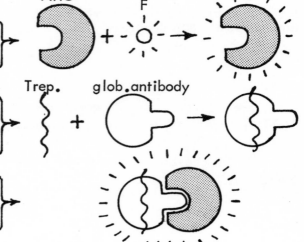

460

GENITAL TUBERCULOSIS

This infection appears in the tubes and endometrium and may spread downwards, but primary lesions in cervix, vagina or vulva are very rare.

Clinical Features

The patient is usually a young woman and the commonest complaints are primary infertility or abdominal pain and menstrual disturbances.

Examination may reveal some pelvic swelling but often no abnormality is felt.

At least half of these patients will give a history suggestive of previous tuberculosis, usually in the respiratory or renal tract.

Appearances

The tubes may be almost normal (endosalpingitis) or show swelling, adhesions and distortions, even tuberculous pyosalpinx. In such cases the ovaries are often involved. Small pinhead tubercles appear on the serosa - accretions of tubercle follicles. (Talc granulomata and secondary spread from ovarian cancer may give a similar appearance.)

Pathology

Genital tuberculosis is nearly always a blood-borne infection, but spread may occur from adjacent viscera. Ascending infection per vaginam is a theoretical possibility and may be the explanation of the exceedingly rare occurrence of cervical infection without involvement of the tubes or endometrium. In the United Kingdom the human variety of Myco. Tuberculosis is almost the rule. Infection begins in the tubes and spreads thence to the endometrium.

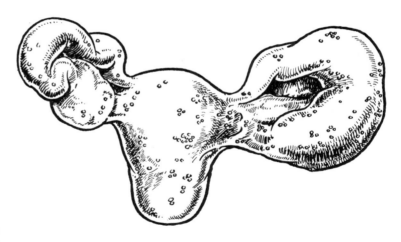

The endometrium also shows tubercle follicles although these are shed at menstruation (if occurring) and they are best seen in premenstrual endometrium.

GENITAL TUBERCULOSIS

Diagnosis

Genital tuberculosis has a reputation for appearing unexpectedly; but any woman with a complaint suggestive of pelvic inflammation, and especially if she is infertile, should be regarded with suspicion. Tuberculosis is a common disease.

1. Histological evidence from endometrial curettings. This is the most easily obtained evidence and when seen it is assumed that the tubes are also infected. But: (a) the curette may have missed the infected area or (b) the biopsy may have been taken at the wrong time or (c) the infection may not yet have spread from the tubes.

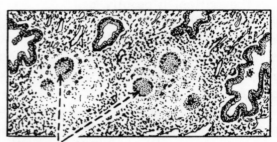
Giant cells
Tuberculous Endometritis

2. Bacteriological evidence should always be looked for and curettings sent for Ziehl-Neelsen staining, culture, and guinea-pig inoculation. Growth is slow and six weeks at least must be allowed. The guinea pig should show signs of illness within a month and is usually sacrificed after six weeks.

3. Biopsy should be made of any ulcerated area in cervix, vagina or vulva.

4. If all findings are negative but clinical suspicion remains, a laparotomy and biopsy of any infected areas should be carried out.

5. Once evidence of genital infection is obtained, a search should be made for signs of active tuberculosis elsewhere, particularly the respiratory and urinary tracts.

Chemotherapy

There are various systems, for example: Streptomycin 1g daily for three months, PAS 12g and isoniazid 300mg. for 18-24 months depending on progress. Such a regime must be altered if side-effects appear such as vestibular nerve damage, or allergy; and if the disease does not appear to be responding. Curettage is repeated at 6 and 12 months.

GENITAL TUBERCULOSIS

Indications for Surgical Treatment

1. Failure of chemotherapy which occurs in about one quarter of patients. Failure means in most cases the persistence of tubercle follicles in the endometrium, or the persistence of abdominal pain and a tender pelvic swelling.

2. As a primary treatment combined with chemotherapy in the patient over 40 who is psychologically prepared to lose her uterus and ovaries. Conservation of one ovary would be a justifiable compromise if the patient were a young woman, but complete clearance is considered the operation of choice. Tuberculous tissue does not heal and inadequate surgery may result in the development of a bowel or bladder fistula.

Tuberculosis and Infertility

Failure to conceive is probably the most important consequence of genital tuberculosis, and 90% of the women presenting with the disease will never have had a pregnancy. This is probably due to blocking or distortion of the lumen of the tubes.

Pregnancy after treatment may be looked for in about 10% of patients, but the frequency of ectopic gestation is very high (about 50%) and it may be advisable to acquaint the patient of this risk.

VENOUS THROMBOSIS

This complication was formerly regarded as rather rare but is now believed to occur in about one in three post-operative patients. Classical signs and symptoms are often absent but the risk of pulmonary embolism remains.

Causes of Thrombosis

1. Lesions in the vascular intima
2. Changes in the rate of blood flow
3. Changes in composition of the blood

These factors are called 'Virchow's Triad' and all are affected by the operative and post-operative situations.

Lesions in the Venous Intima

These may be caused by infection local or blood-borne, or by prolonged pressure on the calf-veins.

Changes in Rate of Flow

Venous flow in the legs is much reduced in the post-operative period of inactivity, restricted respiratory movements and poor muscle tone in the legs.

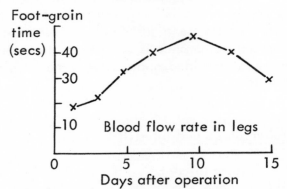

Blood flow rate in legs

Changes in the Blood

Platelet count and platelet 'stickiness' and fibrinogen levels are all increased. Fortunately there is a compensating increase in fibrinolytic activity so that most thrombi are naturally broken down.

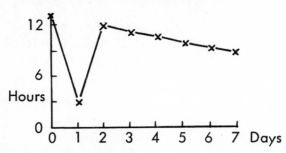

Post-operative decrease in clot-lysis time, showing increased plasmin activity.

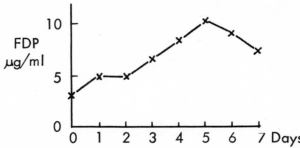

Post-operative increase in fibrin degradation products (FDP) as a result of thrombus destruction.

SITES OF THROMBOSIS FORMATION

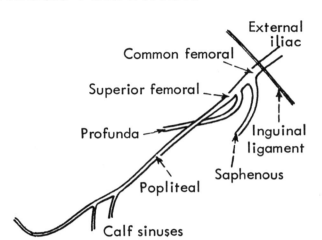

1. Calf veins (often extending to the popliteal vein).

2. Common femoral vein.

3. Iliofemoral (perhaps extending to the vena cava).

4. Saphenous vein at or above the knee.

5. Superficial thrombosis in varices.

Emboli may come from any of these sites except the last. Saphenous thrombosis is clinically the most obvious (Gk. saphes; clear, obvious) and is often called thrombophlebitis. This term was formerly applied to a thrombosis which was thought to be due to sepsis and very unlikely to detach and embolize, while phlebothrombosis implied the absence of sepsis and a great risk of embolus. This distinction is now known to be invalid, and the terms are less used.

Formation of the Clot

The platelets 'stick' to damaged endothelium and the liberated thromboplastins initiate the process of coagulation. The mesh of fibrin so formed is filled with haemolysed red cells and leucocytes. The plasminogen-plasma system normally lyses the thrombus but if the balance is upset (for reasons unknown) the clot may extend up the vein.

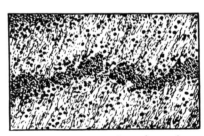

Low power view of a thrombus

'Propagated' clot tends to be unattached and may break off as an embolus.

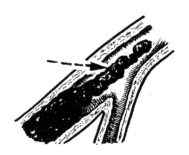

CLINICAL FEATURES OF VENOUS THROMBOSIS

Elderly patients undergoing major surgery are most at risk. There is often no complaint at all, but examination of the legs either as a routine or in search of a cause for a slight pyrexia may reveal signs.

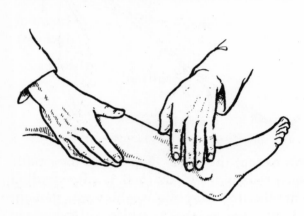

Palpation of the calf demonstrates tenderness and oedema.

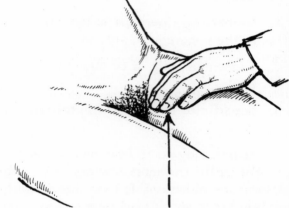

The femoral vein must also be palpated in the groin.

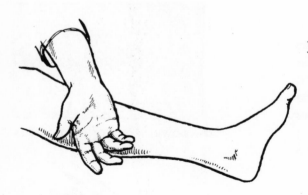

The affected leg may feel warmer to the back of the hand.

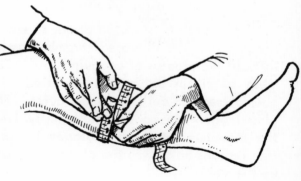

Careful measurement may reveal some swelling compared with the other leg.

CLINICAL FEATURES OF VENOUS THROMBOSIS

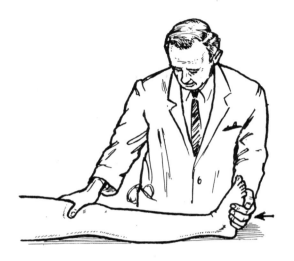

Homan's sign

Homan's sign is elicited by dorsi-flexing the foot. Calf tenderness indicates a positive response; but this test is not specific for thrombosis, nor does a negative response exclude thrombosis.

Phlegmasia alba dolens (painful white inflammation) and phlegmasia caerulea dolens are old terms for the appearance of the leg when the femoral vein is completely blocked. This is not characteristic of post-operative thrombosis.

Phlegmasia alba

There is a diffuse lymphangitis causing a solid oedema which does not pit on pressure. The superficial veins give a marbled appearance, but the arterial supply is not affected. The condition is very painful and some enlargement usually persists.

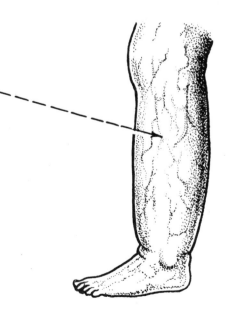

Phlegmasia caerulea

The whole leg is cyanosed and swollen by a severe pitting oedema. This pressure may affect the arterial supply causing a degree of gangrene. This is a very painful and serious condition.

DIAGNOSING VENOUS THROMBOSIS

Clinical methods as described make a reliable diagnosis in only about 50% of patients who actually have thrombi (most of which it must be remembered are naturally broken down). In recent years various techniques have been developed for detecting thrombosis more accurately.

Phlebography

This is the most reliable method but takes time and experience.

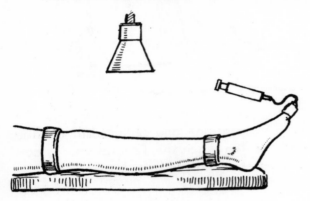

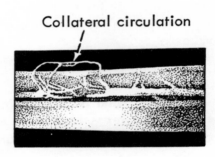

Collateral circulation

Contrast medium is injected into a vein near the big toe. Two inflated cuffs force it into the deep veins where its progress can be watched on image intensification apparatus.

A filling defect indicates the site of thrombosis. Note the opening of the collateral circulation.

Isotopic Diagnosis

A small amount of ^{125}I-labelled fibrinogen is injected before operation after the thyroid has been blocked with sodium iodide to prevent uptake of the isotope. In the post-operative period a scintillation counter is applied to the legs and an increase in radioactivity suggests thrombus formation.

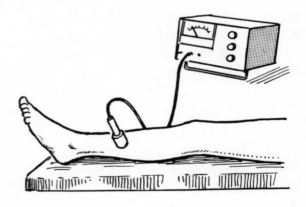

DIAGNOSING VENOUS THROMBOSIS

Ultrasonic Diagnosis

This technique makes use of the Doppler flowmeter, an apparatus developed for the purpose of foetal heart auscultation in obstetrics.

The flowing movements of blood in a vein produce characteristic sounds when picked up by a transducer held over the vessel. If the flow is accelerated the frequency and amplitude of the sounds are increased.

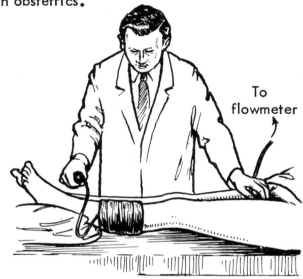

To flowmeter

The transducer is placed over the groin and the thigh or calf squeezed with an inflatable cuff. The increased sound is easily heard, and its absence suggests that the blood flow is being impeded by a thrombus.

COMPLICATIONS OF DEEP VEIN THROMBOSIS

1. Pulmonary Embolism

This is dealt with on page 474 et seq. Embolism can be mild or severe, single or recurrent, arising during treatment or weeks or months later.

2. Post-phlebitic Syndrome

This is a result of the damage sustained by the vein, in particular the loss of functioning valves. It includes swelling, varicose veins, eczema, varicose ulceration.

Treatment of deep vein thrombosis therefore must have three objectives:
1. Relief of the acute condition.
2. Prevention of pulmonary embolism.
3. Restoration as far as possible of normal vein function.

TREATMENT OF VENOUS THROMBOSIS

Improvement in Blood Flow

The leg is elevated with pillows and protected by a cage. A firm crepe bandage is applied and exercises begun under the instruction of the physiotherapist. This can only be done when pain and tenderness are sufficiently reduced to allow movement.

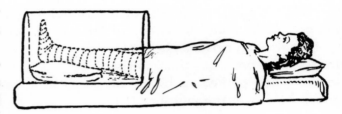

Prevention of Further Thrombosis by Anticoagulants

<u>Heparin</u> should be used for the first 48 hours because of its rapidity of action. Heparin acts on several of the blood-clotting enzymes and its effect is monitored by the clotting time which should be above 20 minutes. The dosage is 12,500 I.U. every 6 hours intravenously or by infusion.

<u>Warfarin</u> This is the best of the coumarin drugs. An initial dose of 30mg orally will produce a therapeutic level in about 48 hours and maintenance is about 2-5mg daily. Monitoring is by estimation every second day of the 'prothrombin time' which should be below 15%.

Coumarin drugs interfere with the synthesis of vitamin K which is essential for factors, II, VII, IX and X.

<u>Arvin</u> Venom from the Malayan pit viper which defibrinates the blood by combining with fibrinogen. It is possible that Arvin has some fibrinolytic action as well for fibrin degradation products (FDP) are found in the blood during treatment. Monitoring is by observing blood for absence of clot formation. This drug is still in the hands of specialists and experience is limited.

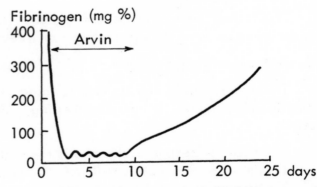

Fibrinogen levels return slowly to normal after treatment is stopped.

COMPLICATIONS OF ANTICOAGULANTS

Toxic reactions are rare and the main hazard is haemorrhage from the operation site or elsewhere. Dosage must always be monitored and the urine inspected for occult haematuria. Antidotes must be available.

Antidotes   Heparin: 5ml of 1% protamine sulphate intravenously.

              Warfarin: 25mg intravenously or 50mg orally of Vit.K$_1$. This may take up to 12 hours to produce an increase in prothrombin time.

              Arvin: 1ml of a specific antivenom.

Duration of Treatment

There is usually a good response and in mild cases it is usually necessary to maintain anticoagulant drugs for only about 14 days, after which they should be gradually withdrawn. If there is no clinical improvement, treatment must be continued and may have to be maintained for several weeks or months until recanalisation is considered to have occurred.

PREVENTION OF THROMBOSIS

1. Routine anticoagulant treatment causes too much haemorrhage but small doses of heparin (1000 units every 6 hours) have recently been found to reduce platelet adhesiveness and this scale of dosage may be found worth while.

2. Fibrinolytic activity can be stimulated by the pre-operative administration of phenormin (an oral hypoglycaemic) and ethyloestrenol (an anabolic steroid). But the drugs must be given for a period of 6 weeks before operation.

3. Pre- and post-operative physiotherapy, tight bandaging, elevation of the legs etc. These measures are to some degree adopted by every gynaecologist. They are expensive in terms of skilled personnel, but even 'early ambulation' amounting to no more than getting the patient out of her bed on the day after operation and keeping her on the move, is better than nothing.

SURGICAL TREATMENT OF VENOUS THROMBOSIS

There are two basic procedures, thrombectomy (removal of the thrombus) and ligation of the vein above the thrombosis to prevent embolism. The place of surgery is at present controversial.

Against Surgery

1. It is the common experience that most patients with post-operative deep vein thrombosis will respond well to anticoagulant treatment.

2. Surgery is the precipitating factor in post-operative thrombosis and it seems illogical to inflict further trauma.

3. Experience with thrombolytic drugs is increasing (see p 470) and they are beginning to appear as a possibly superior alternative to surgery.

For Surgery

1. Anticoagulants do not destroy thrombi, but only prevent their propagation. They cannot be relied on to prevent embolism.

2. It is recognised that while 'clinical' post-operative thrombosis is rather rare, 'silent' thrombosis is not. There is no way of identifying those patients with thrombosis who are most likely to develop embolism.

3. There have been many reports of reduced incidence of embolism and post-phlebitis morbidity when surgery and anticoagulant treatment are combined.

Suggested Scheme of Treatment of Post-Operative Thrombosis

1. Assiduous physiotherapy before and after operation, including muscle exercises, elastic bandages during operation and early ambulation especially in the elderly or obese.

2. Careful examination of the legs in the post-operative period, and the use of any ancillary screening method that may be available.

3. Determined anticoagulant treatment if a diagnosis is made.

4. Consult a specialist in vascular surgery if there is no improvement after a week of anticoagulant treatment or if there appears to be a complete blockage at ilio-femoral or vena cava level.

SURGICAL TREATMENT OF VENOUS THROMBOSIS

SURGICAL OPERATIONS FOR THROMBOSIS

(These are best left to a surgeon experienced in vascular work).

Thrombectomy

1. The exact site of the thrombus must be demonstrated by phlebography.

2. Venous flow is controlled above and below the site by rubber tubes or clips.

3. The vein is opened at the site of blockage and the clot removed proximally by suction and the passage of balloon catheters (Fogarty technique).

The catheter used is essentially a very fine Foley's catheter. It is passed along the vein, inflated and pulled back, bringing the clot with it.

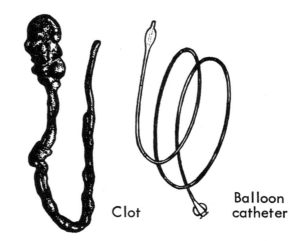

Clot   Balloon catheter

Ligation or Plication of Veins

Ligation is almost guaranteed to prevent embolism and is a good practice provided the collateral circulation is adequate (p 468). Superficial or deep femoral veins may be ligated, but ligating the common femoral or vena cava is followed by considerable morbidity. To avoid this, high ligation has been superseded by vena cava plication. The vena cava is approached trans- or extra-peritoneally and converted by a series of silk sutures into several parallel small channels which allow blood flow but entrap migrating emboli. Plication is usually combined with thrombectomy.

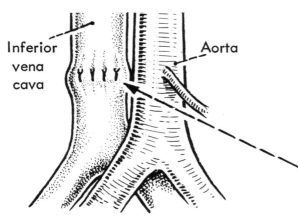

Inferior vena cava   Aorta

PULMONARY EMBOLISM

The migration of a venous thrombus from a leg or pelvic vein along the vena cava to the right ventricle and thence to the pulmonary artery. Cardiac output is at once reduced and the right ventricle exhibits signs of failure.

The lungs are an area of very active fibrinolysis and have a considerable capacity for disposing of thrombi. Embolism is not now considered an isolated catastrophe but a semi-continuous process, and survival depends on a balance between the number and size of the emboli reaching the lungs and the rate at which they are broken down.

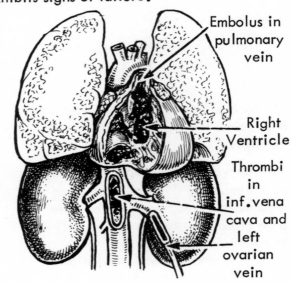

Embolus in pulmonary vein

Right Ventricle

Thrombi in inf.vena cava and left ovarian vein

Clinical Features

A large embolus lodging in the pulmonary artery produces signs of shock and circulatory failure, and in about 40% of cases the patient will die within 15 minutes. The survivors may be unconscious, hypotensive, with tachycardia and peripheral constriction.

A small embolus possibly recurrent will manifest itself by the signs of pulmonary infarction – chest pain, dyspneoa, haemoptysis, perhaps some degree of shock.

Diagnosis

Other causes of collapse and dyspnoea must be excluded. The ECG will reflect ventricular strains and is helpful. Chest X-ray is usually done with portable apparatus on a collapsed patient and is of little help.

Lung Scanning

Labelled albumin is injected and a scintillation counter passed over the chest will indicate areas of poor perfusion.

Pulmonary Arteriography

The contrast medium is injected through a catheter in the right ventricle and this carries an added risk for the ill patient. It is however diagnostic, and the catheter is also used for injecting fibrinolytic agents.

MANAGEMENT OF PULMONARY EMBOLISM

Large Emboli

The gynaecologist should initiate treatment for shock (p 427) and then if possible transfer the patient to a cardiology unit. At present the best treatment appears to be the administration of fibrinolytic drugs under strict laboratory control with surgery in reserve if the patient fails to respond.

Fibrinolytic Drugs

These are enzymes which activate plasminogen and thus initiate fibrinolysis. Streptokinase is produced by haemolytic streptococci, urokinase is extracted from human urine. They are extremely expensive and powerful and their chief complication is haemorrhage especially from wound sites. Both are inhibited by EACA (ξ-amino caproic acid).

Pulmonary arteriography

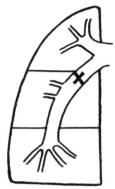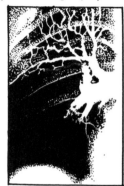

Only the upper lobe arteries are seen. The embolism has lodged at **X**.

Trendelenburg's Operation

This consists of median sternotomy, opening the pulmonary artery and sucking out the clot. This operation had become almost obsolete because of its high mortality, but has been brought back into use in recent years with the development of rapid and efficient cardio-respiratory by-pass techniques.

Small Emboli

Shock is absent or minimal and there is time to attack the source of the embolism. Anticoagulant treatment should be started at once; and as small emboli are often recurrent the advice of a vascular surgeon should be taken on the need for phlebography and perhaps thrombectomy and vein ligation.

INDEX

Abdomen, 71, 356 et seq.
Abdominal pregnancy, 354
Abdomino-vaginal hysterectomy, 228
Abortion, 412 et seq.
  Act, 413, 414
  causes, 424
  cervical suture, 425
  classification, 414
  curettage, 415–417
  criminal, 413, 426, 409
  following biopsy, 182, 183
  fibroids, 424, 425
  habitual, 424, 425
  history-taking, 66
  hysterotomy, 418
  incompetent cervix, 424, 425
  incomplete, 412, 417
  inevitable, 412
  injection of paste, 422
  intra-amniotic injection, 420. 421
  missed, 92, 413
  prostaglandins, 413, 423
  recurrent, 424, 425
  septic, 413, 426–428
  Shirodkar's repair, 425
  shock, 427, 428
  therapeutic, 413, 422
  threatened, 412
  uterine anomalies, 424, 425
  vacuum aspiration, 419
Abrasives (in hirsutism), 115
Absence of vagina, 128, 169, 170
Accessory horn, 127
Acromegaly, 93
Actinomycin D, 440
Adenoacanthoma, 242
Adenocarcinoma (see organ affected)
Adenoma malignum, 242
Adenomyosis, 91, 240
Adnexae, 36
Adrenal gland, 62, 92, 93, 94, 97–100, 103, 104, 113, 431
Adreno-genital syndrome, 98 et seq., 113

Afterloading technique (in radio-therapy) 216
Ahumada-del Castillo syndrome, 101
Aldridge's operation, 298, 299
Alkylating agents, 379, 440
Allantois, 3, 8
Alpha particles, 202
Amenorrhoea, 92 et seq.
  adrenal, 93, 94, 97, 98 et seq.
  anorexia nervosa, 92
  causes, 92, 93
  Chiari-Frommel syndrome, 101
  cryptomenorrhoea, 112
  genital hypoplasia, 95
  genetic causes, 93, 95, 105 et seq., 113
  haematocolpos, 112
  hirsutism, 114, 115
  hormone treatment, 95, 104, 109, 111
  investigation, 94
  Klinefelter's syndrome, 110
  lactation-amenorrhoea syndrome, 101
  laparoscopy, 94, 113
  missed abortion, 92
  ovarian, 93, 94, 97, 102 et seq., 113
  pituitary, 93, 96, 97, 113
  polycystic ovary disease, 102, 114
  pregnancy, 92, 94
  primary, 92
  pseudopregnancy, 92
  psychological, 92
  secondary, 92
  Stein-Leventhal syndrome, 102, 114
  systemic diseases, 93
  testicular feminisation, 111
  thyroid, 93, 94, 97
  Turner's syndrome, 109
  vaginal cytology, 94, 111, 113
  virilism, 113, 114
  wedge resection, 104
Amniotic cavity, 3

Ampulla (of tube), 36, 350, 351
Anaemia, 87, 95, 352, 438
  oral contraceptives and, 402
Anal membrane, 8, 9
Anal sphincter, 20, 22, 154, 156
Anal triangle, 16
Androgens
  adrenogenital syndrome, 98–100
  amenorrhoea, 93
  dysfunctional bleeding, 87
  hirsutism, 114
  ovarian tumours, 375, 380–383
  polycystic ovary disease, 102–104
  pre-menstrual tension, 121
  testicular feminisation, 111
  virilism, 113
Anorexia nervosa, 92
Anovular bleeding, 85
Anterior colporrhaphy, 272, 273
Anticoagulants, 470, 471
Antifibrinolytic agents, 87
Antimetabolites, 379, 440
Anuria, 427, 428
Anus, 9, 13, 16, 23, 129
Apareunia, 399
Appendicitis, 353, 363, 449
Arbor vitae, 31
Argentaffinoma, 383
Arcuate uterus, 424
Arrhenoblastoma, 381, 382
Arteries
  aorta, 3
  common iliac, 42
  endometrial, 54
  external iliac, 33, 42
  femoral, 44
  internal iliac, 42, 222, 223
  ovarian, 37, 51
  pelvic, 42, 43
  pelvic collateral, 44
  pudendal, 43, 46
  ureteric, 310, 311
  uterine, 32, 33, 37, 42, 43, 221
  vaginal, 42, 43
Arteriography, 439
Artificial isotopes, 209

Artificial menopause, 90, 132
Arvin, 470, 471
Ascites, 73, 359, 366
Atypical hyperplasia, 242
Aveling's repositor, 261
Axial rotation of pedicle, 363, 365
Ayre's spatula, 180

Bacillus coli, 162, 426, 450
Backache, 116, 255, 268
Baldy-Webster operation, 258
Ball's operation, 303
Barr bodies, 108, 110
Bartholin's gland, 9, 16, 18, 19
  abscess, 138, 139
  carcinoma, 139
  cyst, 138, 139, 269
  gonorrhoea, 454, 455
  palpation, 74
Basal cell carcinoma, 143
Basal temperature, 389
Basculation, 256
Bastiaanse's operation, 339
Beta particles, 202, 203
Betatron, 201
Bicornuate uterus, 127
Bimanual pelvic examination, 75
Biopsy of cervix, 175, 182, 183, 190
Bivalve speculum, 76
Bladder
  anatomy, 26, 29, 32, 309
  cystometry, 293
  development, 7
  displacement, 263, 264, 268, 272,
    273, 283, 315
  ectopia vesicae, 129
  endometriosis, 446
  electrical control, 305, 306
  fistula, 316, 318, 324 et seq.
  frequency, 291
  nervous control, 287
  neurological disease, 290
  overflow incontinence, 290
  physiology, 286, 288
  post-operative, 283
  radiation dosage, 215
  stress incontinence, 289
  tuberculosis, 463
  urgency incontinence, 290
  urethrocystography, 294

Boari operation, 318
Bowel
  atonicity, 120
  endometriosis, 446
  ileal conduit, 322
  obstruction, 363
  radiation damage to, 219
  tuberculosis, 463
Breasts
  examination, 70
  galactorrhoea, 101
  hirsutism, 114
  hormone effects, 60
  Klinefelter's syndrome, 110
  lactation-amenorrhoea syn-
    drome, 101
  menstruation, 67
  precocious puberty, 165
  premenstrual tension, 121
  Sheehan's syndrome, 97
  testicular feminisation, 111
  Turner's syndrome, 109
  virilism, 113
Bremsstrahlung, 199
Brenner tumour, 373
Broad ligament, 33, 37
  cysts, 362
Broders' classification, 220
Bulbospongiosus muscle, 19, 20,
  138, 335
Buttressing operation, 297

Caesium-137, 209
Call-Exner body, 375
Canal
  of Nuck, 141
  pudendal, 22, 43, 46
Candida albicans, 68, 162, 163
Carcinogenesis
  oral contraceptives and, 403
Carcinoid tumour, 383
Carcinoma
  Bartholin's gland, 139
  bladder, 167, 325
  bowel, 167, 376
  breast, 167, 376
  cervix, 184
  clitoris, 143
  endometrium, 241
  fallopian tube, 344

Carcinoma (continued)
  in situ, 191
  ovary, 376
  pain in, 230, 231
  stomach, 376, 377
  urethra, 153
  uterus, 241
  vagina, 167
  vulva, 143
  with pessary, 270
Carcinoma in situ, 180, 191
  cervix, 180
  colposcopy, 232
  cone biopsy, 175
  examination, 180, 181
  histology, 178–181
  pregnancy, 183
  treatment, 182
  uterus, 242
  vulva, 135
Carcinoma of cervix, 184 et seq.
  adenocarcinoma, 184, 186
  aetiology, 187
  biopsy, 190
  clinical staging, 191, 192
  coitus, 187, 189
  colposcopy, 232
  differential diagnosis, 190, 260
  fistula, 325
  histology, 185, 186
  incidence, 187
  lymphatic spread, 188
  microcarcinoma, 183
  pain in, 230, 231
  pelvic exenteration, 226–228
  radiotherapy, 193, 196, 197, 205
    et seq.
  results of treatment, 194
  Schauta's hysterectomy, 224,
    225, 228
  Schiller's test, 179
  stump carcinoma, 197
  surgical treatment, 193, 195–
    197, 221 et seq.
  symptoms, 189
  Wertheim's hysterectomy, 221–
    223, 228
Carcinoma of endometrium, 235,
  238, 241 et seq., 344
  adenoacanthoma, 242
  adenoma malignum, 242
  aetiology, 245

Carcinoma of endometrium (*continued*)
 atypical hyperplasia, 242
 clinical features, 241, 245
 clinical staging, 244
 fractional curettage, 245
 granulosa cell tumour, 380
 histology, 242
 ovarian carcinoma, 376
 progesterone, 248
 radiotherapy, 246, 247
 recurrence, 248
 spread, 243
 squamous metaplasia, 242
 surgery, 246, 247
 treatment, 246
Carcinoma of ovary (see Ovarian
 tumours)
Carcinoma of vulva
 clinical features, 143
 complications, 149
 pathology, 143
 prognosis, 149
 radical vulvectomy, 145–148
 radiotherapy, 149
 spread, 144
Cardinal ligaments, 25, 34, 262
Carneous mole, 413
Caruncle, urethral, 151
Carunculae myrtiformes, 18
Cellulitis, pelvic, 451–453
Central venous pressure, 429, 430
'Cervical cascade', 390
Cervix, cervical
 amputation, 275
 anatomy, 30–34
 arbor vitae, 31
 biopsy, 175, 182, 183, 462
 carcinoma (see Carcinoma of
  cervix)
 carcinoma in situ, 180 et seq.
 cauterisation, 175
 cervicitis, 68
 chancre, 177, 190, 456
 changes with age, 41
 chronic cervicitis, 174, 176, 190
 colposcopy, 232
 cone biopsy, 175, 182, 183
 congenital abnormalities, 127,
  128
 conisation, 175
 cytological examination, 180,
  181

Cervix (*continued*)
 diathermy, 175
 dilatation, 117, 415, 416, 419
 discharge, 390, 395
 displacement, 253
 dysplasia, 179
 ectropion, 174
 erosion, 173, 175, 401
 examination, 75, 77
 glands, 455
 Hegar's sign, 71
 histology, 35
 hysterectomy, 88, 89, 182
 incompetent, 424, 425
 injury, 416, 421, 426
 mucus, 390, 395
 Nabothian follicles, 176
 nulliparous, 31
 oral contraceptives and, 173,
  400, 401
 parous, 31, 409
 pinhole os, 117
 polyps, 176, 190, 269
 post-partum, 409
 prolapse, 264, 266
 smear, 180
 squamous metaplasia, 178
 subtotal hysterectomy, 90
 suture, 425
 trachelorrhaphy, 174
 tuberculosis, 177, 190, 461, 462
Chancre, 456
Chancroid, 458
Chemotherapy, 379, 441, 462
Chiari-Frommel syndrome, 101
Chlorotrianisene, 394
Chocolate cyst, 445, 450
Chorio-adenoma destruens, 436
Choriocarcinoma (chorionepithe-
 lioma), 375, 437 et seq.
 of ovary, 383
Choriodecidual space, 413
Chromosomes
 additions, 110
 analysis, 94, 108
 Barr body, 108, 109
 drumsticks, 108
 mosaicism, 107, 109, 110
 non-disjunction, 106
 partial deletion, 107, 109
 sex, 105–111
Chronic inversion of uterus, 240, 259–61

Circumcision, 187
Climacteric, 62, 63
Clinical staging of
 carcinoma of cervix, 191, 192
 carcinoma of endometrium, 244
 carcinoma of vagina, 167
 ovarian tumours, 378

Clitoris
 anatomy, 17
 carcinoma, 143
 development, 9
 enlargement, 98, 113

Cloaca, 6, 8 12
 congenital abnormalities, 129
Clomiphene, 101, 104, 394
Cloquet, lymph node of, 144
Clostridium welchii, 426, 427
Coagulation of blood, 464, 465
Cobalt-60, 205, 209
Coccygeus muscle, 23
Coitus
 apareunia, 169, 399
 candida albicans, 161
 carcinoma of cervix, 187, 195
 carcinoma of vagina, 168
 frequency, 397
 gonadotrophins, 396
 hymen, 18
 infertility, 387
 interruptus, 407
 post-operative, 169, 170, 284
 post-radiation, 217
 rape, 408
 tests following, 390
 trichomonas, 163
 with pessary, 270
Colchicine, 108
Collateral circulation
 in thrombosis, 468
 of pelvis, 44
Colostomy, 226
Colostrum, 70
Colpocleisis, 333
Colpoperineorrhaphy, 276
Colporrhaphy, 273
Colposcopy, 232
Colpostat, 211, 214, 216
Complete tear of perineum, 154,
 156
Condom, 407
Condylomata acuminata, 142

Condylomata lata, 457
Cone biopsy, 175, 182, 183
Congenital abnormalities, 125 et seq., 349
Congestive dysmenorrhoea, 116
Continuous spectrum X-rays, 199
Contraceptives, 400–407
  coitus interruptus, 407
  condom, 407
  IUCD, 404 et seq.
  oral, 400 et seq.
  rhythm method, 407
  sheath, 407
  spermicides, 406
  vaginal diaphragm, 406
Cordotomy, 231
Corona radiata, 52
Corpus albicans, 40, 53
Corpus luteum, 40, 53
Coumarin drugs, 470, 471
Cowper's glands, 19
Criminal abortion, 409, 413, 426
Cruciate anastomosis, 44
Cryptomenorrhoea, 112, 127
Culdocentesis, 353
Culdoscopy, 80
Curettage, 101, 415–417
Curette
  biopsy, 389
  suction, 419
  Vabra, 86
Cusco's speculum, 76
Cushing's syndrome, 98
Cyclical hormone therapy, 87, 95, 104
Cyclophosphamide, 379
Cyst
  Bartholin's 138, 139, 269
  broad ligament, 342, 362
  chocolate, 445, 450
  corpus luteum, 57, 58, 364
  dermoid, 374
  epoophoron, 37, 342
  fimbrial, 37, 166
  follicular, 102, 103
  Gartner's duct, 166, 342
  hydatid of Morgagni, 166
  inclusion, 141, 166
  Kobelt's tubules, 37, 166, 342
  lutein, 433
  ovarian, 71, 73, 355 et seq.
  paroophoron, 37

Cyst (continued)
  parovarian, 342
  sebaceous, 141
  Skene's duct, 152, 269
  tarry, 445, 450
  traumatic, 166
  vaginal, 166, 269
  vestigial, 37
Cystic glandular hyperplasia, 85, 91
Cystitis, 218, 219, 282, 283, 291, 326, 327
Cystocele, 264, 273, 274, 279
Cystometry, 293
Cystoscopy, 192, 327, 328
Cytology
  cervical, 180, 232
  vaginal, 61, 63, 94, 391
Cytotoxic drugs, 379, 440
Cytotrophoblast, 383, 432, 437

Defaecation, difficult, 268
Dalkon shield, 404
Decidua, 353
Decidual cast, 350
Deep transverse perineal muscle, 20, 21
Deep vein thrombosis, 464 et seq.
Deficient perineum, 154, 155
Delayed puberty, 92, 96
Depilatories, 115
Depression, 62, 88
Dermoid cyst, 374
Development of
  bladder, 8
  corpus luteum, 51, 52
  external genitalia, 8–13
  fallopian tubes, 6, 7
  ovary, 3–5
  testis, 10, 11, 13
  uterus, 6, 7
  vagina, 7
Dexamethasone, 104, 113
Diabetes, 74, 245, 402
Diaphragm, vaginal, 406
Diathermy, 115, 119, 346
Dienoestrol cream, 63
Dilatation and curettage, 117, 415–417
Dilator
  cervical, 415

Dilator (continued)
  vaginal, 399
Discharge
  cervical, 160, 390, 395
  vaginal, 160 et seq. (See also Vaginal discharge.)
Diuretics, 121
Diverticulitis, 363, 447, 449
Doderlein's bacillus, 28
Donald-Fothergill operation, 274
Donovan bodies, 459
Dorsal position, 74
Dosimeter, 215
Double vagina, 128
Double vulva, 129
Douglas, pouch of, 27, 265, 280, 351, 352
Drumsticks, 108
Ducrey's bacillus, 458
Duct
  Bartholin's gland, 18
  ejaculatory, 10
  Gartner's, 37
  mesonephric (Wolffian), 3, 7, 10, 37
  paramesonephric (Mullerian), 6, 7, 10
  para-urethral (Skene's), 18
Dutch cap, 406
Dydrogesterone, 87, 447
Dysfunctional uterine bleeding, 84–87
Dysgerminoma 373, 374
Dysmenorrhoea, 116 et seq.
  congestive, 116, 118
  cryptomenorrhoea, 112
  dilatation of cervix, 117
  endometriosis, 118, 446
  history-taking, 69, 116
  hormone therapy, 117
  hypoplastic uterus, 117
  IUCD, 119
  membranous, 119
  metritis, 448
  mittelschmerz, 116, 119
  normal, 69
  pelvic inflammation, 449
  pregnancy, 117
  presacral neurectomy, 117, 120
  primary, 116, 117
  retroversion, 118, 255
  salpingitis, 118

Dysmenorrhoea (*continued*)
    treatment, 117, 119, 120
    uterine polyp, 119
Dyspareunia, 69, 398, 399
    after repair, 284
    endometriosis, 446
    history-taking, 69
    infertility, 386
    interposition operations, 304
    kraurosis, 132
    pelvic inflammation, 449, 452
    retroflexion, 255
    vaginal cysts, 166
    vaginal discharge, 161, 386
    with pessary, 270
Dysplasia of cervix, 179
Dystrophia adiposo-genitalis, 96
Dystrophy, vulval, 132
Dysuria, 151, 283, 291

EACA, 475
Early ambulation, 471
E. Coli, 450
Ectopia vesicae, 129
Ectopic anus, 129
Ectopic kidney, 362
Ectopic pregnancy, 69, 349 et seq.
    accessory horn, 127
    aetiology, 349
    anaemia, 352
    clinical features, 352
    culdocentesis, 353
    differential diagnosis, 364, 449
    laparoscopy, 80, 353
    lithopaedion, 354
    pain, 352
    pathology, 349–351
    pregnancy, 352
    rupture, 351
    sterilisation, 346
    treatment, 353, 354
    tuberculosis, 463
Ectropion, 174
Ejaculate, 255, 390, 397
Ejaculatory duct, 10
Electrical control of bladder, 305, 306
Electrolysis, 115
Electrolyte balance, 100, 321
Embolism, 474, 475
    cellulitis, 452
    choriocarcinoma, 439

Embolism (*continued*)
    CVP monitoring, 430
    diagnosis, 474
    fibrinolytic drugs, 475
    paste injection, 422
    post-operative, 88, 229, 282, 346
    Trendelenberg's operation, 476
Embryology, 1 et seq.
Endometriosis, 91, 167, 445–447
    adenomyosis, 91, 240
    dysmenorrhoea, 118
    vulva, 140
Endometritis, 448, 462
Endometrium (endometrial), 30
    action of hormones, 60, 87, 401
    atypical hyperplasia, 85
    biopsy, 86, 245, 389
    carcinoma, 241 et seq. (See Carcinoma of endometrium)
    cyclic changes, 54
    cystic glandular hyperplasia, 85
    histology, 35
    hypoplastic, 85
    in dysfunctional bleeding, 84 et seq.
    oral contraceptives, 400, 401
    polyp, 86, 91, 235
    pseudo-atrophy, 401
    sarcoma, 249, 250
    senile, 41
    squamous metaplasia, 242
    'Swiss cheese' pattern, 85
    tuberculosis, 461–463
Endosalpingitis, 461
Enlargement of vaginal orifice, 154, 157
Enterocele, 265, 266
    repair, 277, 278
Epididymis, 10
Epimenorrhoea, 84
Epiphyseal fusion, 111
Epithelioma (see Carcinoma)
Epoophoron, 37, 342
Erythema ab igne, 97
Esthiomène, 458
Ethinyl oestradiol, 87, 400
Examination, 66–81
    abdomen, 71–73
    Bartholin's gland, 74, 138
    bimanual, 75
    breast, 70
    colposcopy, 232

Examination (*continued*)
    cystometry, 293
    cystoscopy, 192, 327, 328
    gynaecography, 81
    hysterosalpingography, 392, 393
    intravenous pyelogram, 217, 311
    laparoscopy, 78–80, 118, 353, 446
    lymphography, 81
    small children, 165
    speculum, 76, 77
    tubal insufflation, 388
    ultrasound, 360, 435
    urethrocystography, 294
    vulva, 74
Exenteration, pelvic, 226–228
Exercises, 296, 472
External urethral sphincter, 286, 287

Faecal fistula, 215, 219, 339
Fallopian tube
    anastomosis, 348
    anatomy, 36, 37
    carcinoma, 344
    coagulation, 346
    congenital abnormalities, 125, 126, 349
    cyclic changes, 55
    development, 6, 7
    dye injection, 78
    gonorrhoea, 455
    haematosalpinx, 112, 450
    implantation, 348
    infection, 346, 386, 449, 450, 455, 461–463
    infertility, 386
    insufflation, 388
    ligation, 345
    Mulligan's operation, 347
    paste injection, 422
    pregnancy in, 346, 349 et seq.
    salpingectomy, 346, 354
    salpingostomy, 347
    tuberculosis, 386, 461–463
Fascia, pelvic, 21, 22, 25
Feminisation, testicular, 111
Femoral canal, 25
Ferning test, 390
Fibrin degradation products, 464

Fibrinolytic drugs, 475
Fibroids, 236 et seq., 360
  causing inversion, 259
  in abortion, 424, 425
  myomectomy, 239
  torsion, 364
Fibroma
  of ovary, 366, 373
  of vulva, 140
Fibromyomata (see Fibroids)
Fibrosis uteri, 448
Fimbria (of tube), 36, 347
Fimbrial cyst, 37, 166
Fistula, 323 et seq. (See also
  Urinary fistula)
  aetiology, 219, 229, 312, 313,
    324, 325, 463
  classical repair, 331
  cystoscopy, 328
  faecal, 215, 219, 339
  flap-splitting technique, 332
  intestinal, 219, 463
  methylene blue test, 327
  radiation, 219, 335, 339
  rectovaginal, 219, 330 et seq.
  transvesical repair, 340
  tuberculous, 463
  ureteric, 229, 319
  ureterovaginal, 327
  urethral, 334
  urethrovaginal, 325
  urinary, 219
  vesicovaginal, 77, 325
Fletcher colpostat, 214
Fluid thrill, 73
Fluocinolone, 135, 136
Fluorescent tests for syphilis, 460
Fogarty technique (in thrombectomy), 473
Folic acid antagonists, 440
Follicle
  atretic, 40
  Graafian, 40, 52, 401
  primitive, 4
Follicle stimulating hormone
  (FSH), 57, 59, 395
Forceps, biopsy, 79
Fornix, vaginal, 26, 27
Fossa
  ischiorectal, 22, 26, 43
  navicular, 18
Fothergill suture, 275

Fourchette, 17
Fractional curettage, 245
Frankenhauser's plexus, 47
Frei's intradermal test, 458
Frenulum of clitoris, 17
Frequency of micturition, 291
Frigidity, 121, 398
Fröhlich's syndrome, 96
Full bladder, 359

Galactorrhoea, 101
Gamma rays, 202 et seq.
Gartner's duct, 37, 166, 342
Genetic amenorrhoea, 105 et seq.
Genital hypoplasia, 95
Genital ridge, 3–5
Genital swelling, 9, 12
Genital tubercle, 8, 9, 12
Genitalia, development, 8, 9
Germ cell tumours, 373 et seq.
Germ cells, 3, 4
Germinal epithelium, 51
Gilliam's operation, 258, 304
Gland(s). (See also specific organs)
  adrenal, 93, 98 et seq., 403
  Bartholin's, 9, 16, 18, 19, 74, 454
  bulbo-urethral (see Cowper's)
  cervical, 35
  Cowper's, 19
  greater vestibular (see Bartho-
    lin's)
  para-urethral (see Skene's)
  pituitary, 59, 62, 92–94, 97, 101,
    102, 395, 396
  Skene's, 9, 18, 454
  thyroid, 93, 95, 403
  uterine, 35, 242
Glucksman and Spear's method,
  220
Gonadal dysgenesis, 109
Gonadoblastoma, 375
Gonadotrophins, 58, 87, 104, 395,
  396
Gonorrhoea, 450, 454, 455
Graafian follicle, development, 58
Gracilis muscle interposition, 336,
  337
Granuloma inguinale, 459
Granulomatous caruncle, 151
Granulosa cell tumour, 90, 375,
  380

Green-Armytage cannula, 392
Gubernaculum, 5, 11, 33, 126
Guinea pig inoculation, 462
Gumma, 457
Gynaecography, 81
'Gynaecological' perineum, 16
Gynatresia, 128, 169, 170

Habitual abortion, 424, 425
Haematocele, pelvic, 351, 354
Haematocolpos, 112
Haematoma
  post-operative, 302
  rectus sheath, 361
  vulva, 140
Haematometra, 112
Haematosalpinx, 112, 450
Haematuria, 291, 446
Haemorrhage
  abortion, 419, 422
  ectopic pregnancy, 352
  fibrinolytic drugs, 475
  follicular cyst, 396
  hydatidiform mole, 435, 436
  IUCD, 405
  radical surgery, 229
  Sheehan's syndrome, 97
  shock, 430, 431
  uterine, abnormal 84–91
  vaginal hysterectomy, 280
Hair distribution, 114
Hair follicle, 115
Haultain's operation, 261
Hegar's sign, 71, 359
Heparin, 470
Hernia, 141, 147
Herpes simplex, 177
  carcinoma of cervix and, 187
Hidradenoma, 142
Hilum, 39
Hilus cell tumour, 381, 382
Hind gut, 3
Hirsutism, 98, 114, 115
History taking, 66
  infertility, 387
Hodge pessary, 257
Homan's sign, 467
Hormone assays
  ovulation and, 391
Hormones (see also specific
  glands)

Hormones (*continued*)
 adrenal, 92–94, 97–100, 113, 115, 165, 431
 androgens, 87, 102, 103, 113, 114, 117, 121, 381–383
 carcinogenesis, 245, 403
  chorionic gonadotrophin, 395, 396, 433 et seq.
 clomiphene, 101, 104, 394
 corpus luteum, 40, 53–63, 92, 94, 102, 390
 cyclic treatment, 87, 95, 104, 117
 dexamethasone, 104, 113
 dienoestrol, 63
 dydrogesterone, 87, 447
 ethinyl oestradiol, 87, 95, 109, 400
 fluocinolone, 135, 136
 menopause, 62, 63, 90
 metyrapone, 113
 norethisterone, 95, 400
 oestrogens, 63, 119, 133, 135, 137, 164, 165, 380
 oral contraceptives, 87, 400–403
 ovarian tumours, 380 et seq.
 ovary, production in, 102
 Pergonal 395, 396
 pituitary, 57–63, 92–97, 102–104, 391, 395, 396
 polycystic ovary, 102
 progestogens, 119, 121, 165, 248
 serotonin, 383
 thyroid, 87, 92, 93, 95
'Hot flushes', 63, 67
Human chorionic gonadotrophin, 395, 433, 435
Human menopausal gonadotrophin, 57, 395
Human pituitary gonadotrophin, 395
Hydatid of Morgagni, 37
Hydatidiform mole, 432 et seq.
Hydrocele of Canal of Nuck, 141
Hydrosalpinx, 450
Hydrothorax, 366, 373
Hymen
 anatomy, 18
 development, 7
 imperforate, 112, 128
 tough, 399
Hyperchloraemic acidosis, 321

Hyperpituitarism, 93
Hyperstimulation syndrome, 396
Hypertension
 oral contraceptives and, 402
Hyperthecosis, 102 et seq.
Hypogastric plexus, 47, 120
Hypopituitarism, 93, 96
Hypothalamus, 59, 62, 92, 101, 102, 400
Hypothyroidism, 87, 93
Hysterectomy
 abdomino-vaginal, 228
 carcinoma in situ, 182
 carcinoma of endometrium, 246
 complications, 88, 229
 dysfunctional bleeding, 87
 fibroids, 239
 fistula, 88, 229, 312–314
 hydatidiform mole, 436
 ovarian tumours, 368, 369
 pelvic inflammation, 448, 452
 Schauta, 224, 225
 subtotal, 90
 total, 88, 89, 312, 313
 tuberculosis, 463
 vaginal, 279, 280
 Wertheim, 221–223, 246, 314
Hysteria, 66
Hysterosalpingography, 392, 393
Hysterotomy, 418

Ileal bladder, 226
Ileal conduit, 322
Ileus, 229
Iliac vessels, 33, 42, 44
Iliococcygeus muscle, 24
Immunoglobulin
 oral contraceptives and, 402
Immunological factors
 in infertility, 386
Imperforate hymen, 112, 128
Impotence, 399
Inclusion cyst, 141
Incompetent cervix, 424, 425
Incomplete abortion, 412, 417
Incontinence (see also Stress incontinence)
 faecal, 154
 urinary, 289, 290

Inevitable abortion, 412
Infantile uterus, 41, 117
Inferior vena cava, 473
Infertility, 102, 386 et seq.
 causes, 386, 397, 462
 cervix, 255, 390
 clomiphene, 394
 coitus, 397
 endometriosis, 446
 ferning test, 390
 gonadotrophins, 395, 396
 hormone assays, 391
 hyperstimulation, 396
 hysterosalpingography, 392, 393
 immunological factor, 397
 laparoscopy, 78 et seq.
 male, 397
 post-coital test, 390
 retroversion, 255
 seminal analysis, 397
 sperm invasion test, 390
 spinnbarkeit, 390
 temperature changes, 389
 tubal insufflation, 388
 tuberculosis, 462, 463
Infundibulopelvic ligament, 33
Infundibulum (of tube), 36
Inguinal canal, 25
Inguinal glands, 45, 144, 153, 456, 458
Inguinal hernia, 141, 147
Injection of paste, 422
Insufflation of tube, 388
Intercourse (see Coitus)
Intermenstrual bleeding, 91
Interposition operations
 for stress incontinence, 304
 in fistula, 335, 336
Interstitial (part of tube), 36, 351
Intra-amniotic injection, 420, 421
Intracavitary irradiation, 210–216, 218, 219
Intra-epithelial carcinoma (see Carcinoma in situ)
Intra-uterine contraceptive device, 119, 404–405
Invasive mole, 436
Inversion of uterus, 259 et seq., 269
Iron-dextran, 87
Irradiation (see also Radiotherapy)
 alpha particles, 202

Irradiation (continued)
 beta particles, 203, 206
 betatron, 201
 biological effects, 204
 bremsstrahlung, 199, 203
 caesium-137, 209
 characteristic X-rays, 199
 cobalt-60, 209
 cobalt beam applicator, 205
 continuous spectrum X-rays, 199
 gamma rays, 202, 203, 205
 isotopes, 203, 209
 linear accelerator, 200
 neutrino, 203
 rad, 206
 radium, 203
 radon, 203
 rontgen, 206
 X-rays, 198–201, 205
Ischiorectal fossa, 22
Isoniazid, 462
Isotopes, 462
Isotopic diagnosis, 468
Isthmus (of tube), 36, 351, 352
Isthmus uteri, 30
IUCD, 119, 404 et seq.

Kelly's operation, 297
Kidney
 blood supply, 310, 311
 damage to ureter, 316–322
 ectopic, 362
 hydronephrosis, 267, 319
 nephrostomy, 317
 palpation, 72
Klinefelter's syndrome, 110
Kobelt's tubules, 37
Kraurosis, 132, 133
Krukenberg tumour, 377

Labium majus, 9, 17, 335
Labium minus, 9, 17
Lactation-amenorrhoea syndrome, 101
Lactogenic bacilli, 160
Laparoscopy, 78 et seq., 353
 diathermy coagulation and, 346
 in amenorrhoea, 94, 113

Lapides' operation, 303
Latzko's operation, 333
Le Fort's operation, 281
Leiomyoma, 236
Leukoplakia, 134, 135
Levator ani muscle, 20, 23, 24, 262
Leydig cells, 111, 381
Lichen planus, 136
Lichen simplex, 137
Ligament(s)
 broad, 33, 37
 cardinal, 36
 infundibulopelvic, 33
 Mackenrodt's, 34
 of uterus, 33, 34
 ovarian, 29, 33
 pubocervical, 273
 round, 29, 33
 sacrospinous, 23
 sacrotuberous, 16, 22
 suspensory (of ovary), 5
 transverse cervical, 34
 triangular, 21
 uterosacral, 34
Linear accelerator, 200
Lipoid cell tumour, 381, 382
Lipoma, 140, 362
Lippes' loop, 404
Lithopaedion, 354
Liver
 oral contraceptives, 402
 palpation, 72
Lorain-Levi syndrome, 96
Louros' operation, 304
Lumbar plexus, 230
Lung scanning, 474
Lung, endometriosis, 406
Lutein cyst, 433
Luteinising hormone (LH), 57, 58, 395
Luteotrophic hormone (LTH), 57, 58
Lymphatic drainage of pelvis, 45
Lymphatic nodes, 45, 144, 153, 207, 223, 243, 456, 458
Lymphocyst formation, 229
Lymphogranuloma inguinale, 458
Lymphography, 81

Mackenrodt's ligament, 34
Male infertility, 397

Male sterilisation, 407
Manchester method, 213
Manchester operation, 274
Marshall-Marchetti-Kranz operation, 302, 334
Marsupialisation, 139
Martius' operation, 334, 335
Masculinovoblastoma, 382
Mastopathia, 121
Maturation of germ cells, 105 et seq.
McIndoe–Bannister operation, 169
Meatitis, urethral, 151
Medico-legal problems, 408, 409
Meigs' syndrome, 366, 373
Melanoma of vulva, 143
Membrane
 anal, 8
 perineal, 21
 urogenital, 8
Membranous dysmenorrhoea, 119
Menarche, 67
Menopause, 62, 63
 anatomical changes, 41
 delayed, 237, 245
 early, 93
 history taking, 67
 radiation, 90
Menorrhagia
 clinical features, 86
 definition, 84
 differential diagnosis, 91
 fibroids, 238
 history, 68
 inflammation, 449
 retroversion, 255
 treatment, 87–90
Menstruation (menstrual)
 abnormal, 83 et seq., 380
 antifibrinolytic agents, 87
 blood loss, 67
 dysmenorrhoea, 116 et seq.
 epimenorrhoea, 84
 histological cycle, 54, 55, 60
 hormonal cycle, 56–61
 hormone treatment, 87
 infertility, 389–391
 irregular shedding, 84
 menarche, 67
 menopause, 62, 63, 67
 menorrhagia, 68, 84
 molimina, 67

Menstruation (*continued*)
  normal, 67
  oral contraceptives, 400
  precocious, 165
  pre-menstrual tension, 121
  rhythm, 67
  vaginal smear, 61
Mercaptopurine, 379
Mesoderm, 4
Mesonephric (Wolffian) duct, 3, 7,
  10, 37
Mesonephros, 3 et seq.
Mesosalpinx, 342
Mesovarium, 38
Metanephros, 3
Methotrexate, 379, 440
Methyl testosterone, 121
Metritis, 448
Metronidazole, 163
Metropathia haemorrhagica, 85,
  91
Metrorrhagia, 68, 91
Metyrapone, 113
Microcarcinoma, 183
Micturition
  dysuria, 151, 283, 291
  electrical control, 305
  exercises, 296
  frequency, 291
  haematuria, 291, 446
  physiology, 286–288
  urethrocystography, 294
Mid-cycle bleeding, 91
Millin's operation, 301
Missed abortion, 92, 354, 413, 414
Mittelschmerz, 116, 119
Mixed mesodermal tumour, 250
Moir's operation, 300
Mole
  carneous, 413
  hydatidiform, 432 et seq.
  invasive, 436
Monilia albicans, 162, 163
Monilial vaginitis, 68
Mons pubis, 17
Montgomery's tubercles, 70
Morgagni, hydatid of, 37
Mosaicism, 107, 109, 110
Mucinous cystadenocarcinoma,
  371
Mucinous cystadenoma, 371
Mullerian duct, 6, 7, 10, 125

Mulligan's operation, 347
Multiple pregnancy, HPG and, 396
Muscles
  bulbospongiosus, 20, 335
  coccygeus, 20, 23, 24
  gluteus maximus, 22
  gracilis, 336, 337
  iliococcygeus, 24
  ischiocavernosus, 20
  ischiococcygeus, 24
  levator ani, 20, 22, 24
  obturator, 23, 24, 26
  perineal, 20, 21
  pelvic, 23, 24
  piriformis, 24
  pubococcygeus, 24
  rectus, 338, 361
  sphincter ani, 20, 22, 23
  sphincter urethrae, 21
  transversus perinei, 20
Mycobacterium tuberculosis, 388
Myohyperplasia, 240, 448
Myoma, 236 (see Fibroid)

Nabothian follicles, 176
Nephrostomy, 317
Nerve(s)
  autonomic, 47
  bladder, 287
  erigentes, 47
  obturator, 46
  ovarian, 47
  pelvic, 46
  pre-sacral, 47, 120
  pudendal, 22, 23, 46
  sacral, 22, 23, 46
Nervous control of micturition,
  287
Neurodermatitis, 137
Neurological incontinence, 290
Neurological operations for pain,
  230, 231
Neutrino, 203
Non-disjunction, chromosomal,
  106
Norethisterone, 95, 400
Nulliparous uterine prolapse, 266
Nystatin, 163

Obesity
  abdomen, 73

Obesity (*continued*)
  amenorrhoea, 95
  carcinoma of uterus, 245
  Fröhlich's, 96
  hysterectomy, 88, 195
  menopause, 62
  ovarian tumours, 357, 361
  polycystic ovary disease, 102
  prolapse, 262
Obturator foramen, 25
  muscle, 23, 24, 26
  nerve, 46
Oestradiol, 56
Oestriol, 56
Oestrogen(s)
  action, 60
  assays, 391
  blood vessels, 60
  breast, 40, 60
  carcinoma of endometrium, 245
  changes in genital tract, 41
  corpus luteum, 40
  cyclical therapy, 95
  dysfunctional bleeding, 84, 85,
  87
  dysmenorrhoe, 117
  endometrium, 41, 51
  fallopian tube, 55
  ferning, 390
  follicular atresia, 40
  frigidity, 398
  hydatidiform mole, 433
  kidney, 60
  kraurosis, 132, 133
  leukoplakia, 135
  menopause, 62, 63, 164
  menstrual cycle, 56
  oral contraception, 400
  ovarian tumours, 245, 380, 383
  ovulation, 53, 57–59, 390, 394
  polycystic ovary disease, 102
  post-radiation, 219
  pre-menstrual tension, 121
  pre-pubertal vaginitis, 164
  scleroderma, 137
  senile vaginitis, 164
  testicular feminisation, 111
  uterus, 41, 60
  vagina, 41, 55, 60, 61, 94
Oestrone, 56
Oligomenorrhoea, 102, 113
Omental fat interposition, 339

Oophorectomy, 90, 368, 370
Oophoritis, 118, 450
Operation(s)
  Aldridge, 298
  Baldy–Webster, 258
  Ball, 303
  Bastiaanse, 339
  Boari, 318
  colporrhaphy, 272
  currettage, 415
  dilatation, 415
  Donald-Fothergill, 274
  Gilliam, 258
  Haultain, 261
  hysterectomy
    abdomino-vaginal, 228
    Schauta, 224
    subtotal, 90
    total, 88
    vaginal, 279
    Wertheim, 221
  hysterotomy, 418
  injection of paste, 422
  interposition
    bulbospongiosus, 335
    gracilis, 336
    omentum 339
    rectus, 338
    uterine, 304
  intra-amniotic injection, 420
  Kelly, 297
  Lapides, 303
  Latzko, 333
  Le Fort, 281
  Louros, 304
  McIndoe–Bannister, 169
  Manchester, 274
  Marshall–Marchetti–Kranz, 302
  Martius, 335
  Millin, 301
  Moir, 300
  Mulligan, 347
  presacral neurectomy, 117
  repair of fistula, 331
  repair of prolapse, 272
  salpingectomy, 346
  salpingostomy, 347
  Shirodkar, 425
  sterilisation, 345
  Trendelenberg, 475
  tubal implantation, 348
  tubal ligation, 345

Operation(s) (*continued*)
  vacuum aspiration, 419
  ventro-suspension, 258
  vulvectomy
    radical, 145
    simple, 150
Oral contraceptives, 165, 400 et seq.
  cervical erosion and, 173
  for dysfunctional bleeding, 87
Ovarian cachexia, 356
Ovarian cyst, tapping, 309
Ovarian steroids, 59
Ovarian tumour(s), 73, 91, 356 et seq.
  adrenal-like, 382
  amenorrhoea, 93
  argentaffinoma, 383
  arrhenoblastoma, 381, 382
  ascites, 73, 359, 366
  Brenner, 373
  broad ligament, 362, 367
  carcinoid, 383
  carcinoma, 376
  carcinoma of endometrium, 243
  choriocarcinoma, 375, 383, 437
  clinical features, 356
  clinical staging, 378
  cystadenocarcinoma, 371, 372
  cytotoxic drugs, 379, 440
  dermoid, 374
  differential diagnosis, 91, 254, 353, 359–362
  dysgerminoma, 373, 374
  ectopic kidney, 362
  ectopic pregnancy, 364
  examination, 73, 357, 365
  fibroids, 360, 364
  fibroma, 373
  germ cell, 373
  gonadoblastoma, 375
  granulosa cell, 380
  haemorrhage, 363
  hilus cell, 382
  hydrothorax, 366
  infection, 367
  Krukenberg's, 377
  lipoid cell, 382
  malignancy, features of, 366
  masculinovoblastoma, 382
  Meigs' syndrome, 366, 373
  mucinous cystadenocarcinoma, 371

Ovarian tumour(s) (*continued*)
  mucinous cystadenoma, 371
  obesity, 73
  oestrogen-producing, 380
  pedicle, 363, 370
  pelvic inflammation, 358, 361, 364
  polycystic, 102–104, 433
  pregnancy, 359, 365
  pseudomyxoma peritonei, 366
  radiotherapy, 378
  rectus sheath haematoma, 361
  retroperitoneal, 362, 367
  rupture, 365
  serous cystadenocarcinoma, 372
  serous cystadenoma, 372
  'signet ring' cell, 377
  struma ovarii, 383
  surgical treatment, 368–370
  tapping, 369
  teratoma, 374, 375
  thecoma, 380
  torsion of pedicle, 363
  ultrasound, 360
  virilism, 114, 381, 382
Ovariotomy, 368
Ovary (ovarian)
  absent, 125
  amenorrhoea, 93
  anatomy, 38–40
  artery, 44, 47
  biopsy, 79, 396
  carcinoma (see Ovarian tumours)
  carcinoma of endometrium, 243
  changes with age, 41
  corpus luteum, 40, 53
  cyst (see Ovarian tumours)
  development, 4, 5
  dysgenesis, 109, 110
  endometriosis, 446
  examination, 73, 75
  follicle, 52
  gubernaculum, 7
  histology, 39, 40
  hormones, 53, 56, 58, 60, 61, 94, 391
  infertility, 391, 394–396
  irradiation, 90
  ligament, 29, 30
  nerves, 47
  oophorectomy, 90, 368, 370

Ovary (continued)
  oophoritis, 118, 450
  oral contraception, 401
  ovulation, 53, 57–59, 389–391
  pedicle, 370
  physiology, 51–53, 57
  polycystic, 81, 102–104
  prolapsed, 398
  streak, 109, 125
  tumour (see Ovarian tumour)
  vestigial, 125
  wedge resection, 104, 368
Overflow incontinence, 290
Ovulation
  bleeding, 364
  cervical changes, 390
  clomiphene, 394
  control, 57, 59
  corpus albicans, 40
  corpus luteum, 40
  follicular atresia, 40
  gonadotrophins, 395, 396
  Graafian follicle, 39, 51, 52
  hormonal changes, 53, 56, 58
  hypothalamus, 57, 59
  induction, 394–396
  infertility, 386
  mittelschmerz, 116, 119
  oral contraception, 400
  physiology, 51–53
  pituitary, 56, 57, 59
  rupture of follicle, 52
  temperature changes, 389
  tests for, 389–391
  vaginal smear, 391
'Oyster' ovary, 103

Pain
  cordotomy in, 231
  dysmenorrhoea, 116
  endometriosis and, 446
  history taking, 69
  in ectopic pregnancy, 69, 352
  in pelvic cancer, 230
  intrathecal phenol, 230
  IUCD and, 405
Paracentesis (of cyst), 369
Paramesonephric duct, 6, 7
Parasitic tumour, 363
Parasympathetic nerves, 47, 287

Paraurethral ducts, 18, 151, 152
Paris method (in radiotherapy), 211
Paroophoron, 37
Parovarian cysts, 342 et seq.
Partial deletion, 107, 109
PAS, 462
'Peg' cells, 36
Pelvis (pelvic)
  abscess, 453
  anatomy, 15–47
  blood vessels, 42–44
  cellulitis, 451–453
  congestion, 116, 118, 119
  diaphragm, 24
  examination, 75
  exenteration, 226 et seq.
  exercises, 296
  fascia, 25
  haematocele, 351, 354
  inflammation, 91, 361, 364, 448, et seq.
  kidney, 362
  lymphadenectomy, 223
  lymphatic drainage, 45
  muscles, 22–24
  nerves, 46, 47, 120
Penicillin, 455
Penis
  contraception, 407
  development, 11–13
  dyspareunia, 255, 398
  impotence, 399
  pruritus, 161
Perforation
  bowel, 80
  uterus, 405, 416, 426
Perineal body, 21
Perineal membrane, 21
Perineoplasty, 157
Perineum
  anatomy, 16 et seq.
  complete tear, 154, 156
  deficient, 154, 155
  enlargement of vaginal orifice, 154, 157
  operations, 154 et seq.
Peritonitis, 450, 461
Pessary
  antibiotic, 163
  bakelite, 271
  carcinoma, 370

Pessary (continued)
  electrode, 306
  Hodge, 257
  indication, 270
  lactic acid, 164
  nystatin, 163
  polythene, 271
  spermicidal, 406
  stem, 271
  vinyl, 271
Pessary test, 255, 257, 258
Phallus (see Penis)
Phenol, intrathecal, 230
Phenormin, 471
Phlebography, 468, 473
Phlebothrombosis, 465
Phlegmasia alba dolens, 467
Physiology of micturition, 286 et seq.
Physiology of reproductive tract, 49 et seq.
Physiotherapy, 296, 471
Pigmentation
  oral contraceptives and, 403
Piperazine, 164
Piriformis muscle, 24
Pituitary gland
  adrenogenital syndrome, 100
  amenorrhoea, 92, 93
  carcinoma of uterus, 245
  corpus luteum, 57, 58
  dysfunctional bleeding, 87
  galactorrhoea, 101
  gonadotrophins, 57, 58, 62, 395, 396
  hypopituitarism, 96, 97
  hypothalamus, 59, 92, 102
  infertility, 395, 396
  menopause, 62
  ovarian hormones. 58
  ovulation, 57–59, 102, 395, 396
  Sheehan's syndrome, 97
  Simmonds' disease, 97
  tumour, 94, 101
Plasminogen, 87
Plexus(es)
  Frankenhauser's, 47
  hypogastric, 47
  lumbar, 230
  sacral, 23, 46, 230
Plication, vena cava, 473
Polycystic ovary disease, 102 et seq.

Polyp
  cervical, 91, 176, 269
  mucous, 235
  placental, 235
  uterine, 86
'Positive' smear in pregnancy, 183
Post-coital bleeding, 68
Post-coital test, 390
Post-menopausal bleeding, 68
Post-partum necrosis, 97
Post-phlebitic syndrome, 469
'Potato' ovary, 103
Pouch of Douglas, 27, 265, 280, 351, 352
Precocious puberty, 165
Pregnancy
  abdominal examination, 71
  abortion, 412 et seq.
  amenorrhoea, 92
  ectopic, 349
  dysmenorrhoea, 117
  Hegar's sign, 71, 359
  hydatidiform mole, 432
  hysterography, 393
  positive smear, 183
  retroversion, 255
  rupture of cyst, 365
  signs of recent delivery, 409
  sterilisation, 345
  tuberculosis, 463
Pregnanediol, 391
Pregnanetriol, 100
Pre-invasive carcinoma (see Carcinoma in situ)
Pre-menstrual tension, 67, 121
Prepuce of clitoris, 17
Pre-sacral neurectomy, 117, 120
Primary amenorrhoea, 92
Primitive follicle, 4
Primordial follicle, 51
Procaine penicillin
  in gonorrhoea, 455
  in syphilis, 457
Processus vaginalis, 11
Procidentia, 263
Progesterone
  action, 60
  adrenogenital syndrome, 100
  blood vessels, 60
  breast, 60
  carcinoma of endometrium, 248
  cervix, 60

Progesterone (continued)
  cyclical changes, 53–56
  dysfunctional bleeding, 85
  endometrium, 60
  ferning test, 390
  hormonal changes, 56
  kidney, 60
  menopause, 62
  ovulation, 53, 57–59
  precocious puberty, 165
  vagina, 60, 61
  vaginal smear, 61
Progestins, 40
Progestogens
  carcinogenesis, 403
  corpus luteum, 40
  cyclical treatment, 95, 104
  dysfunctional bleeding, 87
  dysmenorrhoea, 119
  endometriosis, 447
  norethisterone, 95, 400
  oral contraception, 400
  pre-menstrual tension, 121
Prolapse, 262–284
  anterior colporrhaphy, 272, 273
  causes, 262
  cervical, 266
  cervicovaginal, 264
  clinical features, 268
  complications, 283, 284
  cystocele, 264, 272, 273
  differential diagnosis, 269
  Donald-Fothergill operation (see Manchester operation)
  enterocele, 265, 277, 278
  Le Fort's operation, 281
  Manchester operation, 274, 275, 277, 278
  nulliparous, 266
  pessary treatment, 270, 271
  posterior colporrhaphy, 276
  procidentia, 263
  rectocele, 265, 276
  ulceration, 267
  ureter in, 263, 267, 315
  urethral, 152
  urethrocele, 264
  uterovaginal, 262, 263, 274, 275, 279, 280
  vaginal hysterectomy, 279, 280
Prostaglandins, 413, 423
Prostate, development, 11

Prostatic utricle, 11
Pruritus
  leukoplakia, 135
  lichen planus, 136
  kraurosis, 133
  penile, 161
  vaginal discharge, 161
Pseudomucinous cystadenoma, 371
Pseudomyxoma peritonei, 366
Pseudopregnancy, 92, 447
Puberty
  delayed, 192
  menarche, 167
  precocious, 165
Pubocervical ligament, 273
Pubococcygeus muscle, 24
Pudendal canal, 22, 43
Puerperal infection, 66
Pulmonary arteriography, 474, 475
Pulmonary embolism, 469, 474 et seq.
Pulmonary metastases, 438
Pyometra, 219, 448
Pyosalpinx, 450

Rad, 206
Radiation menopause, 87, 90
Radical surgery
  abdomino-vaginal, 228
  carcinoma in situ, 182
  cervix, 221
  complications, 229
  endometrium, 221, 246
  exenteration, 226, 227
  preparation for, 228
  Schauta, 224, 225
  vulva, 145 et seq.
  Wertheim, 221–223
Radical vaginal hysterectomy, 224, 225
Radical vulvectomy, 145 et seq.
  complications, 149
Radioresistance, 193, 195, 204, 220
Radiosensitivity, 204, 220
Radiotherapy (see also Irradiation)
  Broders' classification, 220
  carcinoma of cervix, 191, 193–197, 210–219
  carcinoma of endometrium, 246, 247

Radiotherapy (*continued*)
  carcinoma of ovary, 369, 378
  carcinoma of tube, 344
  carcinoma of urethra, 153
  carcinoma of vagina, 168
  carcinoma of vulva, 149
  cellulitis, 451, 452
  colpostat, 214–216
  combined with surgery, 196, 246, 247, 369, 378
  complications, 218, 219
  dosimeter, 215
  external, 205, 207, 208, 378
  Glucksman and Spear's classification, 220
  intracavitary, 168, 205, 206, 210–216, 246, 247
  Manchester method, 213
  menopause, 90
  Paris method, 211
  preparation of patient, 217
  protection of tissues, 214, 215
  radioresistance, 204, 220
  radiosensitivity, 204, 220
  sarcoma of uterus, 250
  Stockholm method, 212
  tandem, 211, 213, 214, 216
Radium, 203, 209
Rape, 408
Rectal bladder, 321
Rectocele, 265, 276
Rectovaginal examination, 75
Rectus muscle interposition, 338
Rectus sheath haematoma, 361
Recurrent abortion, 424
Reiter's test, 460
Releasing factors, 59, 62, 92, 102, 400
Repair
  anterior colporrhaphy, 272
  complete tear, 154, 156
  cystocele, 272
  deficient perineum, 154, 155
  enterocele, 277
  fistula, 329 et seq.
  incompetent cervix, 425
  posterior colporrhaphy, 276
  rectocele, 276
  ureter, 316 et seq.
  uterovaginal prolapse, 274
Reproductive physiology, 51 et seq.

Restoring tubal patency, 347, 348
Retroflexion, 253, 424
Retroperitoneal tumours, 362
Retroposition, 253
Retroversion, 253, 254
  correction, 256
  dysmenorrhoea, 118
  dyspareunia, 255, 398
  infertility, 255, 386
  operations, 258
  pessary treatment, 258
Rhizotomy, 231
Rhythm method, 407
Ring biopsy, 182
Ring pessary, 270, 271
Rontgens, 206
Round ligament, 33, 126, 258
Ruptured cyst, 363, 365, 366

Sacral plexus, 46, 230
'Safe period', 407
Saf-T-Coil, 404
Salpingectomy, 346, 354
Salpingitis, 118, 346, 349, 461–463
Salpingo-oophoritis, 118, 450
Salpingostomy, 347
Sarcoma botryoides, 250
Sarcoma of uterus, 249, 250
Sarcoma of vulva, 140, 143
Schauta's operation, 224, 225
Schiller's test, 179
Schuchardt's incision, 224
Scleroderma, 137
Scrotum, 12, 13, 99
Sebaceous cyst of vulva, 141
Secondary amenorrhoea, 92
Seminal fluid, 397
Seminal vesicle, 10
Senile vaginitis, 63, 133, 269
Septate uterus, 127, 424, 425
Septate vagina, 128
Septic abortion, 413, 426, 431
Septic shock, 413, 426–428, 431
Serous cystadenoma, 372
Sex and gender, 105 et seq.
Sex chromosomes, 105 et seq.
Sexual problems, 386 et seq.
Shaving, 115
Sheath (contraceptive), 407
Sheehan's syndrome, 93, 97
Shirodkar's repair, 425

Shirodkar's suture, 425
Shock
  postpartum, 97
  pulmonary embolism, 474
  septic, 427, 428
'Signet ring' cells, 377
Simmonds' disease, 93, 97
Simple vulvectomy, 150
Sims' position, 77
Sims' speculum, 77
Skene's duct (gland), 9, 18
  cyst, 152, 269
  gonorrhoea, 454
Skin
  hirsutism, 114
  pigmentation, 403
  radiation damage, 219
Sling operations
  urethral, 298–301
  uterine, 258
'Snail track' ulcers, 457
Soft sore, 458
Solid teratoma, 375
Spasmodic dysmenorrhoea, 116, 117
Speculum
  bi-valve, 76
  Cusco's, 76
  Sims', 77
Spermatozoa
  cervical mucus, 30, 390
  contraception, 407, 408
  count, 397
  invasion test, 390
  retroversion, 255
Sphincter
  ani, 20, 22
  urethrae, 21, 22
Spinnbarkeit, 61, 390
Spleen, palpation of, 72
Squamous epithelioma (see Carcinoma)
Squamous metaplasia
  cervix, 178
  endometrium, 242
Stein–Leventhal syndrome, 102 et seq.
Stem pessary, 271
Sterilisation, 345, 346
  cauterisation, 79, 80
Sterility, gonorrhoea and, 455
  (See also Infertility)

Stilboestrol, 117, 165
Stockholm method, 212
'Streak' ovary, 125
Streptokinase, 475
Streptomycin, 462
Stress incontinence
　after repair, 268, 284, 334
　Aldridge's operation, 298
　Ball's operation, 303
　causes, 289
　cystometry, 293
　differential diagnosis, 290, 291
　electrical control, 305, 306
　interposition operations, 304
　investigation, 292–294
　Kelly's operation, 297
　Lapides', 303
　Louros', 304
　Marshall – Marchetti – Kranz
　　operation, 302
　Millin's, 301
　Moir's, 300
　physiotherapy, 296
　sling operations, 298–301
　urethrocystography, 294
　vaginal urethroplasty, 297
Struma ovarii, 383
'Stump' carcinoma, 197
Subinvolution, 448
Subtotal hysterectomy, 90
Super-female, 110
Superior vena cava, 429
Sympathetic nerves, 47, 287
Syndrome
　adrenogenital, 98–100
　Ahumada-del Castillo, 101
　Chiari-Frommel, 91
　Fröhlich's, 96
　hyperstimulation, 396
　Klinefelter's, 110
　lactation-amenorrhoea, 91
　Lorain–Levi, 96
　Meigs', 366, 373
　Sheehan's, 97
　Stein–Leventhal, 102
　Turner's, 109
Syphilis, 456–460
　diagnostic tests, 460
　of cervix, 177

Tapping (of cyst), 369

Temperature changes
　ovulation and, 389
Teratoma, 374
Testicular feminisation, 111
Testis, 10, 11, 111
Theca externa, 52
Theca interna, 52
Thecoma, 382
Therapeutic abortion
　Act, 414
　definition, 413
　hysterotomy, 418
　injection of paste, 422
　intra-amniotic injection, 420,
　　421
　prostaglandins, 423
　vacuum aspiration, 419
Threadworms, 164
Threatened abortion, 412
Threshold bleeding, 84
Thrombectomy, 472, 473
Thrombophlebitis, 465
Thrombosis, 464 et seq.
　oral contraceptives and, 402
　pelvic cellulitis and, 452
Thyroid gland
　amenorrhoea, 92, 93
　hormone, 87
Torsion of cyst pedicle, 363,
　365
Total hysterectomy, 88, 89
　in carcinoma in situ, 182
Trachelorrhaphy, 174
Tranexamic acid, 87
Transverse cervical ligaments, 25,
　34, 262
Transvesical repair of fistula, 340
Trendelenberg's operation, 475
Treponemal immobilisation test,
　460
Triangular ligament, 21
Trichomonal vaginitis, 68
Trichomonas vaginalis, 162, 163
Trophoblastic tumours, 432 et
　seq.
Tube, tubal (see Fallopian tube)
Tuberculosis of genital tract, 177,
　461–463
Tumour, (see organ involved)
Tunica albuginea, 39
Tunica vaginalis, 11
Turner's syndrome, 109

Ultrasonography
　fibroid, 360
　hydatidiform mole, 435
　ovarian cyst, 360
　thrombosis, 469
Umbilicus, endometriosis of, 446
Undescended testis, 111
Unicornuate uterus, 127
Urachus, 8
Ureter, ureteric
　anatomy, 29, 32, 307–309
　blood supply, 310
　damage during operation, 88,
　　221, 280, 311 et seq.
　displacement, 311, 343
　fistula, 319
　histology, 310
　in prolapse, 263, 267, 315
　obstruction, 219
　prevention of injury, 313 et seq.
　repair, 316 et seq.
Uretero-colic anastomosis, 226,
　320
Ureterostomy, 317
Urethra
　anatomy, 18, 26
　carcinoma, 153
　caruncle, 151
　development, 12, 13
　fistula, 334
　glands, 9, 18
　gonorrhoea, 455
　internal pressure, 286
　meatitis, 151
　meatus, 74
　prolapse, 152
　sling operations, 298–303
　sphincter, 21, 286–289
　urethrocele, 152, 264
　vaginal urethroplasty, 297
Urethrocystography, 294
Urethro-vaginal fistula, 325
Urgency incontinence, 290
Urinary diversion operations, 226,
　320 et seq.
Urinary fistula (see also Fistula)
　bulbospongiosus muscle, 335
　causes, 324
　clinical features, 327, 328
　colpocleisis, 333
　flap-splitting, 332
　gracilis muscle, 336, 337

Urinary fistula (*continued*)
  interposition operations, 335–339
  Latzko's operation, 333
  omentum, 339
  pathology, 326
  radiation, 196, 215, 218, 219, 339
  rectus muscle, 338
  saucerisation, 331
  sites, 325
  transvesical repair, 340
  treatment, 329 et seq.
  urethral, 334
  vault fistula, 333
Urinary tract
  diversion, 226
  haematuria, 291
  infection, 72
  pain, 291
Urogenital diaphragm, 21, 22, 26
Urogenital sinus, 8
Urogenital triangle, 16
Urokinase, 475
Uterosacral ligament, 25, 34, 262
Uterotubal implantation, 348
Uterus, uterine
  absent, 111, 126, 128
  accessory horn, 127
  adenomyosis, 91, 240
  adult, 41
  anatomy, 29 et seq.
  artery, 32 et seq.
  atrophy, 41, 97, 101
  bicornis, 127
  carcinoma (see Carcinoma of endometrium)
  chronic inversion, 240, 259 et seq.
  congenital abnormalities, 110, 126, 127, 424, 425
  development, 6, 7
  didelphys, 127, 393
  displacements, 253 et seq.
  dysfunctional bleeding, 84
  ectopic pregnancy, 350
  endometriosis, 446
  fibroids, 91, 236 et seq.
  haematometra, 112
  histology, 35
  hypoplastic, 117
  hysteria, 66
  hysterography, 392

Uterus (*continued*)
  infantile, 41
  isthmus, 30
  IUCD, 404
  ligaments, 262
  measurements, 29, 30
  myohyperplasia, 240
  palpation, 75
  perforation, 405, 416, 426
  polyps, 86, 235
  pregnancy, 71, 350, 393, 409, 434
  prolapse, 262 et seq., 274, 275
  pubertal, 41
  pyometra, 219, 448
  retroflexion, 253
  retroposition, 253
  retroversion, 253
  rupture, 421
  sarcoma, 238, 249, 250
  senile, 41
  sling operations, 258
  torsion, 364
  tuberculosis, 462
  unicornis, 127

Vabra curette, 86
Vacuum aspiration, 419
Vagina, vaginal
  absent, 128, 169
  adhesions, 284
  anatomy, 26–28
  anus, 129
  artery, 42
  artificial, 169, 170
  carcinoma, 167, 168
  changes with age, 41
  congenital abnormalities, 128
  cyclic changes, 55, 61
  cysts, 166, 269
  cytology, 61, 63, 94, 391
  development, 7, 41
  diaphragm, 406
  dilator, 399
  discharge
    abnormal, 161–163
    carcinoma and, 167, 189, 245, 344
    dyspareunia, 161, 386
    examination, 68, 161, 162
    gonorrhoea, 454, 455

Vagina (*continued*)
  in the child, 164
  monilial, 68, 161–163
  non-specific, 161–163
  normal, 160
  pessary, 164, 270
  postmenopausal, 63, 164
  radiotherapy, 218
  senile, 63, 133, 164, 269
  trichomonal, 68, 161–163
  yeasts, 68, 161–163
  double, 128
  endometriosis, 446
  enlargement of orifice, 154, 157, 284
  examination, 76, 165, 168
  fistula, 324 et seq.
  fistula of vault, 333
  fornices, 27
  foreign body, 165
  haematocolpos, 112
  histology, 28
  hormonal effects, 55
  hysterectomy, 279, 280
  imperforate, 112
  leucorrhoea, 68
  lymphatic drainage, 168
  prolapse, 77, 262 et seq.
  secretion, 28
  septate, 128
  smear, 61, 65, 94, 391
  spermicides, 406
  urethroplasty, 297
  vault prolapse, 265, 266
Vaginismus, 399
Vaginitis, (see also Vaginal discharge)
  children, 165
  monilial, 68, 161–163
  non-specific, 161–163
  senile, 63, 133, 164, 269
  trichomonal, 68, 161–163
Varicocele, 397
Vas deferens, 11
Vasectomy, 407
Vasodilator drugs, 431
Vasomotor disturbances, 63
Vault fistula, 333
Vault prolapse, 265, 266
Vena cava
  inferior, 473
  superior, 429

Venereal infections, 454-460
Venous ligation, 472, 473
Ventrosuspension, 258
Vesico-vaginal fistula, 325 et seq.
Vesicular mole (see Hydatidiform
    mole)
Vestibular anus, 129
Vestibular glands, 16, 18, 19 (see
    also Bartholin's glands)
Vestibule
    anatomy, 18, 19
    examination of, 74
Vestigial cysts, 37
Virchow's triad, 464
Virilism
    adreno-genital syndrome, 98–
        100
    amenorrhoea, 93
    causes, 113
    clinical features, 113, 381
    hirsutism, 114, 115, 381
    hormone estimations, 113
    investigation, 113
    ovarian tumours, 381, 382
    voice changes, 113
Vulva, vulval
    absent, 129
    anatomy, 16–18
    basal cell carcinoma, 143
    blood supply, 46
    carcinoma, 143 (see Carcinoma
        of vulva)

Vulva (continued)
    changes with age, 41
    condylomata acuminata, 142
    condylomata lata, 457
    congenital abnormalities, 129
    cysts, 141
    development, 9
    double, 129
    dystrophy, 132
    ectopia vesicae, 129
    endometriosis, 140
    enlargement of vaginal orifice,
        154, 157
    examination of, 74
    fibroma, 140
    granuloma, 451
    haematoma, 140
    hidradenoma, 142
    hydrocele, 141
    inclusion cyst, 141
    kraurosis, 132, 133
    leukoplakia, 134
    lichen planus, 136
    lichen simplex, 137
    lipoma, 140
    lymphatic drainage, 45, 144
    lymphogranuloma, 458
    melanoma, 143
    nerve supply, 46
    neurodermatitis, 137
    pruritus, 133, 135, 136
    sarcoma, 140, 143

Vulva (continued)
    scleroderma, 137
    sebaceous cyst, 141
    simple tumours, 140
    simple vulvectomy, 150
    tuberculosis, 461
Vulvitis, diabetic, 74

Warfarin, 470, 471
Warts, 142, 457
Wasserman reaction, 460
Wedge resection of ovaries, 104,
    368
Wertheim's hysterectomy, 221
    et seq.
'White line', 23
William's operation, 170
Wolffian duct, 6, 10

X chromosome, 105, 108
X-rays, 198 et seq.

Y chromosome, 105
Yeasts, 162

Zona pellucida, 51, 52